Teen Health Series

Sports Injuries Information For Teens, Third Edition

Sports Injuries Information For Teens, Third Edition

Health Tips About Acute, Traumatic, And Chronic Injuries In Adolescent Athletes

Including Facts About Sprains, Fractures, And Overuse Injuries, Treatment, Rehabilitation, Sport-Specific Safety Guidelines, Fitness Suggestions, And More

Edited by Zachary Klimecki and Elizabeth Bellenir

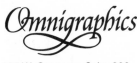

155 W. Congress, Suite 200
Detroit, MI 48226

Bibliographic Note

Because this page cannot legibly accommodate all the copyright notices, the Bibliographic Note portion of the Preface constitutes an extension of the copyright notice.

Edited by Zachary Klimecki and Elizabeth Bellenir

Teen Health Series

Karen Bellenir, *Managing Editor*
David A. Cooke, M.D., *Medical Consultant*
Elizabeth Collins, *Research and Permissions Coordinator*
Cherry Edwards, *Permissions Assistant*
EdIndex, *Services for Publishers, Indexers*

* * *

Omnigraphics, Inc.
Matthew P. Barbour, *Senior Vice President*
Kevin M. Hayes, *Operations Manager*

* * *

Peter E. Ruffner, *Publisher*
Copyright © 2012 Omnigraphics, Inc.
ISBN 978-0-7808-1265-9
E-ISBN 978-0-7808-1266-6

Library of Congress Cataloging-in-Publication Data

Sports injuries information for teens : health tips about acute, traumatic, and chronic injuries in adolescent athletes including facts about sprains, fractures, and overuse injuries, treatment, rehabilitation, sport-specific safety guidelines, fitness suggestions, and more / edited by Zachary Klimecki and Elizabeth Bellenir. -- 3rd ed.
    p. cm. -- (Teen health series)
  Summary: "Provides basic consumer health information for teens about sports-related injury prevention, treatment, and rehabilitation. Includes index and resource information"-- Provided by publisher.
  Includes bibliographical references and index.
  ISBN 978-0-7808-1265-9 (hardcover : alk. paper) 1. Sports injuries. 2. Teenagers--Wounds and injuries--Prevention. 3. Wounds and injuries. I. Klimecki, Zachary. II. Bellenir, Elizabeth.
  RD97.S689 2012
  617.1'027--dc23

2012018884

Table of Contents

Preface

Part Three: Diagnosing And Treating Common Sports Injuries

Part Four: Caring For Injured Athletes

Part Five: If You Need More Information

Preface

About This Book

Participating in sports is great for teens—physically, socially, and mentally, and according to the National Institute of Arthritis and Musculoskeletal and Skin diseases, more than 30 million young people participate in organized sports in the United States. While sports participation is beneficial in many ways, it also carries risk. One recent study found that 20% of all children and teens participating in sports will be injured, and one in four sports injuries is considered serious. By observing proper training practices and using appropriate protective gear, however, young athletes can help minimize the risks they face.

Sports Injuries Information For Teens, Third Edition, offers teens a comprehensive, fact-based guide to being a healthy athlete. It includes guidelines for participating safely in sports and avoiding injury. It also discusses how to deal with injuries when they do occur. It explains diagnostic and treatment procedures and discusses issues related to rehabilitation, including suggestions for making decisions about returning to play. The book concludes with directories of resources for more information about sports-related injuries and fitness.

How To Use This Book

This book is divided into parts and chapters. Parts focus on broad areas of interest; chapters are devoted to single topics within a part.

Part One: Health Tips For Student Athletes focuses on the important choices sports participants make about healthy lifestyles. It discusses choosing the right sports, sports physicals, basic nutrition, emotional issues, and substance abuse among athletes.

Part Two: Sports Safety And Injury Prevention summarizes guidelines for achieving and maintaining a level of fitness necessary to help avoid injuries. It describes the proper use of important protective equipment, including various types of helmets, eye protectors, and mouthguards. This part also offers specific safety tips for many popular sports.

Part Three: Diagnosing And Treating Common Sports Injuries explains the differences between acute and chronic injuries, and it discusses problems associated with extreme heat conditions. It also describes the symptoms, treatment, and management of injuries that may occur among athletes, including sprains, strains, broken bones, concussions, and other injuries to the body's musculoskeletal system and soft tissues.

Part Four: Caring For Injured Athletes offers facts about the rehabilitation process, beginning with immediate care during the first moments after injury. It describes the important role of athletic trainers in helping assess and prevent injuries, offers suggestions for choosing a doctor and making medical decisions, and provides tips for caring for casts and splints. Guidelines for returning to play are presented, and the part concludes with information about the connection between sports injuries and the potential for the later development of arthritis.

Part Five: If You Need More Information offers resource directories of organizations able to provide more information about traumatic and chronic sports-related injuries and fitness and exercise.

Bibliographic Note

This volume contains documents and excerpts from publications issued by the following government agencies: Centers for Disease Control and Prevention (CDC); Federal Citizen Information Center; National Eye Institute; National Institute of Alcohol Abuse and Alcoholism; National Institute of Arthritis and Musculoskeletal and Skin Diseases; National Institute of Diabetes and Digestive and Kidney Diseases; National Institute of Neurological Disorders and Stroke; National Institute on Drug Abuse; National Library of Medicine; President's Council on Fitness, Sports, and Nutrition; Ready.gov; U.S. Consumer Product Safety Commission; U.S. Department of Health and Human Services; U.S. Department of Labor; U.S. Public Health Service; and the Weight-control Information Network.

In addition, this volume contains copyrighted documents and articles produced by the following organizations, publications, and individuals: About.com; Amateur Endurance; American Academy of Orthopaedic Surgeons; American Association of Adapted Sports Programs; American Association of Endodontists; American College of Sports Medicine; American Council on Exercise; American Institute for Preventative Medicine; American Orthopaedic Foot and Ankle Society; American Orthopaedic Society for Sports Medicine; American Podiatric Medical Association, Inc.; Ann and Robert H. Lurie Children's Hospital of Chicago; California Office of the Patient Advocate; Canadian Society for Exercise Physiology; Children's Hospital Colorado; Coastal Physiotherapy and Sports Injury Clinic; CRC Health Group; Tim Durta, DPM, MS; Fairview Health Services; Guthrie Sports Medicine; HMP Communications; Ian Tilmann Foundation; International Food Information Council Foundation; Los Angeles County Department of Public Health Injury and Violence Prevention Program; MEYou Health, LLC; MomsTeam.com; Heather Nakamura, MPE, MS,

RD; National Center for Sports Safety; National Federation of State High School Associations; Nationwide Children's Hospital; Nemours Foundation; *Podiatry Today*; Prevent Blindness America; Safe Kids Canada; Safe Kids Worldwide; Singapore Sports Council; Smart Play (Sports Medicine Australia); SportsMD Media, Inc.; SportsMed Web; St. John's Hospital; United States Olympic Committee; and Utah State University Cooperative Extension.

The photograph on the front cover is from Stockbyte/Thinkstock.

Full citation information is provided on the first page of each chapter. Every effort has been made to secure all necessary rights to reprint the copyrighted material. If any omissions have been made, please contact Omnigraphics to make corrections for future editions.

Acknowledgements

In addition to the organizations listed above, special thanks are due to Liz Collins, research and permissions coordinator; Karen Bellenir, managing editor; Lisa Bakewell, verification assistant; and WhimsyInk, prepress services provider.

About The Teen Health Series

At the request of librarians serving today's young adults, the *Teen Health Series* was developed as a specially focused set of volumes within Omnigraphics' *Health Reference Series*. Each volume deals comprehensively with a topic selected according to the needs and interests of people in middle school and high school.

Teens seeking preventive guidance, information about disease warning signs, medical statistics, and risk factors for health problems will find answers to their questions in the *Teen Health Series*. The *Series*, however, is not intended to serve as a tool for diagnosing illness, in prescribing treatments, or as a substitute for the physician/patient relationship. All people concerned about medical symptoms or the possibility of disease are encouraged to seek professional care from an appropriate health care provider.

If there is a topic you would like to see addressed in a future volume of the *Teen Health Series*, please write to:

Editor
Teen Health Series
Omnigraphics, Inc.
155 W. Congress, Suite 200
Detroit, MI 48226

A Note about Spelling and Style

Teen Health Series editors use *Stedman's Medical Dictionary* as an authority for questions related to the spelling of medical terms and the *Chicago Manual of Style* for questions related to grammatical structures, punctuation, and other editorial concerns. Consistent adherence is not always possible, however, because the individual volumes within the *Series* include many documents from a wide variety of different producers and copyright holders, and the editor's primary goal is to present material from each source as accurately as is possible following the terms specified by each document's producer. This sometimes means that information in different chapters or sections may follow other guidelines and alternate spelling authorities. For example, occasionally a copyright holder may require that eponymous terms be shown in possessive forms (Crohn's disease *vs.* Crohn disease) or that British spelling norms be retained (leukaemia *vs.* leukemia).

Locating Information within the Teen Health Series

The *Teen Health Series* contains a wealth of information about a wide variety of medical topics. As the *Series* continues to grow in size and scope, locating the precise information needed by a specific student may become more challenging. To address this concern, information about books within the *Teen Health Series* is included in *A Contents Guide to the Health Reference Series*. The *Contents Guide* presents an extensive list of more than 16,000 diseases, treatments, and other topics of general interest compiled from the Tables of Contents and major index headings from the books of the *Teen Health Series* and *Health Reference Series*. To access *A Contents Guide to the Health Reference Series*, visit www.healthreferenceseries.com.

Our Advisory Board

We would like to thank the following advisory board members for providing guidance to the development of this *Series*:

Dr. Lynda Baker, Associate Professor of Library and Information Science, Wayne State University, Detroit, MI

Nancy Bulgarelli, William Beaumont Hospital Library, Royal Oak, MI

Karen Imarisio, Bloomfield Township Public Library, Bloomfield Township, MI

Karen Morgan, Mardigian Library, University of Michigan-Dearborn, Dearborn, MI

Rosemary Orlando, St. Clair Shores Public Library, St. Clair Shores, MI

Medical Consultant

Medical consultation services are provided to the *Teen Health Series* editors by David A. Cooke, M.D. Dr. Cooke is a graduate of Brandeis University, and he received his M.D. degree from the University of Michigan. He completed residency training at the University of Wisconsin Hospital and Clinics. He is board-certified in internal medicine. Dr. Cooke currently works as part of the University of Michigan Health System and practices in Ann Arbor, MI. In his free time, he enjoys writing, science fiction, and spending time with his family.

Part One
Health Tips For Student Athletes

Chapter 1

Choosing The Right Sport For You

Corey and Angie, twin brother and sister, enjoy playing all kinds of outdoor games and sports with their friends. They especially love playing pickup games of basketball and touch football. On particularly nice days, Corey and Angie have been known to kick around the soccer ball, toss around the baseball, or go on long runs.

In just a month the twins will be high school freshmen and neither can figure out which sport to try out for in the fall. Corey is deciding between football, soccer, and cross-country. Angie is debating whether to try her hand at a sport she has never played, like field hockey, or go with one she knows, like soccer or cross-country. They're facing a dilemma a lot of teens face—which sports to play and which sports to give up.

So Many Sports, Only One You

For some people, choosing which sports to pursue throughout high school is hard because they have never really played an organized sport before and aren't sure what they'll most enjoy. For others it's a tough decision because their friends don't like to play the same sports.

No matter what your sports dilemma is, you have to make the decision that is best for you. If you're great at soccer but would rather play football because you think it's more fun, then give the pigskin a go (just make sure it's cool with mom and dad).

About This Chapter: "Choosing the Right Sport for You," January 2011, reprinted with permission from www .kidshealth.org. Copyright © 2011 The Nemours Foundation. This information was provided by KidsHealth, one of the largest resources online for medically reviewed health information written for parents, kids, and teens. For more articles like this one, visit www.KidsHealth.org or www.TeensHealth.org.

Sports are meant to be fun. If there is a sport you really enjoy but you aren't sure if you can make the team, try out anyway. What's the worst that can happen? If you get cut you can always try another sport. And sports like cross-country and track don't typically cut participants from the team. You can still participate even if you're not on the meet squad.

Table 1.1. When Most Organized Sports Land On The School Calendar

Fall	Winter	Spring
• Cheerleading	• Basketball	• Badminton
• Cross-Country	• Cheerleading	• Baseball (Boys)
• Dance Team	• Dance	• Golf
• Field Hockey (Girls)	• Gymnastics	• Lacrosse
• Football (Guys)	• Ice Hockey	• Rugby
• Soccer	• Indoor Track and Field	• Softball (Girls)
• Volleyball	• Swimming and Diving	• Tennis
• Water Polo	• Wrestling	• Track and Field

Every Now And Then There Is An "I" In Team

Some sports, like lacrosse or field hockey, require every person on the field to be on the same page. Sure, certain people stand out more than others but superstars don't necessarily make a good team.

Sports like tennis, track and field, cross-country, swimming, gymnastics, and wrestling are all sports where individual performances are tallied into team scores. Of course there are exceptions, like relays in track and swimming, but for the most part it's possible to win a solo event in these sports and still have your team lose or vice-versa.

No one knows you better than you do. Maybe you enjoy the spotlight. Maybe you get annoyed by the way teammates act when they are über-competitive. Or maybe you just don't like competing with friends for a spot in the starting lineup. For whatever reason, team sports might not be your thing—and that's fine. Luckily, there are many individualized sports to choose from.

You Aren't Under Contract

If you try a sport for a season and you don't enjoy it, or it's not what you expected, it's OK to try out for another sport the next year. Don't let parents or coaches persuade you to stick with something you don't want to—ultimately it's your decision.

If Your School Doesn't Have Your Sport

Some schools are limited in resources—a city school may not have a lot of fields, for example, while a rural school may not have enough students to make up a team for every sport.

A school's geographic region can also play a role. If you live in a climate where it snows from the fall to the spring, your school may not be able to participate in a lot of outdoor sports.

If your school doesn't have your sport, don't let it get you down. You can always try out for a different sport during the same season or look into whether your local town has a recreational league that you can join.

If You Don't Have It, Start It

If you are interested in a sport, and your school doesn't have it, maybe you and some friends can talk to the administration and start a club or intramural team. With enough willing participants and the school's permission you could have a high school cricket team.

If Organized Sports Aren't Your Thing

Many people are attracted to the competition and popularity that can come with team sports. Others love the camaraderie and unity that are present in a team atmosphere. But for some people, teams are just frustrating and another form of cliques. If you're not the biggest fan of organized sports, where you have to follow someone else's schedule and rules, many other fun and exciting options are out there for you.

You might already have an exercise routine or activity you like to do in your free time, but if you're looking for something that will both keep you busy and allow you to blow off steam, try some of these activities:

Climb To The Top: Did you love scaling trees and walls when you were younger? Rock climbing offers participants one of the best all-around workouts possible. As a rock climber, you work your hands, arms, shoulders, back, stomach, legs, and feet—all at once.

Take A Hike (And Bring Your Bike): Hiking and trail biking are two great ways to learn about nature while still getting your heart rate up. Even if you're just going to a local trail, bring at least one other person along in case something happens. If you're going for an intense multi-day hike, you should bring someone who is experienced and trained in hiking.

Water World: The water is the perfect place to give yourself new challenges. There are plenty of water activities for all levels of difficulty and energy. Besides swimming, try canoeing, kayaking, fishing, rowing, sailing, wakeboarding, water skiing, windsurfing, and, if you're feeling particularly daring, surfing.

Find Your Inner Self

Many activities can be relaxing and taxing at once. These three activities strengthen you physically and mentally:

- Yoga can improve flexibility, strength, balance, and stamina. In addition to the physical benefits, many people who practice yoga say that it reduces anxiety and stress and improves mental clarity.

- Pilates is a body conditioning routine that seeks to build flexibility, strength, endurance, and coordination without adding muscle bulk. Pilates also increases circulation and helps to sculpt the body and strengthen the body's "core" or "powerhouse" (torso). People who do Pilates regularly feel they have better posture and are less prone to injury.

- T'ai chi is an ancient Chinese martial art form that is great for improving flexibility and strengthening your legs, abdominal or core muscles, and arms.

> ## Hiker's Gear List
>
> The American Red Cross has a huge list of supplies for hiking. Here are some of the basics you should throw in your bag:
>
> - Cell phone
> - Extra clothing
> - Compass
> - First-aid kit
> - Extra food
> - Flashlight
> - Bug spray
> - Maps
> - Any prescriptions
> - Radio with batteries
> - Sunscreen
> - Water
> - Whistle
> - Poncho or trash bag to make a poncho

Take An Off-Season—But Not A Season Off

Whether you choose one sport or three, make sure you give yourself a break from intense competition with some cross-training activities. Through cross training you can take a rest from your sport or sports while still getting a workout and staying in shape.

Two examples of cross training are swimming and cycling. They not only help build cardiovascular fitness, but also work your muscles. Swimming can really help tone your upper body, while cycling strengthens your legs.

> ## Benefits Of Strength Training
> - Increases endurance and strength for sports and fitness activities
> - Improves focus and concentration, which may result in better grades
> - Reduces body fat and increases muscle mass
> - Helps burn more calories even when not exercising
> - May reduce the risk of short-term injuries by protecting tendons, bones, and joints
> - Helps prevent long-term medical problems such as high cholesterol or osteoporosis (weakening of the bones) when you get older.

You can also try outdoor bike rides and runs on nice days, stopping periodically to do sit-ups and push-ups. These simple exercises can work and tone your core muscles.

That time between seasons is also the perfect opportunity to get into a strength-training routine. Before starting strength training, consult your doctor and school's strength and conditioning coach. Your doc will be able to give you health clearance to participate in the different types of physical activities, and your strength coach can come up with a workout to help you prepare for your specific sports.

Chapter 2

Sports For Students With Disabilities

The American Association of AdaptedSPORTS Programs works in partnership with education agencies in the U.S. to establish programs, policies, procedures, and regulations in interscholastic adapted sports for students with physical disabilities to enhance educational outcomes. While students must have some type of orthopedic or physical disability they need not use a wheelchair for mobility to be eligible to participate.

What is the adaptedSPORTS® Model?

The American Association of Adapted Sports Programs (AAASP) employs athletics through a system called the adaptedSPORTS® Model. This award-winning model is an interscholastic structure of multiple sports seasons that parallels the traditional interscholastic athletic system and supports the concept that school-based sports are a vital part of the education process and the educational goals of students.

The sports featured in the adaptedSPORTS Model have their origin in Paralympic and adult disability sports; however, they are innovative in that they are cross-disability in nature. AAASP has adapted these sports for the student-athlete based on their functional ability. By providing standardized competition rules, it is possible for the widespread implementation of an interscholastic adapted athletic system. Additionally, student athletes are developing the skills that can lead to participation at the collegiate, community, and elite levels.

About This Chapter: Text in this chapter is excerpted and adapted from information available from the American Association of Adapted Sports Programs, Inc. (AAASP) website, online at www.adaptedsports.org. © 2012; reprinted with permission.

What core sports are sanctioned?

AAASP sanctions the following core sports:

Wheelchair Handball: Wheelchair handball kicks off the AAASP sports year in August. Wheelchair handball is a fast-paced game that is easily played by students using either manual or power wheelchairs. The ball, which is a Tachikara Official SV–5W loose bladder constructed white leather volleyball, is easier for children in the early stages of learning fundamental sports skills and enables them to achieve higher levels of confidence and success; therefore they are motivated to continue playing. The sport is played inside on a basketball court and many of the same skills required for wheelchair basketball are used.

Eligible participants, whose primary disability must be physical, are boys and girls attending grades 1–12. They are able to walk unassisted, with devices, or use manual or power wheelchairs. All participants must compete in a manual or power wheelchair.

Wheelchair Basketball: Wheelchair basketball is one of the most widely recognized sports for athletes with disabilities and is one of two AAASP sports organized during the winter.

The wheelchair is considered part of the body, offensive players are allowed four seconds in the lane and there is no double dribble. Teams play within either junior varsity or varsity division. Junior varsity teams use an 8½-foot hoop and a NCAA's women's basketball, and the varsity teams use a standard 10-foot hoop and a NCAA men's basketball.

Eligible participants, whose primary disability must be physical, are boys and girls attending grades 1–12. Although they are able to walk unassisted, with devices, or use manual propelled wheelchairs, all participants must compete in a manual wheelchair. Power wheelchairs are not permitted.

Sports Seasons

The American Association of Adapted SPORTS Programs sanctions the following core sports in the following seasons.

- **Fall:** Wheelchair handball
- **Winter:** Wheelchair basketball and power soccer
- **Spring:** Wheelchair football, track and field, and beep baseball

Just as in able–bodied high school sports, all sport rules have been adapted to support positive educational outcomes.

Power Wheelchair Soccer: Power wheel chair soccer is the second AAASP sport organized during the winter. The season starts in December and runs through March. Power wheelchair soccer is a game that is played by students using power wheelchairs. The sport is played inside on a basketball court. Each team has four players on the court during the game. Many of the rules for soccer are used along with adaptations for the wheelchair. The players must learn to move, pass, dribble and shoot the ball. Temporary foot guards are used to move the ball and to protect the wheelchair. Goals are scored when the ball crosses the goal line.

Eligible participants, whose primary disability must be physical, are boys and girls attending grades 1–12. All participants must compete in a power wheelchair.

Wheelchair Football: Wheelchair football, which is played in the spring, is a fast-paced sport that is best played when athletes are in maximum physical condition and at the top of their game in teamwork, strategy, and wheelchair handling skills. The game is played on a standard basketball court with all players using either a manual or a power wheelchair. Players in manual chairs have successfully tackled an opponent when they tag the opponent with two hands on the body and above the knees. Players in power chairs will have made a successful tackle when they tag the opponent with one hand on the opponent's body or chair. A team has six attempts to score once they receive the ball. Teams may pass or "run" the ball into the end zone. Field goals, kick-offs, and punts are thrown. A running game clock (no time-outs for incomplete passes, etc.) is used, as well as a play clock. Scoring is the same as in stand-up football, with one exception. A team that passes for the point-after-touchdown (PAT) will receive two points. Field goals are scored when the ball is thrown through the first two vertical uprights that support the hanging basket.

Eligible participants, whose primary disability must be physical, are boys and girls attending grades 1–12. They may walk unassisted, with devices, or use manual or power wheelchairs. All participants must compete in a wheelchair.

Track And Field: All high school students in Florida, Georgia, and Kentucky with a permanent, physical disability may be eligible to participate on their school's track and field team. Students must meet all eligibility requirements. They will have the opportunity to compete in the wheelchair races and the shot put.

Students will be members of the school's track and field team and will compete at all the school's meets (regardless of the number of wheelchair competitors). The athletes must complete in their school's team uniform. The top eight (8) qualifiers over the entire track season in each event will advance to compete at the State Track Meet.

Athletes who wish to compete must contact their high school coach. Coaches and high school athletes can call the adaptedSPORTS office at 404-294-0070 for more information.

Beep Baseball: Beep baseball season begins in the spring. This sport was developed for athletes who are blind or visually impaired, with the ideal field being a flat grassy surface. The field setup is traditional, with a few modifications—three bases are used instead of four (home, first, and third).

Beep baseball also requires some special equipment. The balls are large, 16-inch softballs with an implanted electronic beeping device so that players can gauge the location and movement of the ball. Bases are columns of foam rubber, four-feet tall, and at least seven inches across. Each base has a buzzer placed three-feet high that faces home plate and is operated remotely from behind home plate. The buzzer is an auditory indicator for the players. Blindfolds are also an essential component of the equipment list. They must incorporate a nose pad to eliminate the ability to peak down the side of the nose. Each player must be blindfolded, regardless of the extent of their visual impairment.

When a batter hits the ball, he or she will run to either first or third base, depending on which base has been remotely activated. This is done in random order; the batters are never sure which base to run to until they hear it beeping. A sighted fielder, who calls out the number of the fielder closest to where the ball was hit, assists the fielders. A run is scored if the runner touches the base before the fielder locates and lifts the ball. It is an "out" of the fielder gets the ball before the runner touches the base. After the run or out, the runner returns to the dugout while the next batter takes his or her turn at bat.

Eligible participants are blind or visually impaired boys and girls who are attending grades 1–12.

Chapter 3

Sports Physicals

You already know that playing sports helps keep you fit. You also know that sports are a fun way to socialize and meet people. But you might not know why the physical you may have to take at the beginning of your sports season is so important.

What Is A Sports Physical?

In the sports medicine field, the sports physical exam is known as a preparticipation physical examination (PPE). The exam helps determine whether it's safe for you to participate in a particular sport. Most states actually require that kids and teens have a sports physical before they can start a new sport or begin a new competitive season. But even if a PPE isn't required, doctors still highly recommend getting one.

The two main parts to a sports physical are the medical history and the physical exam.

Medical History

This part of the exam includes questions about:

- serious illnesses among other family members
- illnesses that you had when you were younger or may have now, such as asthma, diabetes, or epilepsy
- previous hospitalizations or surgeries
- allergies (to insect bites, for example)

About This Chapter: "Sports Physicals," August 2009, reprinted with permission from www.kidshealth.org. Copyright © 2009 The Nemours Foundation. This information was provided by KidsHealth, one of the largest resources online for medically reviewed health information written for parents, kids, and teens. For more articles like this one, visit www.KidsHealth.org or www.TeensHealth.org.

- past injuries (including concussions, sprains, or bone fractures)

- whether you've ever passed out, felt dizzy, had chest pain, or had trouble breathing during exercise

- any medications that you are on (including over-the-counter medications, herbal supplements, and prescription medications)

The medical history questions are usually on a form that you can bring home, so ask your parents to help you fill in the answers. If possible, ask both parents about family medical history.

Looking at patterns of illness in your family is a very good indicator of any potential conditions you may have. Most sports medicine doctors believe the medical history is the most important part of the sports physical exam, so take time to answer the questions carefully. It's unlikely that any health conditions you have will prevent you from playing sports completely.

Answer the questions as well as you can. Try not to guess the answers or give answers you think your doctor wants.

Physical Examination

During the physical part of the exam, the doctor will usually:

- record your height and weight

- take a blood pressure and pulse (heart rate and rhythm) reading

- test your vision

- check your heart, lungs, abdomen, ears, nose, and throat

- evaluate your posture, joints, strength, and flexibility

Although most aspects of the exam will be the same for males and females, if a person has started or already gone through puberty, the doctor may ask girls and guys different questions. For example, if a girl is heavily involved in a lot of active sports, the doctor may ask her about her period and diet to make sure she doesn't have something like female athlete triad.

A doctor will also ask questions about use of drugs, alcohol, or dietary supplements, including steroids or other "performance enhancers" and weight-loss supplements, because these can affect a person's health.

At the end of your exam, the doctor will either fill out and sign a form if everything checks out OK or, in some cases, recommend a follow-up exam, additional tests, or specific treatment for medical problems.

Why Is A Sports Physical Important?

A sports physical can help you find out about and deal with health problems that might interfere with your participation in a sport. For example, if you have frequent asthma attacks but are a starting forward in soccer, a doctor might be able to prescribe a different type of inhaler or adjust the dosage so that you can breathe more easily when you run.

Your doctor may even have some good training tips and be able to give you some ideas for avoiding injuries. For example, he or she may recommend specific exercises, like certain stretching or strengthening activities, that help prevent injuries. A doctor also can identify risk factors that are linked to specific sports. Advice like this will make you a better, stronger athlete.

When And Where Should I Go For A Sports Physical?

Some people go to their own doctor for a sports physical; others have one at school. During school physicals, you may go to half a dozen or so "stations" set up in the gym; each one is staffed by a medical professional who gives you a specific part of the physical exam.

If your school offers the exam, it's convenient to get it done there. But even if you have a PPE at school, it's a good idea to see your regular doctor for an exam as well. Your doctor knows you—and your health history—better than anyone you talk to briefly in a gym.

If your state requires sports physicals, you'll probably have to start getting them when you're in ninth grade. Even if PPEs aren't required by your school or state, it's still smart to get them if you participate in school sports. And if you compete regularly in a sport before ninth grade, you should begin getting these exams even earlier.

Getting a sports physical once a year is usually adequate. If you're healing from a major injury, like a broken wrist or ankle, however, get checked out after it's healed before you start practicing or playing again.

You should have your physical about six weeks before your sports season begins so there's enough time to follow up on something, if necessary. Neither you nor your doctor will be very happy if your PPE is the day before baseball practice starts and it turns out there's something that needs to be taken of care before you can suit up.

What If There's A Problem?

What happens if you don't get the OK from your own doctor and have to see a specialist? Does that mean you won't ever be able to letter in softball or hockey? Don't worry if your

15

doctor asks you to have other tests or go for a follow-up exam—it could be something as simple as rechecking your blood pressure a week or two after the physical.

Your doctor's referral to a specialist may help your athletic performance. For example, if you want to try out for your school's track team but get a slight pain in your knee every time you run, an orthopedist or sports medicine specialist can help you figure out what's going on. Perhaps the pain comes from previous overtraining or poor running technique. Maybe you injured the knee a long time ago and it never totally healed. Or perhaps the problem is as simple as running shoes that don't offer enough support. Chances are, a doctor will be able to help you run without the risk of further injury to the knee by giving you suggestions or treatment before the sports season begins.

It's very unlikely that you'll be disqualified from playing sports. The ultimate goal of the sports physical is to ensure safe participation in sports, not to disqualify the participants. Most of the time, a specialist won't find anything serious enough to prevent you from playing your sport. In fact, fewer than 1% of students have conditions that might limit sports participation, and most of these conditions are known before the PPE takes place.

Do I Still Have To Get A Regular Physical?

In a word, yes. It may seem like overkill, but a sports physical is different from a standard physical.

The sports physical focuses on your well-being as it relates to playing a sport. It's more limited than a regular physical, but it's a lot more specific about athletic issues. During a regular physical, however, your doctor will address your overall well-being, which may include things that are unrelated to sports. You can ask your doctor to give you both types of exams during one visit; just be aware that you'll need to set aside more time.

Just as professional sports stars need medical care to keep them playing their best, so do teenage athletes. You can give yourself the same edge as the pros by making sure you have your sports physical.

Remember

Even if your sports physical exam doesn't reveal any problems, it's always wise to monitor yourself when you play sports. If you notice changes in your physical condition—even if you think they're small, such as muscle pain or shortness of breath—be sure to mention them to a parent or coach. You should also inform your Phys. Ed. teacher or coach if your health needs have changed in any way or if you're taking a new medication.

Chapter 4

Nutrition For Student Athletes

Sports Nutrition For Student Athletes

Student athletes encounter many challenges during their season. Busy schedules often result in skipped meals or snacks and eating on the run. Late nights doing homework limit sleep before another morning workout. Athletes in weight-related sports often focus on "dieting" and consume too few calories to fuel their workouts. As a result, many suffer from impaired concentration and limited energy, performance, and recovery. If you're a student athlete or have one in your household, use the following guidelines to develop a more optimal sports nutrition plan.

Don't Skip Breakfast

Skipping breakfast is common among student athletes, but starting the day with a good breakfast is the key to maintaining optimal energy and achieving ideal weight. Eating a balanced breakfast increases metabolism, improves concentration, and provides energy for the morning hours. If time is an issue, try one of the following quick and portable breakfast combinations:

- Whole grain bagel with peanut butter, banana, and milk

- Yogurt smoothie with a whole grain cereal bar

- Instant oatmeal (buy prepared cups and add boiling water) with fruit and milk

About This Chapter: This chapter begins with "Sports Nutrition for Student Athletes," by Heather Nakamura, MPE, MS, RD. © 2009. Reprinted with permission. For additional information, visit www.targetgoodhealth.com. It continues with excerpts from "Fast Facts about Sports Nutrition," an undated document produced by the President's Council on Fitness, Sports, and Nutrition (www.fitness.gov), accessed January 22, 2012. The chapter concludes with information from "Questions Most Frequently Asked About Sports Nutrition," President's Council on Fitness, Sports, and Nutrition, January 23, 2012.

- Breakfast burrito (heat in microwave and go) with orange juice
- Yogurt parfait (yogurt, fruit and cereal in a cup)

Eat A Balanced Lunch

Many student athletes use lunch break as a social hour instead of fueling their bodies for afternoon classes and sports practice. They report feeling uncomfortable consuming a balanced lunch, while friends graze on fries, chips, and sweets. When they complain of low energy and trouble getting through practice, they should remember that eating a balanced lunch will help solve these issues. For a balanced lunch, include foods from each of the groups listed in Table 4.1.

Plan A Pre-Workout Snack

Athletes should eat every three to four hours to maintain promote optimal energy. Planning a pre-event snack can help athletes sustain energy throughout their practice session. Students can either purchase snacks at school or bring them from home. Here are some suggestions for healthy pre-event snacks that will provide long-term energy:

- Yogurt parfait (also available at Starbucks and McDonalds)
- String cheese and whole grain crackers
- Energy bar and yogurt smoothie
- Peanut butter crackers and milk
- Fresh fruit and bag of mixed nuts
- ½ peanut butter sandwich and fruit

Table 4.1. Food For A Balanced Lunch

Starches/Grains	Meat/Protein	Fruits/Vegs	Milk/Dairy
Bread/Pita	Lunchmeat/Tuna	Raw Veggies	Milk
Pasta	Chicken/Fish	Steamed veggies	Parmesan cheese
Tortilla	Beans	Salsa	Shredded cheese
Bagel	Peanut butter	Banana	Chocolate milk
Pizza	Canadian bacon	Pineapple/Tomato	Cheese
Bun	Chicken burger	Tomato/lettuce	Cheese

Eat A Balanced Dinner

Many athletes experience a decreased appetite after a hard workout, and prefer to graze on snacks instead of eating a balanced dinner. This can limit both nutrition and recovery. Involve student athletes in the meal planning process and allow them to help select menu choices. They often have higher calories needs than the rest of the family, so include plenty of carbohydrate-rich options. (especially in families where people are following low-carbohydrate diets for weight loss). For a balanced dinner, include one to two servings from each of the food groups listed in Table 4.2.

Table 4.2. Food For A Balanced Dinner

Starches/Grains	Meat/Protein	Fruits/Vegs	Milk/Dairy
Bread/Pita	Lunchmeat	Raw Veggies	Milk
Pasta	Meatballs	Tomato Sauce	Parmesan cheese
Tortilla	Beans/chicken	Salsa	Shredded cheese
Bagel	Peanut butter	Banana	Chocolate milk
Pizza	Canadian bacon	Pineapple/Tomato	Cheese
Bun	Chicken/Beef Burger	Tomato/Lettuce	Sliced Cheese
Rice	Chicken	Steamed Veggies	Milk

Fuel And Hydrate During Workouts

Student athletes need to maintain optimal hydration by having water and/or sports drinks available during workouts. Aim to consume about 16–24 ounces of fluid per hour during practices lasting 60 minutes or more. For workouts lasting more than 90 minutes, include a source of carbohydrate in the form of sports drinks, sports bars, gels or high-carbohydrate foods (that is, fig bars, sliced fruit, sliced bagels, etc.).

Plan Ahead... It's The Key

Student athletes looking for a winning edge should plan ahead for optimal nutrition by focusing on the following strategies:

- Eat a balanced breakfast in the morning or on the way to school.

- Pack or purchase a balanced lunch and make time to eat it.

- Plan a pre-event snack and eat it 30–60 minutes before practice.

- Hydrate and fuel during activity as recommended.

- Eat a balanced dinner to help refuel your body and promote recovery.

Best wishes for a safe, healthy and successful season.

Water, Water Everywhere

You can survive for a month without food, but only a few days without water.

- Water is the most important nutrient for active people.

- When you sweat, you lose water, which must be replaced. Drink fluids before, during, and after workouts.

- Water is a fine choice for most workouts. However; during continuous workouts of greater than 90 minutes, your body may benefit from a sports drink.

- Sports drinks have two very important ingredients—electrolytes and carbohydrates

- Sports drinks replace electrolytes lost through sweat during workouts lasting several hours.

- Carbohydrates in sports drinks provide extra energy. The most effective sports drinks contain 15 to 18 grams of carbohydrate in every eight ounces of fluid.

Source: From "Fast Facts About Sports Nutrition," an undated document produced by the President's Council on Fitness, Sports, and Nutrition (www.fitness.gov).

Fast Facts About Sports Nutrition

Rev Up Your Engine With Carbohydrates

Carbohydrates are your body's main source of energy.

- Carbohydrates are sugars and starches, and they are found in foods such as breads, cereals, fruits, vegetables, pasta, milk, honey, syrups, and table sugar.

- Sugars and starches are broken down by your body into glucose, which is used by your muscles for energy.

- For health and peak performance, more than half your daily calories should come from carbohydrates.

- Sugars and starches have four calories per gram, while fat has nine calories per gram. In other words, carbohydrates have less than half the calories of fat.

- If you regularly eat a carbohydrate-rich diet you probably have enough carbohydrate stored to fuel activity. Even so, be sure to eat a precompetition meal for fluid and additional energy. What you eat as well as when you eat your precompetition meal will be entirely individual.

Flexing Your Options To Build Bigger Muscles

It is a myth that eating lots of protein and/or taking protein supplements and exercising vigorously will definitely turn you into a big, muscular person.

- Building muscle depends on your genes, how hard you train, and whether you get enough calories.
- The average American diet has more than enough protein for muscle building. Extra protein is eliminated from the body or stored as fat.

Score With Vitamins And Minerals

Eating a varied diet will give you all the vitamins and minerals you need for health and peak performance.

- Exceptions include active people who follow strict vegetarian diets, avoid an entire group of foods, or eat less than 1800 calories a day. If you fall into any of these categories, a multi-vitamin and mineral pill may provide the vitamins and minerals missing in your diet.
- Taking large doses of vitamins and minerals will not help your performance and may be bad for your health. Vitamins and minerals do not supply the body with energy and, therefore are not a substitute for carbohydrates.

Popeye And All That Spinach

Iron supplies working muscles with oxygen.
- If your iron level is low, you may tire easily and not have enough stamina for activity.
- The best sources of iron are animal products, but plant foods such as fortified breads, cereals, beans and green leafy vegetables also contain iron.
- Iron supplements may have side effects, so take them only if your doctor tells you to.

No Bones About It, You Need Calcium Everyday

Many people do not get enough of the calcium needed for strong bones and proper muscle function.

- Lack of calcium can contribute to stress fractures and the bone disease, osteoporosis.

- The best sources of calcium are dairy products, but many other foods such as salmon with bones, sardines, collard greens, and okra also contain calcium. Additionally, some brands of bread, tofu, and orange juice are fortified with calcium.

Questions Most Frequently Asked About Sports Nutrition

What diet is best for athletes?

It's important that an athlete's diet provides the right amount of energy, the 50-plus nutrients the body needs and adequate water. No single food or supplement can do this. A variety of foods are needed every day. But, just as there is more than one way to achieve a goal, there is more than one way to follow a nutritious diet.

Do the nutritional needs of athletes differ from non-athletes?

Competitive athletes, sedentary individuals and people who exercise for health and fitness all need the same nutrients. However, because of the intensity of their sport or training program, some athletes have higher calorie and fluid requirements. Eating a variety of foods to meet increased calorie needs helps to ensure that the athlete's diet contains appropriate amounts of carbohydrate, protein, vitamins and minerals.

What do muscles use for energy during exercise?

Most activities use a combination of fat and carbohydrate as energy sources. How hard and how long you work out, your level of fitness and your diet will affect the type of fuel your body uses. For short-term, high-intensity activities like sprinting, athletes rely mostly on carbohydrate for energy. During low-intensity exercises like walking, the body uses more fat for energy.

What are carbohydrates?

Carbohydrates are sugars and starches found in foods like breads, cereals, fruits, vegetables, pasta, milk, honey, syrups, and table sugar. Carbohydrates are the preferred source of energy for your body. Regardless of origin, your body breaks down carbohydrates into glucose that your blood carries to cells to be used for energy. Carbohydrates provide four calories per gram, while fat provides nine calories per gram. Your body cannot differentiate between glucose that comes from starches or sugars. Glucose from either source provides energy for working muscles.

Is it true that athletes should eat a lot of carbohydrates?

When you are training or competing, your muscles need energy to perform. One source of energy for working muscles is glycogen which is made from carbohydrates and stored in your muscles. Every time you work out, you use some of your glycogen. If you don't consume enough carbohydrates, your glycogen stores become depleted, which can result in fatigue. Both sugars and starches are effective in replenishing glycogen stores.

When and what should I eat before I compete?

Performance depends largely on the foods consumed during the days and weeks leading up to an event. If you regularly eat a varied, carbohydrate-rich diet you are in good standing and probably have ample glycogen stores to fuel activity. The purpose of the pre-competition meal is to prevent hunger and to provide the water and additional energy the athlete will need during competition. Most athletes eat two to four hours before their event. However, some athletes perform their best if they eat a small amount 30 minutes before competing, while others eat nothing for six hours beforehand. For many athletes, carbohydrate-rich foods serve as the basis of the meal. However, there is no magic pre-event diet. Simply choose foods and beverages that you enjoy and that don't bother your stomach. Experiment during the weeks before an event to see which foods work best for you.

Will eating sugary foods before an event hurt my performance?

In the past, athletes were warned that eating sugary foods before exercise could hurt performance by causing a drop in blood glucose levels. Recent studies, however, have shown that consuming sugar up to 30 minutes before an event does not diminish performance. In fact, evidence suggests that a sugar-containing pre-competition beverage or snack may improve performance during endurance workouts and events.

What is carbohydrate loading?

Carbohydrate loading is a technique used to increase the amount of glycogen in muscles. For five to seven days before an event, the athlete eats 10-12 grams of carbohydrate per kilogram body weight and gradually reduces the intensity of the workouts. (To find out how much you weigh in kilograms, simply divide your weight in pounds by 2.2.) The day before the event, the athlete rests and eats the same high-carbohydrate diet. Although carbohydrate loading may be beneficial for athletes participating in endurance sports which require 90 minutes or more of non-stop effort, most athletes needn't worry about carbohydrate loading. Simply eating a diet that derives more than half of its calories from carbohydrates will do.

As an athlete, do I need to take extra vitamins and minerals?

Athletes need to eat about 1,800 calories a day to get the vitamins and minerals they need for good health and optimal performance. Since most athletes eat more than this amount, vitamin and mineral supplements are needed only in special situations. Athletes who follow vegetarian diets or who avoid an entire group of foods (for example, never drink milk) may need a supplement to make up for the vitamins and minerals not being supplied by food. A multivitamin-mineral pill that supplies 100% of the Recommended Dietary Allowance (RDA) will provide the nutrients needed. An athlete who frequently cuts back on calories, especially below the 1,800 calorie level, is not only at risk for inadequate vitamin and mineral intake, but also may not be getting enough carbohydrate. Since vitamins and minerals do not provide energy, they cannot replace the energy provided by carbohydrates.

Why is iron so important?

Hemoglobin, which contains iron, is the part of red blood cells that carries oxygen from the lungs to all parts of the body, including muscles. Since your muscles need oxygen to produce energy, if you have low iron levels in your blood, you may tire quickly. Symptoms of iron deficiency include fatigue, irritability, dizziness, headaches, and lack of appetite. Many times, however; there are no symptoms at all. A blood test is the best way to find out if your iron level is low. It is recommended that athletes have their hemoglobin levels checked once a year.

The RDA for iron is 15 milligrams a day for women and 10 milligrams a day for men. Red meat is the richest source of iron, but fish and poultry also are good sources. Fortified breakfast cereals, beans and green leafy vegetables also contain iron. Our bodies absorb the iron found in animal products best.

Why is calcium so important?

Calcium is needed for- strong bones and proper muscle function. Dairy foods are the best source of calcium. However, studies show that many female athletes who are trying to lose weight cut back on dairy products. Female athletes who don't get enough calcium may be at risk for stress fractures and, when they're older, osteoporosis. Young women between the ages of 11 and 24 need about 1,200 milligrams of calcium a day. Low-fat dairy products are a rich source of calcium and also are low in fat and calories.

Chapter 5

Preventing Dehydration

What Is Dehydration?

Dehydration is a condition that occurs when someone loses more fluids than he or she takes in. Dehydration isn't as serious a problem for teens as it can be for babies or young children. But if you ignore your thirst, dehydration can slow you down.

Our bodies are about two thirds water. When someone gets dehydrated, it means the amount of water in his or her body has dropped below the level needed for normal body function. Small decreases don't cause problems, and in most cases, they go completely unnoticed. But losing larger amounts of water can sometimes make a person feel quite sick.

Causes Of Dehydration

One common cause of dehydration in teens is gastrointestinal illness. When you're flattened by a stomach bug, you lose fluid through vomiting and diarrhea.

You might also hear that you can get dehydrated from playing sports. In reality, it's rare to reach a level of even moderate dehydration during sports or other normal outdoor activity. But if you don't replace fluid you lose through sweat as you go, you can become dehydrated from lots of physical activity, especially on a hot day.

Some athletes, such as wrestlers who need to reach a certain weight to compete, dehydrate themselves on purpose to drop weight quickly before a big game or event by sweating in saunas or using laxatives or diuretics, which make a person go to the bathroom more. This practice usually hurts more than it helps, though. Athletes who do this feel weaker, which affects performance. They can also have more serious problems, like abnormalities in the salt and potassium levels in the body. Such changes can also lead to problems with the heart's rhythm.

Dieting can sap someone's water reserves as well. Beware of diets or supplements, including laxatives and diuretics that emphasize shedding "water weight" as a quick way to lose weight. Losing water weight is not the same thing as losing actual fat.

Signs Of Dehydration

To counter dehydration, you need to restore the proper balance of water in your body. First, though, you have to recognize the problem.

Thirst is one indicator of dehydration, but it is not an early warning sign. By the time you feel thirsty, you might already be dehydrated. Other symptoms of dehydration include:

- feeling dizzy and lightheaded
- having a dry or sticky mouth
- producing less urine and darker urine

As the condition progresses, a person will start to feel much sicker as more body systems (or organs) are affected by the dehydration.

Preventing Dehydration

The easiest way to avoid dehydration is to drink lots of fluids, especially on hot, dry, windy days. Water is usually the best choice. Drinking water does not add calories to your diet and can be great for your health.

The amount that people need to drink will depend on factors like how much water they're getting from foods and other liquids and how much they're sweating from physical exertion.

Do you need 8 glasses of water a day?

No, but you do need to drink enough to satisfy your thirst, and maybe a little extra if you're sick or if you're going to be exercising.

When you're going to be outside on a warm day, dress appropriately for your activity. Wear loose-fitting clothes and a hat if you can. That will keep you cooler and cut down on sweating. If you do find yourself feeling parched or dizzy, take a break for a few minutes. Sit in the shade or someplace cool and drink water.

Sports And Exercise

If you're participating in sports or strenuous activities, drink some fluids before the activity begins. You should also drink at regular intervals (every 20 minutes or so) during the course of the activity and after the activity ends. The best time to train or play sports is in the early morning or late afternoon to avoid the hottest part of the day.

Gastrointestinal Infections

If you have a stomach bug and you're spending too much time getting acquainted with the toilet, you probably don't feel like eating or drinking anything. But you still need fluids. Take lots of tiny sips of fluids. For some people, ice pops may be easier to tolerate.

Caffeine

Caffeine is a diuretic, meaning it causes a person to urinate (pee) more. It's not clear whether this causes dehydration or not, but to be safe, it's probably a good idea to stay away from too much caffeine in hot weather, during long workouts, or in other situations where you might sweat a lot.

When To See A Doctor

Dehydration can usually be treated by drinking fluids. But if you faint or feel weak or dizzy every time you stand up (even after a couple of hours) or if you have very little urine output, you should tell an adult and visit your doctor. The doctor will probably look for a cause for the dehydration and encourage you to drink more fluids.

If you're more dehydrated than you realized, especially if you can't hold fluids down because of vomiting, you may need to receive fluids through an IV to speed up the rehydration process. An IV is an intravenous tube that goes directly into a vein.

Occasionally, dehydration might be a sign of something more serious, such as diabetes, so your doctor may run tests to rule out any other potential problems.

In general, dehydration is preventable. So just keep drinking that H2O for healthy hydration.

Chapter 6

Sports And Energy Drinks

Questions And Answers About Energy Drinks And Health

Energy drinks have been increasing in popularity, especially among teens and children. Due to several articles in the media about negative health effects experienced by people who consumed too many energy drinks, some parents and school personnel have become concerned about their growing popularity specifically among teens and children.

However, if you are aware of how much caffeine you are consuming, people of all ages can safely consume energy drinks in moderation. Caffeine is the primary ingredient in most energy drinks, and is often blamed for causing the negative health effects some people have experienced after consuming too many energy drinks. However, the majority of the healthy population can safely enjoy moderate amounts of caffeine without experiencing undesirable symptoms.

Staying aware of how much caffeine you are consuming each day from energy drinks, as well as other sources such as coffee, tea, soda, dietary supplements, and medications, is important to stay within moderate, safe intake levels. Learning how to determine the caffeine content of each item, as well as the number of servings per container, will help you to know how to moderate your consumption. You can also help children and teens learn how to moderate consumption so that they can safely enjoy an energy drink or soda responsibly without risking undesirable symptoms.

About This Chapter: "Questions and Answers about Energy Drinks and Health," © 2011 International Food Information Council (www.foodinsight.org). All rights reserved. Reprinted with permission. Although this text addresses parents, teens will also find the information helpful.

Below are some common questions consumers have about energy drinks and how they work to increase feelings of energy, and what you can do to help children and teens consume them in moderation along with a healthful diet.

What are energy drinks?

The term "energy drink" is a popular term used to refer to some beverages that typically contain caffeine as well as other ingredients, such as taurine, guarana, and B vitamins, for the purpose of providing an extra energy boost. It is not a term that is recognized by the U.S. Food and Drug Administration (FDA) or the U.S. Department of Agriculture (USDA).

What are the most common ingredients in energy drinks and what do they do?

Some common ingredients in energy drinks include caffeine, taurine, guarana, ginseng, B vitamins, and L-carnitine. More about what these ingredients are and why they're added to energy drinks is provided below.

Caffeine is included in energy drinks for its potential to improve mental and physical performance and for its taste profile. As it is often the primary ingredient in energy drinks, we will address more questions about caffeine.

Taurine is an amino acid that the body makes from the foods we eat. High levels of taurine are present in animal products (beef, pork, lamb, chicken, etc.), while some fish and shellfish contain the highest amounts of taurine (for example: cod, clams, and oysters). Taurine supports neurological development and helps regulate water and mineral salt levels in the blood. It is included in energy drinks because some studies have suggested that it may improve athletic performance. Additionally, some studies propose caffeine and taurine together may improve athletic performance, and perhaps even mental performance. In a report published in 2003, the European Union's Scientific Committee on Foods (now known as the European Food Safety Authority, or EFSA) concluded that studies have not shown a link between taurine consumption and cancer, and that both taurine and its components occur naturally in humans, and are further broken down and excreted by the body.

Guarana is a plant that comes from South America, and guarana-containing drinks and sodas are widely consumed in Brazil. Guarana contains caffeine, and is actually denser in caffeine than coffee beans. It is therefore added to energy drinks for the same reason as caffeine—to increase feelings of energy and to improve mental and physical performance. Guarana content is not typically listed on energy drink labels and adds only a very small amount of caffeine. Guarana is generally recognized as safe (GRAS) in the U.S. as a natural flavoring substance.

Ginseng is an herb that is thought to provide a number of potential benefits, including increasing a sense of well-being and stamina and improving both mental and physical performance. Other potential benefits include improving the health of people recovering from illness, beneficial effects on immunity, and lowering blood glucose levels. However, most of these studies were small or conducted only in laboratory animals. Therefore, additional research is needed to confirm these potential health benefits.

B vitamins can be found in different foods and help regulate metabolism. Examples of B vitamins include thiamin and cobalamin. These vitamins are often included in energy drinks because they may contribute to the maintenance of mental function.

Carnitine is derived from an amino acid and plays a role in energy production in cells, helping metabolism and energy levels. Some believe carnitine may improve athletic performance; however, there is no consistent research to support this theory. Most people get sufficient amounts of carnitine though the body's natural production, and through the foods we eat, without needing a supplement.

How does the caffeine in energy drinks increase feelings of energy?

Most energy drinks contain caffeine, which evidence has shown can improve both mental and athletic performance. Several studies have also found that moderate amounts of caffeine can increase alertness. In one study, participants used the words "vigor," "efficiency," "energy," and "clear-headedness" to describe their moods after consuming caffeine. Research has also shown that moderate caffeine consumption has the ability to improve memory and reasoning in sleep-deprived individuals. Additionally, caffeine has been shown to improve endurance if consumed before physical activity.

How much caffeine do energy drinks typically contain?

The caffeine content of energy drinks can vary greatly. A 250 milliliter (mL) energy drink (about 8.5 ounces) can have anywhere from 50–160 mg of caffeine. Comparatively, an average 8-ounce cup of coffee has about 100 mg caffeine, and a 12-ounce soft drink has about 40 mg caffeine. To put this into perspective, moderate caffeine consumption for most individuals, including sensitive populations such as pregnant women and children, is about 300 mg per day. Therefore, on average, one energy drink would fall within moderate consumption levels.

As caffeine content can vary between energy drinks, you should look up the caffeine content when trying a new energy drink. Most energy drink manufacturers list the caffeine content of the product on the label, or on the official product website. Also, remember to check the label for the proper serving size—one energy drink container may provide more than one serving, and you could potentially double or even triple your caffeine intake if you consume the full container.

Should I be concerned about the amount of caffeine in energy drinks?

Like all caffeinated foods and beverages, energy drinks can be consumed safely in moderation. The collective evidence from both scientific reviews and clinical studies concludes that moderate consumption of 300 mg caffeine per day is safe, even for more sensitive members of the population, such as children and pregnant women.

However, some people may be more sensitive to caffeine than others. Some may feel the effects of caffeine after only one serving, whereas others may be less sensitive. Symptoms experienced by some people may include excitement, restlessness and nervousness. Most people will adjust their consumption based on the amount of caffeine they can consume without feeling any effects.

Although daily consumption of 200 mg to 300 mg of caffeine has been shown through extensive scientific research not to have adverse effects on pregnancy, pregnant women should monitor their caffeine consumption and talk to their OB/GYN [obstetrician/gynecologist] and/or health care provider about their caffeine consumption.

And, although caffeine has not been found to cause chronic high blood pressure or increase the risk of heart disease, individuals with high blood pressure and/or history of heart attack or stroke should consult their physician about their caffeine intake.

What about reports of calls made to Poison Control Centers from people who were supposedly sent to the hospital from consuming energy drinks?

There has been some recent concern over calls to Poison Control Centers due to "caffeine intoxication," with media articles citing an increase in consumption of energy drinks by teens and children as the culprit. However, the majority of calls were actually related to people consuming dietary supplements containing caffeine, as opposed to energy drinks. Many of the reported effects occurred when caffeine was combined with other herbal and botanical ingredients and then ingested along with other pharmaceuticals.

Although studies suggest that most of these calls to Poison Control Centers are actually not from consuming energy drinks if you have children, you should talk to them about practicing moderation in all aspects of their diet and lives, including consuming moderate amounts of caffeinated foods and beverages. These beverages are designed to provide an extra energy boost, which many teens and children should not need, as they are young and naturally energetic. However, having one energy drink for enjoyment from time to time should not harm a healthy individual.

If you have any concerns or have observed symptoms from consuming just a small amount of caffeine, you should see a health care provider for advice before continuing to consume energy drinks and/or other caffeinated beverages. Also, energy drinks should always be consumed responsibly and should not be combined with alcohol.

With the growing popularity of energy drinks among children, should I be concerned about my child consuming energy drinks?

Caffeine in moderation is safe for the general healthy population, including children. Research shows that children are no more sensitive to caffeine than adults.

Although caffeine is safe for children to consume, many energy drinks include warnings on the label that state they are not intended for children. As with all treats, practice common sense when giving energy drinks to children—low to moderate amounts every once in a while can be enjoyed as part of an overall healthful diet. One way you can do this is by sharing a container with them, pouring the correct serving (according to the label) into a small glass.

At an early age, most of children's liquids should come from beverages containing important nutrients, such as calcium and vitamin D, such as low-fat milk and 100% fruit juice. Additionally, talking to your kids about moderation in all foods and beverages, and teaching them how to read food labels for caffeine content and other vitamins and minerals, can help them to make smart decisions as they get older.

Does caffeine cause children to become hyperactive?

No. There is no evidence that caffeine is associated with hyperactive behavior. In fact, most well designed scientific studies show no effects of caffeine on hyperactivity or attention deficit hyperactivity disorder (ADHD) in children.

Is caffeine addictive?

No, caffeine is not an addictive substance. Depending on the amount of caffeine ingested, it can be a mild stimulant to the central nervous system. Although caffeine is sometimes casually referred to as "addictive," moderate caffeine consumption is safe and should not be classified

Athletes And Sports Drinks

Athletes who exercise for extended periods of time both during training and at events can lose a substantial amount of sweat. When you sweat, you lose both water and sodium, as well as deplete the carbohydrate stores that help fuel your exercise. Sports drinks contain water, carbohydrates, sodium, and other electrolytes such as potassium and calcium

What's in a sports drink?

Carbohydrates provide the fuel for muscles and the brain and they contribute to the palatability of the drink. Ideally the sport drink should have a carbohydrate concentration of 4–8%. Higher carbohydrate concentrations impair gastric emptying and can cause gastric distress.

Sodium is the main electrolyte in sport drinks. It increases fluid uptake, retention and it also helps with salt replacement in heavy or salty sweaters.

Sodium also encourages fluid intake via the thirst mechanism. The sodium concentration of most sport drinks are in the range of 100 mg per eight ounces. If you will be exercising hard in the heat (particularly for more than three hours) and anticipate losing significant a amounts of sweat, consume a salty food within two to four hours pre-exercise to help stimulate thirst and retain the consumed fluids. Immediately post exercise then consume salty foods to help replace the salt lost in the exercise bout.

Other ingredients can be found in sport drinks that assist in flavor, free radical defense, energy metabolism, and recovery. Athletes should read the labels of their sport drinks and make sure they are free of any banned substances on the World Anti-Doping Agency (WADA) Prohibited List.

When should you consume sports drinks?

Sport drinks are typically consumed before, during and post training sessions and competitions. They help maintain hydration status and provide carbohydrate replacement for optimal performance.

What's the best sports drink?

Fluid requirements vary remarkably between athletes and between exercise bouts. Fluid losses are affected by genetics, body composition, fitness, environment and exercise mode and intensity.

The best sport drink also depends on personal taste and tolerance. Choose sports drinks that are 40 to 80 calories (10 to 20 g carb) and 55 to 110 g sodium per eight ounces.

Source: "Sports Drinks," © 2010 United States Olympic Committee. All rights reserved. Reprinted with permission.

with addictive drugs of abuse. People who say they are "addicted" to caffeine are often using the term loosely, like saying they are "addicted" to running, working, or television.

When regular caffeine consumption is stopped abruptly, some individuals may experience mild symptoms such as headache, fatigue, or drowsiness. These effects are usually mild and will subside in a day or two. By gradually reducing caffeine consumption over time, symptoms may be prevented or reduced.

Bottom Line

Energy drinks are safe and can be consumed in moderation along with a healthful diet. Remember to check the number of servings in an energy drink container to determine the total caffeine content, and to include caffeine from other sources, such as soda and coffee, when determining your total for the day. Use common sense and talk to your kids about all foods and beverages, including energy drinks, in moderation.

Chapter 7

Handling Sports Pressure And Competition

Most people play a sport for the thrill of having fun with others who share the same interest. But it's not always fun and games. There can be a ton of pressure in high school sports. A lot of the time it comes from the feeling that a parent or coach expects you to always win.

But sometimes it comes from inside, too: Some players are just really hard on themselves. And individual situations can add to the stress: Maybe there's a recruiter from your No. 1 college scouting you on the sidelines.

Whatever the cause, the pressure to win can sometimes stress you to the point where you just don't know how to have fun anymore.

How Can Stress Affect Sports Performance?

Stress is a feeling that's created when we react to particular events. It's the body's way of rising to a challenge and preparing to meet a tough situation with focus, strength, stamina, and heightened alertness. A little stress or the right kind of positive stress can help keep you on your toes, ready to rise to a challenge.

The events that provoke stress are called stressors, and they cover a whole range of situations—everything from outright danger to stepping up to take the foul shot that could win the game. Stress can also be a response to change or anticipation of something that's about to happen—good or bad. People can feel stress over positive challenges, like making the varsity team, as well as negative ones.

About This Chapter: "Handling Sports Pressure & Competition," October 2010, reprinted with permission from www.kidshealth.org. Copyright © 2010 The Nemours Foundation. This information was provided by KidsHealth, one of the largest resources online for medically reviewed health information written for parents, kids, and teens. For more articles like this one, visit www.KidsHealth.org or www.TeensHealth.org.

Distress is a bad type of stress that arises when you must adapt to too many negative demands. Suppose you had a fight with a close friend last night, you forgot your homework this morning, and you're playing in a tennis match this afternoon. You try to get psyched for the game but can't. You've hit stress overload. Continuous struggling with too much stress can exhaust your energy and drive.

Eustress is the good type of stress that stems from the challenge of taking part in something that you enjoy but have to work hard for. Eustress pumps you up, providing a healthy spark for any task you undertake.

What Can I Do To Ease Pressure?

When the stress of competition starts to get to you, try these techniques to help you relax:

- **Deep Breathing:** Find a quiet place to sit down. Inhale slowly through your nose, drawing air deep into your lungs. Hold your breath for about five seconds, then release it slowly. Repeat the exercise five times.

- **Muscle Relaxation:** Contract (flex) a group of muscles tightly. Keep them tensed for about five seconds, then release. Repeat the exercise five times, selecting different muscle groups.

- **Visualization:** Close your eyes and picture a peaceful place or an event from your past. Recall the beautiful sights and the happy sounds. Imagine stress flowing away from your body. You can also visualize success. People who advise competitive players often recommend that they imagine themselves completing a pass, making a shot, or scoring a goal over and over. Then on game day, you can recall your stored images to help calm nerves and boost self-confidence.

- **Positive Self-Talk:** Watch out for negative thoughts. Whether you're preparing for a competition or coping with a defeat, tell yourself: "I learn from my mistakes!" "I'm in control of my feelings!" "I can make this goal!"

When sports become too stressful, get away from the pressure. Go to a movie or hang out with friends. Put your mind on something completely different.

How Can I Keep Stress In Check?

If sports make you so nervous that you get headaches, become nauseated, or can't concentrate on other things, you're experiencing symptoms of unhealthy stress that's becoming a pattern. Don't keep such stress bottled up inside you; suppressing your emotions might mean bigger health troubles for you later on.

Enjoy The Game

Winning is exhilarating. But losing and some amount of stress are part of almost any sports program—as they are in life. Sports are about enhancing self-esteem, building social skills, and developing a sense of community. And above all, sports are about having fun.

Talk about your concerns with a friend. Simply sharing your feelings can ease your anxiety. Sometimes it may help to get an adult's perspective—someone who has helped others deal with sports stress like your coach or fitness instructor. Here are some other things you can do to cope with stress:

- Treat your body right. Eat well and get a good night's sleep, especially before games where the pressure's on.

- Learn and practice relaxation techniques, like those described in the previous section.

- Get some type of physical activity other than the sport you're involved in. Take a walk, ride your bike, and get completely away from the sport that's stressing you out.

- Don't try to be perfect—everyone flubs a shot or messes up from time to time (so don't expect your teammates to be perfect either). Forgive yourself, remind yourself of all your great shots, and move on.

It's possible that some stress stems only from uncertainty. Meet privately with your coach or instructor. Ask for clarification if his or her expectations seem vague or inconsistent. Although most instructors do a good job of fostering athletes' physical and mental development, you may need to be the one who opens the lines of communication. You may also want to talk with your parents or another adult family member.

If you're feeling completely overscheduled and out of control, review your options on what you can let go. It's a last resort, but if you're no longer enjoying your sport, it may be time to find one that's less stressful. Chronic stress isn't fun—and fun is what sports are all about.

Recognizing when you need guidance to steer yourself out of a stressful situation doesn't represent weakness; it's a sign of courage and wisdom. Don't stop looking for support until you've found it.

Chapter 8

Athletes And Eating Disorders

Eating disorders and subclinical disordered eating behaviors are serious problems that can negatively affect both the health and performance of young athletes. The incidence of young women struggling with eating disorders or disordered eating behaviors may be higher in some sports (for example, in sports like gymnastics, cross country, swimming, and cheerleading). These disorders need to be better understood by both athletes and those working closely with athletes in all sports so that intervention and treatment can be provided early.

The terms "eating disorders" and "disordered eating" are frequently used interchangeably, but they are distinct and should be recognized as such. With that being said, it may be easier to understand the differences if they are placed on a continuum.

Anorexia nervosa can be placed on the far left end of the continuum with subclinical anorexia just to the right of anorexia nervosa, bulimia nervosa on the far right end of the continuum with subclinical bulimia just to the left of bulimia nervosa and normal eating behaviors in the middle. All across the continuum (somewhere between the far ends and normal eating behavior in the middle) lie a host of abnormal eating behaviors.

The definition of eating disorders is that they are "psychiatric disorders that affect individuals' psychological, physical, nutritional, interpersonal, and emotional functioning and are characterized by dysfunctional eating patterns and disturbances or distortions about body size and shape."

About This Chapter: From "Clinical Eating Disorders versus Disordered Eating: A Wide Spectrum of Dangerous Behaviors," by Terry Zeigler. © 2011 Sports MD Media Inc. (www.sportsmd.com). All rights reserved. Reprinted with permission. The complete article, including references, is available online at http://www.sportsmd.com/SportsMD_Articles/id/404/n/clinical_eating_disorders_versus_disordered_eating_a_wide_spectrum_of_dangerous_behaviors.aspx.

According to the *Diagnostic and Statistical Manual of Mental Disorders* (*DSM-IV*), there are three clinical eating disorders. The three include anorexia nervosa, bulimia nervosa, and eating disorders not otherwise specified (EDNOS). The category of EDNOS was designed to describe conditions that meet some but not all of the criteria for anorexia nervosa and bulimia nervosa.

While there are three distinct categories of clinical eating disorders, there is another grouping of disordered eating syndromes that are classified as subclinical eating disorders. This category is used to describe individuals with considerable eating behavior pathology, but who do not meet the clinical criteria for the three identified clinical eating disorders.

Recognizing And Understanding Anorexia Nervosa

It is interesting to note that the term anorexia nervosa originated from the Greek word *anorexia* which means "lack of appetite." Perhaps early on it was thought that these individuals actually had a lack of appetite, but that is not really the case.

In actuality, the individual is always hungry. However hungry, the individual denies her hunger and in the process is starving herself. The criteria for diagnosing anorexia nervosa include the following:

- Refusal to maintain body weight at or above a minimally normal weight for age and height (that is, at least 85% of expected body weight)

- Intense fear of gaining weight or becoming fat, even though underweight

- Disturbance in the way in which one's body weight or shape is experienced, undue influence of body weight of shape on self-evaluation, or denial of the seriousness of the current low body weight

- In postmenarchal females, amenorrhea (that is, the absence of at least three consecutive menstrual cycles)

The Female Athlete Triad

Within the category of anorexia nervosa are two subtypes: the restricting type and the binge-eating/purging type. An individual with the restricting type of anorexia nervosa severely restricts her caloric intake and indulges in excessive exercise to burn the calories that are consumed. An individual with the binge-eating/purging type also restricts her caloric intake and participates in excessive exercise, but may also be involved with binge eating and purging either through self-induced vomiting or laxative/diuretic use to control weight.

Although the appearance of an individual with anorexia nervosa is one of physiological starvation, one has to understand that the disorder is a complex interplay of psychological, physiological, social, and physical systems. The psychological obsession is the focus on losing weight and being thin, but regardless of how much weight the individual loses, the individual still perceives herself as overweight.

Characteristics of an individual with anorexia nervosa may include the following:

- High-achieving
- Goal-oriented
- Perfectionist
- Low self-esteem
- Need for control
- Body dissatisfaction
- Depression
- Lack of assertiveness
- Obsessive-compulsive tendencies
- Anxiety

The characteristics are important to understand because the low self-esteem is what drives these individuals towards achieving their goal of losing weight with the belief that if only the weight is lost, the individual will be successful. The need for control also plays a critical role because controlling the amount of food intake is something that makes this individual feel successful.

The disorder manifests itself in a host of both physiological and psychological problems including decreased cardiac functioning, iron deficiencies, fatigue, increased rate of infection and illness, increased rate of injuries, gastrointestinal complications, endocrine abnormalities, decreased bone density, and psychological stress. Unfortunately, this disorder has an increased fatality rate with individuals dying from cardiac arrest due to weakening of the heart muscle.

Recognizing And Understanding Bulimia Nervosa

Whereas anorexia nervosa is characterized by starvation, bulimia nervosa is characterized by repeated cycles of uncontrollable food consumption followed by behavior to rid the body of the excessive calories including self-induced vomiting, excessive exercise, or laxative or diuretic abuse.

The criteria for diagnosing bulimia nervosa include:

- Recurrent episodes of binge eating. An episode of binge eating is characterized by both of the following:

    1. Eating, in a discrete period of time (that is, within a two-hour period), an amount of food that is definitely larger than most people would eat during a similar period of time and under similar circumstances, and

    2. A sense of lack of control over eating during the episode.

- Recurrent inappropriate compensatory behavior in order to prevent weight gain, such as self-induced vomiting; misuse of laxatives, diuretics, enemas, or other medications; fasting; or excessive exercise.

- The binge eating and inappropriate compensatory behaviors both occur, on average, at least twice a week for three months.

- Self-evaluation is unduly influenced by body shape and weight.

- The disturbance does not occur exclusively during episodes of anorexia nervosa.

Bulimia nervosa is also further divided into subtypes including the purging type and the nonpurging type. An individual with the purging type of bulimia nervosa engages in purging types of behavior including self-induced vomiting and the misuse of laxatives, diuretics, and other medication to purge her body of the excessive calories.

The non-purging type of bulimic individual uses methods that do not immediately rid the body of the excess calories but does so over time including excessive exercise and fasting. This individual may be involved in an episode of binge eating and then exercise for four or five hours followed by a fast for the next several days.

Unfortunately, the extended starvation period only makes the individual want food more. Instead of being able to eat normal portion sizes, the individual will eventually lose control of their appetite and gorge on food once again. This cycle is repeated over and over as the individual tries to gain control of their food obsession while not gaining weight.

The individual with bulimia nervosa tends to have cyclical variations in weight depending on where the person is in the binge-purge cycle. However, this individual's body weight stays in a neutral range unlike the individual suffering from anorexia nervosa. This up and down weight gain can be easily hidden with loose clothes so the condition may be more difficult to spot in athletes.

Along with the somewhat normal body weight of the individual, these individuals are adept at hiding their condition which makes this condition really difficult to identify. These individuals go to great lengths to binge and purge in private so as not to be caught. The fear of being discovered is a constant fear in the life of an individual with bulimia nervosa.

Some of the psychological characteristics or effects of bulimia nervosa include the following:

- Preoccupation with food
- Relentless pursuit of thinness
- Unusual eating habits and behaviors
- Low self-esteem
- Impulsivity or low sense of self-control
- Affective instability (depression, anger, anxiety)
- Difficulty expressing emotion in a direct manner
- Low frustration tolerance
- Absolute thinking
- Significant body dissatisfaction
- High need for approval (fear of disapproval)

Along with psychological characteristics, the individual suffering from bulimia nervosa may experience specific medical problems including menstrual irregularities, dental and gum disease, swollen parotid glands, gastrointestinal problems, and electrolyte abnormalities due to dehydration.

Whereas the individual with anorexia nervosa may suffer physiological effects directly related to starvation, the individual with bulimia nervosa may suffer from a number of physiological effects from purging. For example, dental cavities and tooth erosion are one side effect due to the gastric acid in the mouth from repeated vomiting.

Gastrointestinal problems may also occur including abdominal cramping, bloating, constipation, diarrhea, esophagitis, gastric and duodenal ulcers, slowed gastric emptying, spontaneous or reflex regurgitation, and even stomach rupture.

Last, cardiovascular complications may occur from electrolyte abnormalities and dehydration including water retention, low blood pressure, dizziness, light-headedness, and fainting. Damage to the heart muscle may also occur as a result of the use of emetics to induce vomiting.

Recognizing And Understanding Eating Disorders Not Otherwise Specified (EDNOS)

This fairly new clinical diagnosis was recently added to the *DMS-IV* to describe conditions that don't quite meet the criteria for either anorexia nervosa or bulimia nervosa but are clinically significant. The criteria for the diagnosis of EDNOS include the following:

- All of the criteria for anorexia nervosa are met except amenorrhea.

- All of the criteria for anorexia nervosa are met except that, despite significant weight loss, the individual's current weight is within the normal range.

- All of the criteria for bulimia nervosa are met except that the binge and purge cycles occur at a frequency of less than twice a week for a duration of less than three months.

- An individual of normal body weight regularly uses purging behaviors after eating small amounts of food.

- An individual repeatedly chews and spits out, but does not swallow, large amounts of food.

Recognizing And Understanding Subclinical Eating Disorders

Across the continuum from behaviors of an individual with anorexia nervosa to behaviors of an individual suffering from bulimia nervosa lie a large range of disordered eating behaviors that fall short of the established *DSM-IV* criteria for one of the three clinical conditions. These conditions may include individuals with considerable unhealthy eating behaviors and body weight concerns, but who may not manifest all of the clinical criteria.

The difficulty with individuals who may fall in to the category of subclinical eating disorders is that they may move along the continuum from unhealthy to healthy eating behaviors and back over time. Unhealthy eating behaviors may include the following:

- Excessive dieting
- Fasting
- Extreme body dissatisfaction
- Binge eating
- Compulsive exercising
- Purging

Regardless of where an individual may fall on the continuum of disordered eating behaviors, the behaviors associated with eating disorders and disordered eating are dangerous. The focus of those working with athletes is to be able to recognize that an athlete may be at risk for an eating disorder and to be able to refer the athlete to a team of appropriate medical professionals for intervention and treatment.

Chapter 9

The Female Athlete Triad

Hannah joined the track team her freshman year and trained hard to become a lean, strong sprinter. When her coach told her losing a few pounds would improve her performance, she immediately started counting calories and increased the duration of her workouts. She was too busy with practices and meets to notice that her period had stopped—she was more worried about the stress fracture in her ankle slowing her down.

Although Hannah thinks her intense training and disciplined diet are helping her performance, they may actually be hurting her—and her health.

What Is Female Athlete Triad?

Sports and exercise are part of a balanced, healthy lifestyle. People who play sports are healthier; get better grades; are less likely to experience depression; and use alcohol, cigarettes, and drugs less frequently than people who aren't athletes. But for some girls, not balancing the needs of their bodies and their sports can have major consequences.

Some girls who play sports or exercise intensely are at risk for a problem called female athlete triad. Female athlete triad is a combination of three conditions: disordered eating, amenorrhea, and osteoporosis. A female athlete can have one, two, or all three parts of the triad.

About This Chapter: "Female Athlete Triad," February 2010, reprinted with permission from www.kidshealth.org. Copyright © 2010 The Nemours Foundation. This information was provided by KidsHealth, one of the largest resources online for medically reviewed health information written for parents, kids, and teens. For more articles like this one, visit www.KidsHealth.org or www.TeensHealth.org.

Triad Factor #1: Disordered Eating

Most girls with female athlete triad try to lose weight as a way to improve their athletic performance. The disordered eating that accompanies female athlete triad can range from avoiding certain types of food the athlete thinks are "bad" (such as foods containing fat) to serious eating disorders like anorexia nervosa or bulimia nervosa.

Triad Factor #2: Amenorrhea

Exercising intensely and not eating enough calories can lead to decreases in estrogen, the hormone that helps to regulate the menstrual cycle. As a result, a girl's periods may become irregular or stop altogether. Of course, it's normal for teens to occasionally miss periods, especially in the first year. A missed period does not automatically mean female athlete triad. It could mean something else is going on, like pregnancy or a medical condition. If you are having sex and miss your period, talk to your doctor.

Some girls who participate intensively in sports may never even get their first period because they've been training so hard. Others may have had periods, but once they increase their training and change their eating habits, their periods may stop.

Triad Factor #3: Osteoporosis

Low estrogen levels and poor nutrition, especially low calcium intake, can lead to osteoporosis, the third aspect of the triad. Osteoporosis is a weakening of the bones due to the loss of bone density and improper bone formation. This condition can ruin a female athlete's career because it may lead to stress fractures and other injuries.

Usually, the teen years are a time when girls should be building up their bone mass to their highest levels—called peak bone mass. Not getting enough calcium now can also have a lasting effect on how strong a woman's bones are later in life.

Who Gets Female Athlete Triad?

Many girls have concerns about the size and shape of their bodies. But being a highly competitive athlete and participating in a sport that requires you to train extra hard can increase that worry.

Girls with female athlete triad often care so much about their sports that they would do almost anything to improve their performance. Martial arts and rowing are examples of sports that classify athletes by weight class, so focusing on weight becomes an important part of the training program and can put a girl at risk for disordered eating.

Participation in sports where a thin appearance is valued can also put a girl at risk for female athlete triad. Sports such as gymnastics, figure skating, diving, and ballet are examples of sports that value a thin, lean body shape. Some athletes may even be told by coaches or judges that losing weight would improve their scores.

Even in sports where body size and shape aren't as important, such as distance running and cross-country skiing, girls may be pressured by teammates, parents, partners, and coaches who mistakenly believe that "losing just a few pounds" could improve their performance.

The truth is, losing those few pounds generally doesn't improve performance at all. People who are fit and active enough to compete in sports generally have more muscle than fat, so it's the muscle that gets starved when a girl cuts back on food. Plus, if a girl loses weight when she doesn't need to, it interferes with healthy body processes such as menstruation and bone development.

In addition, for some competitive female athletes, problems such as low self-esteem, a tendency toward perfectionism, and family stress place them at risk for disordered eating.

What Are The Signs And Symptoms?

If a girl has risk factors for female athlete triad, she may already be experiencing some symptoms and signs of the disorder, such as:

- weight loss
- no periods or irregular periods
- fatigue and decreased ability to concentrate
- stress fractures (fractures that occur even if a person hasn't had a significant injury)
- muscle injuries

Girls with female athlete triad often have signs and symptoms of eating disorders, such as:

- continued dieting in spite of weight loss
- preoccupation with food and weight
- frequent trips to the bathroom during and after meals
- using laxatives
- brittle hair or nails
- dental cavities because in girls with bulimia tooth enamel is worn away by frequent vomiting
- sensitivity to cold

- low heart rate and blood pressure

- heart irregularities and chest pain

Tips For Female Athletes

Here are a few tips to help teen athletes stay on top of their physical condition:

- Keep track of your periods. It's easy to forget when you had your last visit from Aunt Flo, so keep a calendar in your gym bag and mark down when your period starts and stops and if the bleeding is particularly heavy or light. That way, if you start missing periods, you'll know right away and you'll have accurate information to give to your doctor.

- Don't skip meals or snacks. If you're constantly on the go between school, practice, and competitions you may be tempted to skip meals and snacks to save time. But eating now will improve performance later, so stock your locker or bag with quick and easy favorites such as bagels, string cheese, unsalted nuts and seeds, raw vegetables, granola bars, and fruit.

- Visit a dietitian or nutritionist who works with teen athletes. He or she can help you get your dietary game plan into gear and find out if you're getting enough key nutrients such as iron, calcium, and protein. And if you need supplements, a nutritionist can recommend the best choices.

- Do it for you. Pressure from teammates, parents, or coaches can turn a fun activity into a nightmare. If you're not enjoying your sport, make a change. Remember: It's your body and your life. You—not your coach or teammates—will have to live with any damage you do to your body now.

How Doctors Help

An extensive physical examination is a crucial part of diagnosing female athlete triad. A doctor who thinks a girl has female athlete triad will probably ask questions about her periods, her nutrition and exercise habits, any medications she takes, and her feelings about her body. This is called the medical history.

Poor nutrition can also affect the body in many ways, so a doctor might order blood tests to check for anemia and other problems associated with the triad. The doctor also will check for medical reasons why a girl may be losing weight and missing her periods. Because osteoporosis can put someone at higher risk for bone fractures, the doctor may also request tests to measure bone density.

Doctors don't work alone to help a girl with female athlete triad. Coaches, parents, physical therapists, pediatricians and adolescent medicine specialists, nutritionists and dietitians, and mental health specialists can all work together to treat the physical and emotional problems that a girl with female athlete triad faces.

It might be tempting to shrug off several months of missed periods, but getting help right away is important. In the short term, female athlete triad may lead to muscle weakness, stress fractures, and reduced physical performance. Over the long term, it can cause bone weakness, long-term effects on the reproductive system, and heart problems.

A girl who is recovering from female athlete triad might work with a dietitian to help reach and maintain a healthy weight while eating enough calories and nutrients for health and good athletic performance. Depending on how much the girl is exercising, she may have to reduce the length of her workouts. Talking to a psychologist or therapist can help her deal with depression, pressure from coaches or family members, or low self-esteem and can help her find ways to deal with her problems other than restricting food intake or exercising excessively.

Some girls may need to take hormones to supply their bodies with estrogen to help prevent further bone loss. Calcium and vitamin D supplementation can also help when someone has bone loss as the result of female athlete triad.

What If I Think Someone I Know Has It?

It's tempting to ignore female athlete triad and hope it goes away. But it requires help from a doctor and other health professionals. If a friend, sister, or teammate has signs and symptoms of female athlete triad, discuss your concerns with her and encourage her to seek treatment. If she refuses, you may need to mention your concern to a parent, coach, teacher, or school nurse.

You might worry about seeming nosy when you ask questions about a friend's health, but you're not: Your concern is a sign that you're a caring friend. Lending an ear may be just what your friend needs.

Chapter 10

Emotional Injuries In Youth Sports

Abuse Defined

Abuse occurs when someone uses his or her power or position to harm you emotionally, physically, or sexually or as a result of neglect.

Emotional Abuse

- Is a verbal attack on a child's self-esteem by a person in a position of power, authority, or trust such as a parent or coach

- Occurs even if the attack is intended as a form of discipline or is not intended by the adult to cause harm

- Takes many forms, including any of the following:

    - Name calling ("Hey, Fatty!" or "Hey, Shorty" or "Hey, Mr. Klutz")

    - Threatening ("If you don't win, you can forget about me buying that new CD you want.")

    - Insulting ("You're stupid," or "You're clumsy," or "You're an embarrassment to our family," or "You don't deserve to wear that uniform.")

    - Bullying or taunting by a teammate

About This Chapter: "Abuse in Youth Sports Takes Many Different Forms," by Brooke de Lench, Founder and Editor-in-Chief of MomsTeam.com: the Trusted Source for Youth Sports Parents. © 2006–2012 MomsTeam.com. All rights reserved. Reprinted with permission.

- Criticizing or ridiculing ("You are a loser," or "I thought you were better than that. I guess I was wrong.")

- Intimidating ("Watch out kid, my son is going to break your nose.")

- Yelling at a child for losing or not playing up to the adult's expectations

- Hazing

- Negative questioning ("Why didn't you win?" or "How could you let that guy beat you?")

- Shunning or withholding love or affection

- Being punished for not playing up to expectations or when your team loses

Physical Abuse

- Occurs when a person in a position of power, authority, or trust such as a parent or coach purposefully injures or threatens to injure a child

- Takes many forms, including any of the following:

  - Slapping

  - Hitting

  - Shaking

  - Throwing equipment

  - Kicking

  - Pulling hair

  - Pulling ears

  - Striking

  - Shoving

  - Grabbing

  - Hazing

  - Punishing "poor" play or rules violations through the use of excessive exercise (extra laps, etc.) or by denying fluids

Sexual Abuse

- Occurs when a person in a position of power, authority, or trust engages in "sexualized" touching or sex with a child

- "Sexualized touching" is where touching, instead of being respectful and nurturing, is done in a sexual manner. Here are some examples:
    - Fondling instead of a hug
    - Long kiss on the lips instead of a peck on the cheek
    - Seductive stroking of any area of the child's body instead of a simple pat on the rear-end for a good play

What Is Harassment?

A child is being harassed when she or he is threatened, intimidated, taunted, or subjected to racial, homophobic, or sexist slurs. Sexual harassment includes comments, contact, or behavior of a sexual nature that is offensive, uninvited, or unwelcome.

Neglect

Neglect is a chronic inattention to the basic necessities of life such as supervision, medical and dental care, adequate rest, safe environment, exercise, and fresh air.

Neglect in a sports setting make take the following forms:

- Injuries are not properly treated
- Athletes are forced to play hurt
- Equipment is inadequate, poorly maintained, or unsafe
- Road trips are not properly supervised
- Allowing bullying by teammates

Surprisingly Common

According to a widely reported 1993 survey conducted by the Minnesota Amateur Sports Commission:

- Almost half (45.3%) of those surveyed (both males and females) said they had been emotionally abused while participating in sports (i.e., called names, yelled at, or insulted).

- Slightly more than one out of six (17.5%) said they had suffered physical abuse while playing sports (i.e., hit, kicked, or slapped.

- More than one in five (21%) said they had suffered neglect while playing sports (pressured to play with an injury).

- One in 12 (8%) said they had been sexually harassed while playing sports (called names with sexual connotations).

- One in 30 (3.4%) said they had been pressured into sex or sexual touching.

Twelve years later, a 2005 study by researchers at the University of Missouri, the University of Minnesota, and Notre Dame University reported in the *Journal of Research in Character Education* found that emotional abuse in youth sports was still widespread:

- More than four in ten coaches have loudly argued with a ref or sport official following a bad call (youth athletes said 48% of coaches engaged in this behavior, although only 20% of parents said they did so).

- Seven out ten youth athletes have heard a fan (most likely a parent) angrily yell at an official.

- Four in ten youth athletes have heard a fan angrily yell at a coach.

- One in eight parents has angrily criticized their child's sports performance (another study, this one conducted in Fall 2005 by Blue Cross and Blue Shield of Minnesota, reported that more than four in ten parents had seen a verbal altercation between a parent and their child that they thought was inappropriate).

- One third of coaches have angrily yelled at a player for making a mistake, a high rate "of significant concern" to the study's authors, who wondered, "What would we think if a third of our teachers yelled at students for making mistakes, and one in ten made fun of a student?"

- One in seven athletes made fun of a less-skilled opponent. About one in ten coaches admitted to making fun a team member. These numbers suggests that on most teams there is a high probability that one or more of the lesser skilled players has been at least mildly victimized.

- More than four in ten youth athletes reported having been teased or yelled at by a fan or seeing a fan angrily yell at or tease another player.

Emotional Abuse: The Damage Is No Less Real

Perhaps because the damage caused by emotional abuse is not obvious, like sexual abuse, or immediately apparent, like a physical injury, its effect is often overlooked and minimized. But, says San Francisco child psychologist Maria Pease, the damage is no less real, and, in fact, may be much more damaging and long-lasting:

- Children are deeply affected by negative comments from parents, coaches and other adults to whom they look up and respect, or even by more skilled teammates (e.g., bullying). One comment can turn a child off to sports forever.

- Children are much more sensitive than adults to criticism: being yelled at, put down, or embarrassed is much more likely to have negative psychological consequences and to cause the child to feel humiliated, shamed, and degraded and to damage her feelings of self-worth and self-esteem.

- If the abuse becomes chronic, a pattern of negative comments can destroy a child's spirit, motivation, and self-esteem. Over time, the young athlete will begin to believe what adults say about him. Abusive comments intended to improve athletic performance are likely to have precisely the opposite effect.

- Children who experience screaming on a regular basis will react in certain ways to protect or defend themselves. This may be adaptive in the moment to survive the screaming, but ultimately be maladaptive and constrict their ability to be psychologically healthy over time.

- A more anxious, sensitive child may be intolerant of screaming very early on and remove himself from the sport (he maybe the lucky one). However, he is also more likely to endure the screaming without telling a parent or responding to the coach directly out of fear of reprisal from the coach. A more sensitive child who stays in this situation may be more affected physiologically with overall heightened arousal levels as discussed above.

- A more secure child will likely have the same physiological responses but be less vulnerable to them. He may find a way to tune out the coach, but this may come at a cost of emotional sensitivity. As the child becomes less sensitive to his own fearful feelings, he can become less sensitive to the feeling of others, leading to loss of empathy. He will also become less sensitive to emotions in general, and have a loss of sensitivity to positive emotions as well. He is also likely to resent the coach for putting him in such a psychologically vulnerable position.

Children involved in sports often make strong connections and develop a special trusting relationship with their coaches and instructors, and if the coaches' power is abused, children can suffer severe psychological injuries that may last a lifetime. In a 2004 study of emotional abuse of elite child athletes in the United Kingdom, for instance, athletes reported that the abuse by their coaches created a climate a fear and made them feel stupid, worthless or upset, lacking in self-confidence, angry, depressed, humiliated, fearful and hurt, and left long-lasting emotional scars.

Chapter 11

Athlete Burnout

Burnout, or overtraining syndrome, is a condition in which an athlete experiences fatigue and declining performance in his/her sport despite continuing or increased training. Overtraining can result in mood changes, decreased motivation, frequent injuries, and infections.

How It Occurs

Burnout is thought to be a result of the physical and emotional stress of training. Many athletes have some initial decrease in performance when they increase their level of training. Generally, however, after a short recovery period the athlete will see an improvement in performance. Overtraining syndrome happens when an athlete fails to recover adequately from training and competition. The symptoms are due to a combination of changes in hormones, suppression of the immune system (which decreases the athlete's ability to fight infection), physical fatigue and psychological changes.

Risk Factors

There are many factors are thought to increase the risk of developing overtraining syndrome including:

- Specializing in one sport
- Sudden and large increases in training
- Participation in endurance sports

About This Chapter: "Burnout in Young Athletes (Overtaining Syndrome)," reprinted with permission from Ann & Robert H. Lurie Children's Hospital of Chicago (www.luriechildrens.org). © 2012. All rights reserved.

- High anxiety level
- Low self esteem
- Pressure from parents/coaches

Signs And Symptoms

In the young athlete, signs and symptoms of burnout can be highly variable and can include:

- Chronic muscle and joint pain
- Weight loss and loss of appetite
- Increased heart rate at rest
- Decreased sports performance
- Fatigue
- Prolonged recovery time
- Lack of enthusiasm
- Frequent illnesses
- Difficulty completing usual routines
- Decreased school performance
- Personality or mood changes
- Increased anger or irritability
- Sleep disturbances (difficulty sleeping, or sleeping without feeling refreshed)

These are warning signs of unhealthy sports participation, which may increase the risk of burnout:

- The athlete is no longer having fun playing sports.
- The athlete's sport is dominating his/her and his/her family's life.
- The only topic of conversation at home or at the dinner table is the child's sports.
- The athlete is rewarded on how they perform in sports.
- The athlete has missed 10% of his/her season and has not yet seen a doctor.
- The only important thing to the athlete or parent is winning.

- A female athlete is now 16 and has not yet started her period.
- The athlete is dieting just to become a faster runner.
- A young athlete only plays one sport and is unwilling to try any others.

Diagnosis

There is no test for overtraining syndrome. The diagnosis is based on an athlete's story, the symptoms that he/she reports, and the absence of an alternative explanation for these symptoms.

Treatment

The only treatment for burnout is rest. The athlete should stop participation in training/competition for a set period of time. The time required varies (generally 4–12 weeks) depending on several factors, including the type of sport, level of skill and competition, and severity of symptoms. During the rest period, the athlete can participate in short intervals of low intensity aerobic exercise to help keep active and fit; this type of activity should be unrelated to his/her sport.

Preventing Burnout

Specific guidelines for trainers/coaches/parents include:

1. Make training fun and interesting with age-appropriate games and workouts.
2. Keep the training regimen flexible with planned breaks one to two days per week and longer breaks every few months to allow for complete recovery.
3. Maintain a supportive environment for the athlete.
4. Teach the athlete to be aware of the cues from their body that indicate a need to slow down or change their training routine. Discuss the importance of overall health and wellness and be open to conversations about these issues.

Specific guidelines for the athlete include:

1. Spend one to two days per week resting from organized sport participation or participating in alternate activities.
2. Allow slightly longer breaks (a couple of weeks) from training and competition every three months. This time could be spent focusing on other activities and cross training without intensive training or competition.
3. Maintain a healthy, balanced diet. Drink plenty of water.
4. Listen to your body. Take a short break or alter your training if your body needs a change.
5. Try to be a well-rounded athlete who participates in many different activities.

Returning To Activity And Sports

When the signs and symptoms of burnout have resolved completely (including physical symptoms, mood changes, sleep disturbances etc.), the athlete may begin slowly to reintroduce training. Athletes should increase the duration of activity before increasing the intensity of activity. If symptoms begin to recur when training is restarted, the athlete should again initiate a rest period and reevaluate the training approach.

Chapter 12

Anabolic Steroids

What are anabolic steroids?

Ever wondered how those bulky weight lifters got so big? While some may have gotten their muscles through a strict regimen of weightlifting and diet, others may have gotten that way through the illegal use of anabolic-androgenic steroids. *Anabolic* refers to a steroid's ability to help build muscle, and *androgenic* refers to their role in promoting the development of male sexual characteristics. Other types of steroids, like cortisol, estrogen, and progesterone, do not build muscle, are not anabolic, and therefore do not have the same harmful effects.

Anabolic-androgenic steroids are usually synthetic substances similar to the male sex hormone testosterone. They do have legitimate medical uses. Sometimes doctors prescribe them to help people with certain kinds of anemia and men who don't produce enough testosterone on their own. But doctors never prescribe anabolic steroids to young, healthy people to help them build muscles. Without a prescription from a doctor, anabolic steroids are illegal.

There are many different anabolic-androgenic steroids. Here's a list of some of the most common ones taken today: Andro, Oxandrin, Dianabol, Winstrol, Deca-Durabolin, and equipoise.

What are the common street names?

Slang words for steroids are hard to find. Most people just say steroids. On the street, steroids may be called "roids" or "juice." The scientific name for this class of drugs is anabolic-androgenic steroids. But even scientists shorten it to anabolic steroids.

About This Chapter: Excerpted from "Anabolic Steroids," National Institute on Drug Abuse (www.nida.nih.gov), June 2009.

How are they used?

Some people who abuse steroids pop pills. Others use hypodermic needles to inject steroids directly into muscles. When people take drugs without regard for their legality or their adverse health effects, they are abusing steroids. People who abuse steroids have been known to take doses 10 to 100 times higher than the amount prescribed by a doctor for medical reasons.

What is the scope of steroid abuse?

Most teens are smart and stay away from steroids. As part of a 2010 NIDA-funded study, teens were asked if they ever tried steroids—even once. Only 1.1% of 8th graders, 1.6% of 10th graders, and 2.0% of 12th graders ever tried steroids. Abuse is well known to occur in a number of professional sports, including bodybuilding and baseball.

How are anabolic steroids abused?

Some people, both athletes and non-athletes, abuse anabolic steroids in an attempt to enhance performance and/or improve physical appearance. Anabolic steroids are taken orally or injected, typically in cycles rather than continuously. *Cycling* refers to a pattern of use in which steroids are taken for periods of weeks or months, after which use is stopped for a period of time and then restarted. In addition, users often combine several different types of steroids in an attempt to maximize their effectiveness, a practice referred to as *stacking*.

How do anabolic steroids affect the brain?

The immediate effects of anabolic steroids in the brain are mediated by their binding to androgen (male sex hormone) and estrogen (female sex hormone) receptors on the surface of a cell. This anabolic-androgenic steroid–receptor complex can then shuttle into the cell nucleus to influence patterns of gene expression. Because of this, the acute effects of anabolic steroids in the brain are substantially different from those of other drugs of abuse. The most important difference is that anabolic steroids are not euphorigenic, meaning they do not trigger rapid increases in the neurotransmitter dopamine, which is responsible for the "high" that often drives substance abuse behaviors. However, long-term use of anabolic steroids can eventually have an impact on some of the same brain pathways and chemicals—such as dopamine, serotonin, and opioid systems—that are affected by other drugs of abuse. Considering the combined effect of their complex direct and indirect actions, it is not surprising that anabolic steroids can affect mood and behavior in significant ways.

Excerpted from "InfoFacts: Steroids (Anabolic-Androgenic)," National Institute on Drug Abuse, July 2009.

What are the effects?

A major health consequence from abusing anabolic steroids can include prematurely stunted growth through early skeletal maturation and accelerated puberty changes. This means that teens risk remaining short for the remainder of their lives if they take anabolic steroids before they stop growing. Other effects include jaundice (yellowish coloring of skin, tissues, and body fluids), fluid retention, high blood pressure, increases in LDL (bad cholesterol), decreases in HDL (good cholesterol), severe acne, trembling, and in very rare cases liver and kidney tumors. In addition, there are some gender-specific side effects:

- **For Guys:** Shrinking of the testicles, reduced sperm count, infertility, baldness, development of breasts, and increased risk for prostate cancer

- **For Girls:** Growth of facial hair, male-pattern baldness, changes in or cessation of the menstrual cycle, enlargement of the clitoris, and a permanently deepened voice

Steroid abuse can also have an effect on behavior. Many users report feeling good about themselves while on anabolic steroids, but researchers report that extreme mood swings also can occur, including manic-like symptoms leading to violence. This is because anabolic steroids act in a part of the brain called the limbic system, which influences mood and is also involved in learning and memory.

Steroids can also lead to other changes in mood, such as feelings of depression or irritability. Depression, which can be life threatening, often is seen when the drugs are stopped and may contribute to the continued use of anabolic steroids. Researchers also report that users may suffer from paranoia, jealousy, extreme irritability, delusions, and impaired judgment stemming from feelings of invincibility.

Can steroid abuse be fatal?

In some rare cases, yes. When steroids enter the body, they go to different organs and muscles. Steroids are not friendly to the heart. In rare cases, steroid abuse can create a situation where the body may be susceptible to heart attacks and strokes, which can be fatal. Here's how: Steroid use can lead to a condition called atherosclerosis, which causes fat deposits inside arteries to disrupt blood flow. When blood flow to the heart is blocked, a heart attack can occur. If blood flow to the brain is blocked, a stroke can result.

Bulking up the artificial way—by using steroids—puts teens at risk for more than cardiovascular disease. Steroids can weaken the immune system, which is what helps the body fight against germs and disease. That means that illnesses and diseases have an easy target in someone who is abusing steroids.

In addition, people who inject anabolic steroids may share non-sterile "works," or drug injection equipment, that can spread life-threatening viral infections such as HIV/AIDS or hepatitis, which causes serious damage to the liver.

Are anabolic steroids addictive?

It is possible that some people who abuse steroids may become addicted to the drugs, as evidenced by their continued use in spite of physical problems and negative effects on social relationships. Also, they spend large amounts of time and money obtaining the drugs and,

Addictive Potential

Animal studies have shown that anabolic steroids are reinforcing—that is, animals will self-administer anabolic steroids when given the opportunity, just as they do with other addictive drugs. This property is more difficult to demonstrate in humans, but the potential for anabolic steroid abusers to become addicted is consistent with their continued abuse despite physical problems and negative effects on social relations. Also, steroid abusers typically spend large amounts of time and money obtaining the drug: this is another indication of addiction. Individuals who abuse steroids can experience withdrawal symptoms when they stop taking anabolic steroids—these include mood swings, fatigue, restlessness, loss of appetite, insomnia, reduced sex drive, and steroid cravings, all of which may contribute to continued abuse. One of the most dangerous withdrawal symptoms is depression— when persistent, it can sometimes lead to suicide attempts.

Research also indicates that some users might turn to other drugs to alleviate some of the negative effects of anabolic steroids. For example, a study of 227 men admitted in 1999 to a private treatment center for dependence on heroin or other opioids found that 9.3% had abused anabolic steroids before trying any other illicit drug. Of these, 86% first used opioids to counteract insomnia and irritability resulting from the steroids.

Treatment Options

There has been very little research on treatment for anabolic steroid abuse. Current knowledge derives largely from the experiences of a small number of physicians who have worked with patients undergoing steroid withdrawal. They have learned that, in general, supportive therapy combined with education about possible withdrawal symptoms is sufficient in some cases. Sometimes, medications can be used to restore the balance of the hormonal system after its disruption by steroid abuse. If symptoms are severe or prolonged, symptomatic medications or hospitalization may be needed.

Excerpted from "InfoFacts: Steroids (Anabolic-Androgenic)," National Institute on Drug Abuse (www.nida.nih.gov), July 2009.

when they stop using them, they experience withdrawal symptoms such as depression, mood swings, fatigue, restlessness, loss of appetite, insomnia, reduced sex drive, and the desire to take more steroids. The most dangerous of the withdrawal symptoms is depression, because it sometimes leads to suicide attempts. Untreated, some depressive symptoms associated with anabolic steroid withdrawal have been known to persist for a year or more after the person stops taking the drugs.

What can be done to prevent steroid abuse?

Research has shown that there is an effective program for preventing steroid abuse among players on high school sports teams. In the ATLAS (for guys) and ATHENA (for girls) programs, coaches and sports team leaders discuss the potential effects of anabolic steroids and other illicit drugs on immediate sports performance, and they teach how to refuse offers of drugs. They also discuss how strength training and proper nutrition can help adolescents build their bodies without the use of steroids. Later, special trainers teach the players proper weightlifting techniques. An ongoing series of studies has shown that this multi-component, team-centered approach reduces new steroid abuse by 50% and, at the same time, produces the kind of athletic performance that the teen desires.

What is the bottom line?

Science proves that there are serious risks associated with the abuse of steroids, and teens should never use anabolic steroids to help them bulk up.

Chapter 13

Alcohol And Marijuana: Problems For Teen Athletes

Teen Athletes More Likely To Drink Alcohol Than Peers

Young athletes are more likely to consume alcohol than their peers, but are less likely to smoke cigarettes, marijuana, or do other drugs, a new study finds.

Reuters reported May 30 [2011] that around 57 percent of athletes drank alcohol at least once in the past month, compared to 45 percent of non-athletes, according to research from the University of Michigan at Ann Arbor.

With cigarettes and marijuana, however, the trend reverses: 25 to 29 percent of exercisers and athletes say they smoked cigarettes in the past month, compared to 38 percent of non-exercisers, while 15 to 17 percent of athletes smoked marijuana in the past month, compared to 23 percent of non-athletes.

Athletes may turn to drink because of their competitive nature, to blow off steam, or because the physical toll of alcohol is not as immediately detrimental to their performance as other recreational substances, experts speculate. High-school drinkers also report drinking more heavily later in life, according to follow-up surveys.

"Individuals who tend to be high drug-users often can't keep up in a really competitive environment," says study author Yvonne Terry-McElrath. "Also, they're likely to get kicked off of teams that do drug testing."

About This Chapter: This chapter begins with "Teen Athletes More Likely to Drink Alcohol than Peers" and "Alcohol and Exercise Relationship Surprises Experts," reprinted with permission from Well-Being Wire, http://wellbeingwire .meyouhealth.com. © 2011 MeYou Health LLC. All rights reserved. Reviewed by David A. Cooke, MD, FACP, April 2012. The chapter concludes with excerpts from "Marijuana: Facts for Teens," National Institute on Drug Abuse, Mach 2011.

But, "if we can encourage an enjoyment in general exercise, we may be able to see a lowering of participation in drug use," she adds.

The study appears online in the journal *Addiction*.

Alcohol Effects

Alcohol affects every organ in the drinker's body. Intoxication can impair brain function and motor skills; heavy use can increase risk of certain cancers, stroke, and liver disease. Alcoholism or alcohol dependence is a diagnosable disease characterized by a strong craving for alcohol, and/or continued use despite harm or personal injury. Alcohol abuse, which can lead to alcoholism, is a pattern of drinking that results in harm to one's health, interpersonal relationships, or ability to work.

Risky Drinking And Summer Sports

Summer is a wonderful time for outdoor activities with family and friends, but drinking impairs both physical and mental abilities, and it also decreases inhibitions—which can lead to tragic consequences. In fact, research shows that half of all water recreation deaths of teens and adults involve the use of alcohol.

Swimmers Can Get In Over Their Heads

Alcohol impairs judgment and increases risk-taking, a dangerous combination for swimmers. Even experienced swimmers may venture out farther than they should and not be able to make it back to shore, or they may not notice how chilled they're getting and develop hypothermia. Surfers could become over-confident and try to ride a wave beyond their abilities. Even around a pool, too much alcohol can have deadly consequences. Inebriated divers may collide with the diving board or dive where the water is too shallow.

Boaters Can Lose Their Bearings

According to research funded by the National Institute on Alcohol Abuse and Alcoholism, alcohol may be involved in 60 percent of boating fatalities, including falling overboard. And a boat operator with a blood alcohol concentration (BAC) over 0.1 percent is 16 times more likely to be killed in a boating accident than an operator with zero BAC. According to the U.S. Coast Guard and the National Association of State Boating Law Administrators, alcohol can impair a boater's judgment, balance, vision, and reaction time. It can also increase fatigue and susceptibility to the effects of cold-water immersion. And if problems arise, intoxicated boaters are ill equipped to find solutions. For passengers, intoxication can lead to slips on deck, falls overboard, or accidents at the dock.

Source: "Alcohol Effects" excerpted from "Alcohol," National Institute on Drug Abuse, 2011. "Risky Drinking And Summer Sports," excerpted from "Risky Drinking Can Put a Chill on Your Summer Fun," National Institute on Alcohol Abuse and Alcoholism (NIAAA), 2011.

Alcohol And Exercise Relationship Surprises Experts

Some animal and human studies have shown that—contrary to expectations—vigorous exercise may actually make you drink more alcohol, and vice-versa, the *New York Times* reported January 5 [2011].

University of Miami researchers who studied health surveys on thousands of Americans concluded that "drinking is associated with a 10.1 percentage point increase in the probability of exercising vigorously" and that "heavy drinkers exercise about 10 more minutes per week than current moderate drinkers and about 20 more minutes per week than current abstainers."

On the other hand, University of Houston scientists found that rats that exercised more had more desire to drink alcohol.

The reasons that people seem to drink more if they exercise more is unclear. Experts say that those who exercise frequently may be sensation-seekers in general, be more likely to take part in social activities where alcohol is served, or may be working out to compensate for their perceived alcohol over-use.

As for the rats, they may have turned to the reward of alcohol after being deprived of their exercise wheels, researchers speculated.

The University of Miami study appeared in the *American Journal of Health Promotion*.

Marijuana: Facts For Teens

How does marijuana exert its effects?

All forms of marijuana are mind-altering (psychoactive). In other words, they change how the brain works. Marijuana contains more than 400 chemicals, including THC (delta-9-tetrahydrocannabinol). Since THC is the main active chemical in marijuana, the amount of THC in marijuana determines its strength or potency and therefore its effects.

Exposure to marijuana may affect the brain, particularly during development, which continues into the early twenties. Effects may include changes to the brain that make other drugs more appealing.

How long does marijuana stay in your body?

The THC in marijuana is rapidly absorbed by fatty tissues in various organs throughout the body. In general, standard urine tests can detect traces (metabolites) of THC several days after use. In heavy users, however, THC metabolites can sometimes be detected for weeks after use stops.

What happens if you smoke marijuana?

Some people feel nothing at all when they smoke marijuana. Others may feel relaxed or high. Some experience sudden feelings of anxiety and paranoid thoughts (more likely with stronger varieties of marijuana). Regular use of marijuana has also been associated with depression, anxiety, and an amotivational syndrome, which means a loss of drive or ambition, even for previously rewarding activities. Marijuana also often makes users feel hungry. Its effects can be unpredictable, especially when other drugs are mixed with it.

In the short-term, marijuana can cause problems with learning and memory; distorted perception (sights, sounds, time, touch); diminished motor coordination; and increased heart rate. But marijuana affects each person differently according to: biology (e.g., his or her genes); marijuana's strength or potency (how much THC it has); the circumstances of its use and expectations of effects; previous experience with the drug; how it's taken (smoked versus ingested); and whether alcohol or other drugs are involved.

Does marijuana affect sports performance or other activities and behaviors?

Sports: Marijuana affects timing, movement, and coordination, which can throw off athletic performance.

Learning: Marijuana's effects on attention and memory make it difficult not only to learn something new, but to do complex tasks that require focus and concentration or the stringing together of a lot of information sequentially.

Judgment: Marijuana, like most abused substances, can alter judgment and reduce inhibitions. This can lead to risky behaviors.

Does smoking marijuana affect the lungs?

Someone who smokes marijuana regularly may have many of the same respiratory problems that tobacco smokers do, such as daily cough, more frequent upper respiratory illnesses, and a greater risk of lung infections like pneumonia. As with tobacco smoke, marijuana smoke consists of a toxic mixture of gases and tiny particles, many of which are known to harm the lungs. Although we don't yet know if marijuana causes lung cancer, many people who smoke marijuana also smoke cigarettes, which do cause cancer—and smoking marijuana can make it harder to quit tobacco use.

Chapter 14

Teen Athletes And The Abuse of Over-The-Counter Drugs

From baseball stars to Olympians, media coverage of elite athletes increasingly includes reports of the use of performance-enhancing drugs to gain an edge over competitors. These substances are usually taken to boost athletic performance, increase muscle mass and strength, and diminish fatigue.

Teen athletes in high school and even middle school are taking these drugs, too. There are many reasons for this, such as frustration over being at a plateau in training or curiosity about the drugs' effects. Some young athletes also may use performance-enhancing drugs if they think that others (especially competitors) are using them—and if they believe that coaches and parents will look the other way regarding the use of such products.

Drug Types

Performance-boosting substances come in both prescription and over-the-counter (OTC) versions. The following are among the most (OTC) performance-enhancing drugs.

Creatine: Creatine is a compound that helps muscles use energy and recover more quickly following exercise. Small amounts of the substance—which is produced by the liver and stored in the skeletal muscles—can be found in red meat and fish. Creatine is also available in supplement form, both as a powder and in capsules. It can be purchased in health food stores, some pharmacies, and online.

Research suggests that supplemental creatine may help boost performance during brief, intense periods of exercise, such as weight lifting or sprinting. It also may help to decrease muscle fatigue by reducing the buildup of lactic acid (an energy waste product) in the body. Some studies have shown an increase in lean muscle mass as a result of creatine intake.

Most studies show that, when taken as directed, creatine is a relatively safe product—however, this supplement may injure the kidneys, liver, and heart, especially when taken in high doses. Some health care professionals believe that because creatine metabolizes into a toxic waste product (formaldehyde), it could cause damage to cells and blood vessels. More research needs to be done to determine the safety of creatine supplements, especially regarding their use by teens.

Steroid Precursors: Steroid precursors are substances that the body converts into anabolic steroids, which are synthetic versions of testosterone. Anabolic steroids are used to build muscle and increase endurance.

Anabolic steroids are illegal without a prescription, as are most steroid precursors. However, one steroid precursor, DHEA, is still available in over-the-counter form. Potential side effects of DHEA are the same as those of anabolic steroids: increased acne, male-pattern baldness, dark facial hair, deepening of the voice, and aggression. Anabolic steroids can also halt bone growth, and may result in a permanently short stature. When used chronically, they can damage the liver and the heart.

Remember

- Teens who feel under pressure to succeed from parents and coaches may feel tempted to use OTC drugs to boost performance.
- The use of a drug to enhance performance is similar to cheating on a test.
- It's also important to talk to your parents about the risks of performance-enhancing drugs.
- Any benefits obtained from these products are minimal compared to the long-term problems that may result from their use.
- Finally, monitor your purchase and use of OTC medications. Check labels for ingredients, even if the products appear to be harmless. Keep in mind that many performance-enhancing drugs may be purchased over the internet.

Ephedra: Ephedra, also called ma huang, is a plant that contains two amphetamine-like stimulants: ephedrine and pseudoephedrine. Athletes use ephedra products to provide quick energy and help with weight loss. But ephedra can cause dangerous side effects such as high blood pressure, irregular heart rhythm, seizure, stroke, and even death. These side effects are intensified when ephedra is combined with caffeine.

The concern about ephedra products was so great that the U.S. Food and Drug Administration (FDA) banned ephedra from being sold in dietary supplements in 2004. The scope of the FDA rule, though, does not pertain to traditional Chinese herbal remedies, so ma huang tea or other herbal products that contain ephedra can still be purchased. Some cold products also contain ephedrine or pseudoephedrine.

Part Two
Sports Safety And Injury Prevention

Chapter 15

Healthy Muscles Matter

Basic Facts About Muscles

Did you know you have more than 600 muscles in your body? These muscles help you move, lift things, pump blood through your body, and even help you breathe.

When you think about your muscles, you probably think most about the ones you can control. These are your voluntary muscles, which means you can control their movements. They are also called skeletal muscles, because they attach to your bones and work together with your bones to help you walk, run, pick up things, play an instrument, throw a baseball, kick a soccer ball, push a lawnmower, or ride a bicycle. The muscles of your mouth and throat even help you talk.

Keeping your muscles healthy will help you to be able to walk, run, jump, lift things, play sports, and do all the other things you love to do. Exercising, getting enough rest, and eating a balanced diet will help to keep your muscles healthy for life.

Different kinds of muscles have different jobs:

- Skeletal muscles are connected to your bones by tough cords of tissue called tendons. As the muscle contracts, it pulls on the tendon, which moves the bone. Bones are connected to other bones by ligaments, which are like tendons and help hold your skeleton together.

- Smooth muscles are also called involuntary muscles since you have no control over them. Smooth muscles work in your digestive system to move food along and push waste out of your body. They also help keep your eyes focused without your having to think about it.

About This Chapter: Excerpted from "Healthy Muscles Matter," National Institute of Arthritis and Musculoskeletal and Skin Diseases (www.niams.nih.gov), January 2011.

- Cardiac muscle. Did you know your heart is also a muscle? You have no control over this muscle. It pumps blood through your body, changing its speed to keep up with the demands you put on it. It pumps more slowly when you're sitting or lying down, and faster when you're running or playing sports and your skeletal muscles need more blood to help them do their work.

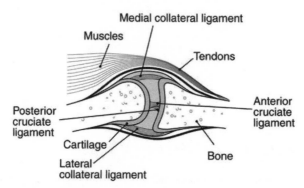

Figure 15.1. A joint showing muscles, ligaments, and tendons.

Why Healthy Muscles Matter To You

Healthy muscles let you move freely and keep your body strong. They help you to enjoy playing sports, dancing, walking the dog, swimming, and other fun activities. And they help you do those other (not so fun) things that you have to do, like making the bed, vacuuming the carpet, or mowing the lawn.

Strong muscles also help to keep your joints in good shape. If the muscles around your knee, for example, get weak, you may be more likely to injure that knee. Strong muscles also help you keep your balance, so you are less likely to get hurt by slipping or falling. Remember, the exercises that make your skeletal muscles strong will also help to keep your heart muscle strong.

What Can Go Wrong?

Injuries

Almost everyone has had sore muscles after exercising or working too much. This is known as muscle strain.

Muscle strains can be mild (the muscle has just been stretched too much) to severe (the muscle actually tears). Maybe you lifted something that was too heavy and the muscles in your arms were stretched too far.

What's It Mean?

Atrophy: Wasting away of the body or of an organ or part, as from defective nutrition, nerve damage, or lack of use.

Cardiac Muscle: The heart muscle. An involuntary or smooth muscle over which you have no control.

Ligament: Tough cords of tissue that connect bones to other bones at a joint.

Skeletal Muscle: Muscles that attach to bones.

Sprain: A stretched or torn ligament. Ankle and wrist sprains are common. Symptoms include pain, swelling, bruising, and being unable to move the joint.

Strain: A stretched or torn muscle or tendon. Twisting or pulling these tissues can cause a strain. Strains can happen suddenly or develop over time. Back and hamstring muscle strains are common. Many people get strains playing sports.

Tendon: Tough cords of tissue that connect muscles to bones.

Voluntary Muscles: Muscles that you can control.

Lifting heavy things in the wrong way can also strain the muscles in your back. This can be very painful and can even cause an injury that will last a long time and make it hard to do everyday things.

The tendons that connect the muscles to the bones can also be strained if they are pulled or stretched too much.

If a ligament (remember, they connect bones to bones) is stretched or pulled too much, the injury is called a sprain. Most people are familiar with the pain of a sprained ankle.

Contact sports like soccer, football, hockey, and wrestling can often cause strains. Sports in which you grip something (like gymnastics or tennis) can lead to strains in your hand or forearm.

Diseases

A number of diseases can affect your muscles. Some, like muscular dystrophy and Pompe disease, affect the muscles directly. Other diseases, like polio and multiple sclerosis, attack the nerves that control the muscles, so that the muscles become weak or paralyzed.

Muscles that are not used can get smaller and weaker. This is known as atrophy. If you have ever had a cast on your arm or leg, you might have noticed that the muscles in that arm or leg were smaller when the cast came off. It's important to exercise your muscles after an injury like this, so that they will grow back to the right size and work the way they should.

How Do I Keep My Muscles Healthy?

Exercise

When you make your muscles work by exercising, they respond by growing stronger. They may even get bigger by adding more muscle tissue. This is how bodybuilders get such big muscles, but your muscles can be healthy without getting that big.

There are lots of things you can do to exercise your muscles. Walking, jogging, lifting weights, playing tennis, climbing stairs, jumping, and dancing are all good ways to exercise your muscles. Swimming and biking will also give your muscles a good workout. It's important to get different kinds of exercise to work all your muscles. And any exercise that makes you breathe harder and faster will help exercise that important heart muscle as well.

Try to get 60 minutes of exercise every day. It doesn't have to be all at once. You can exercise several times during the day, as long as you get 60 minutes worth of exercise by the end of the day.

Eat A Healthy Diet

You really don't need a special diet to keep your muscles in good health. Eating a balanced diet will help manage your weight and provide a variety of nutrients for your muscles and overall health. A balanced diet includes fruits, vegetables, whole grains, and fat-free or low-fat milk and dairy products; protein from lean meats, poultry, fish, beans, eggs, and nuts; and is low in saturated fats, trans fats, cholesterol, salt (sodium), and added sugars.

Prevent Injuries

Here are some tips to prevent sprains, strains, and other muscle injuries:

- Warm up and cool down.
- Wear the proper protective gear for your sport, for example pads or helmets.
- Remember to drink lots of water, especially in warm weather.
- Don't try to "play through the pain." If something starts to hurt, STOP.

Start Now

Keeping your muscles healthy will help you have more fun and enjoy the things you do. Healthy muscles will help you look your best and feel full of energy. Start good habits now, while you are young, and you'll have a better chance of keeping your muscles healthy for the rest of your life.

Chapter 16

The Benefits Of Preseason Conditioning

Over the past few decades the number of recreational and competitive sports programs for children and adolescents has increased dramatically. There are more opportunities for girls to participate in sports, and in some communities children as young as age six can join organized teams and leagues. With qualified coaching and age-appropriate instruction, sports programs can provide young athletes with an opportunity to enhance their physical fitness, improve self-esteem, acquire leadership skills and have fun. However, there is the potential for illness or injury if boys and girls are unfit and ill-prepared to handle the demands of their chosen sport.

Only about half of all young people between the ages of 12 and 21 participate in vigorous physical activity on a regular basis, and daily attendance in physical education classes is unfortunately declining. Further, sedentary pursuits such as television viewing and internet surfing continue to occupy a significant amount of time during childhood and adolescence. In many cases the musculoskeletal system of children and adolescents who enter sports programs may not be prepared to handle the duration and magnitude of force that develops during practice and game situations. While improper footwear, hard playing surfaces, poor nutrition and muscle imbalances are recognized risk factors for sports-related injuries, the background level of physical activity should also be considered. In short, a youngster's participation in sports should not start with competition, but should evolve out of preparatory conditioning that includes strength, aerobic, and flexibility training.

About This Chapter: Written for the American College of Sports Medicine by Avery D. Faigenbaum, Ed.D. and Lyle J. Micheli, M.D., FACSM. Reprinted with permission of the American College of Sports Medicine, "ACSM Current Comment: Preseason Conditioning for Young Athletes." © American College of Sports Medicine. Reviewed by David A. Cooke, MD, FACP, April 2012.

Because aspiring young athletes are often forced to train harder and longer in order to excel in sports, it seems prudent for children and adolescents to participate in at least six to eight weeks of preseason conditioning prior to sports participation. The preparticipation examination may be an opportune time to identify correctable risk factors such as poor flexibility and poor physical condition. If needed, sports medicine physicians, athletic trainers, and qualified youth coaches should prescribe a preseason conditioning program and provide young athletes with information on the type, frequency, intensity, and duration of training. Sharing this information with parents can be helpful; they can reinforce the importance of preseason conditioning at home.

Conditioning Helps Prevent Sports Injuries

Sports activities can result in injuries—some minor, some serious, and still others result in life-long medical problems. Some are from accidents; others can result from poor training practices, improper gear, lack of conditioning, or not warming up or stretching sufficiently.

Many sports injuries can be prevented if people take the proper precautions. You can wear protective gear, use equipment properly, warm up your muscles, follow the rules of the game, and more. The following tips can help prevent an injury or reinjury from occurring:

- Know your limits.
- Avoid playing or exercising when very tired or in pain.
- Do warm-up exercises before you play any sport.
- Always stretch before you play or exercise. When you stretch the Achilles tendon, hamstring, and quadriceps areas, hold the positions—don't bounce.
- Don't twist your knees when you stretch. Keep your feet as flat as you can.
- Wear shoes that fit properly and, provide shock absorption and stability.
- Use the softest exercise surface available—avoid running on hard surfaces like asphalt and concrete.
- Run on flat surfaces. Running uphill may increase the stress on the Achilles tendon and the leg itself.
- When jumping, land with your knees bent.
- Avoid bending knees past 90 degrees when doing half knee bends.
- Use protective gear.
- Follow the rules of the sport.
- Cool down after playing or exercising.
- Don't overdo!

Source: Excerpted from "Sports Health and Safety," Federal Citizen Information Center, April 30, 2010.

Although additional clinical trials are needed to determine the most effective preseason conditioning program for children and adolescents, a combination of strength, aerobic, and flexibility exercises performed two to three times a week on nonconsecutive days seems reasonable.

When preparing young athletes for sports participation, it is important to include multi-joint exercises that require balance, stabilization, and coordination. In addition, due to the potential for lower back injuries, strengthening exercises for the core musculature (lower back and abdominals) should be performed as part of preventive health measures. Over time, the conditioning program should be modified in order to optimize gains in fitness and prevent overtraining.

In addition to knowing the rules of a game, young athletes need to be in shape to play the game. Although some young athletes may want to play themselves into shape, parents and coaches should realize that it is difficult for children and adolescents to gain the specific benefits of physical conditioning (for example, to increase muscle strength) without actually participating in a well-designed conditioning program. In some cases it may be necessary for children and adolescents to decrease the amount of time they spend practicing sport-specific skills in order to allow ample opportunity for preparatory conditioning exercises. That is, preseason conditioning exercises should not simply be added onto a child's exercise regimen, but rather incorporated into a well-rounded program.

ACSM Current Comment

In summary, while there may be many mechanisms for reducing sports injuries, the establishment of general physical fitness should be a prerequisite for youth sports participation. Preseason conditioning programs designed for the needs and abilities of young athletes could offer a protective effect by enhancing the strength and integrity of the musculoskeletal system and developing general fitness abilities. Focusing on sport-specific skills instead of general fitness skills may not only limit the ability of children and adolescents to succeed outside a narrow physical spectrum, but it may also lead to burnout and injury. As health professionals, coaches, teachers and parents, we all bear the shared responsibility of ensuring that aspiring young athletes are prepared for the demands of sports training and competition.

Chapter 17

Warm Up To Work Out

Suppose you were told that you only had to add an extra five to 10 minutes to each of your workouts to prevent injury and lessen fatigue. Would you do it?

Most people would say yes. Then they might be surprised to learn that they already know about those few minutes, which are called a warm-up. If done correctly, a pre-exercise warm-up can have a multitude of beneficial effects on a person's workout and, consequently, his or her overall health.

What Happens In Your Body

When you begin to exercise, your cardiorespiratory and neuromuscular systems and metabolic energy pathways are stimulated. Muscles contract and, to meet their increasing demands for oxygen, your heart rate, blood flow, cardiac output, and breathing rate increase. Blood moves faster through your arteries and veins and is gradually routed to working muscles.

Your blood temperature rises and oxygen is released more quickly, raising the temperature of the muscles. This allows the muscles to use glucose and fatty acids to burn calories and create energy for the exercise. All of these processes prepare the body for higher-intensity action.

Specifically, a gradual warm-up:

- Leads to efficient calorie burning by increasing your core body temperature

- Produces faster, more forceful muscle contractions

- Increases your metabolic rate so oxygen is delivered to the working muscles more quickly

- Prevents injuries by improving the elasticity of your muscles

- Gives you better muscle control by speeding up your neural message pathways to the muscles

- Allows you to comfortably perform longer workouts because all of your energy systems are able to adjust to exercise, preventing the buildup of lactic acid in the blood

- Improves joint range of motion

- Psychologically prepares you for higher intensities by increasing your ability to focus on exercise

Where To Begin

Your warm-up should consist of two phases:

- Progressive aerobic activity that utilizes the muscles that you will be using during your workout

- Flexibility exercises

Choosing which warm-up activity to use is as easy as slowing down what you will be doing during your workout. For example, if you will be running, warm up with a slow jog, or if you will be cycling outdoors, begin in lower gears. An ideal intensity for an aerobic warm-up has yet to be established, but a basic guideline is to work at a level that produces a small amount of perspiration but doesn't leave you feeling fatigued. The duration of the warm-up activity will depend on the intensity of your workout as well as your own fitness level.

After the aerobic warm-up activity, you should incorporate flexibility/stretching exercises. Stretching muscles after warming them up with low-intensity aerobic activity will produce a better stretch, since the rise in muscle temperature and circulation increases muscle elasticity, making muscles more pliable. Be sure to choose flexibility exercises that stretch the primary muscles you will be using during your workout.

Make The Time

To fully reap the benefits of the time you are spending exercising, you must warm up. Taking those extra few minutes to adjust to increased activity will ensure a better performance from your body and, in turn, will make your workout more efficient, productive and, best of all, enjoyable.

Chapter 18

Exercises For Strength And Flexibility

Preparing To Exercise

No matter how old you are or how long you may have been inactive, proper exercise will improve your physical condition. The exercises in this chapter can be done by people who have been inactive for some time. Programs to improve flexibility, strength, and endurance are arranged in three levels of difficulty. It is important to begin any exercise program slowly and build up gradually. Remember, it may take several months to attain the minimal levels of physical fitness identified in Level I activities. Some people will take less time, others more.

Before beginning an exercise program, have a physical examination and discuss the program with your doctor. In addition, if your mobility is limited as a result of a chronic or disabling condition, be sure to review these exercises with your doctor. Keep in mind your level of ability and endurance so that you don't risk discomfort or injury. If you experience pain while exercising, stop that particular movement and ask your doctor about it on your next visit.

Stick with it, and you will see results.

Warming Up

Preparing the body for exercise is important for people at all fitness levels. A warm-up period should begin with slow, rhythmic activities such as walking or jogging in place.

Gradually increase the intensity until your pulse rate, respiration rate, and body temperature are elevated, which is usually about the time that you break a light sweat. It also is advisable

About This Chapter: This chapter includes excerpts and illustrations adapted from "Pep Up Your Life: A Fitness Book for Mid-Life And Older Persons," President's Council on Fitness, Sports, and Nutrition (www.fitness.gov), 1998. Reviewed by David A. Cooke, MD, FACP, April 2012.

to do some easy stretching exercises (such as the ones described later in this chapter) before moving on to the strength and endurance activities.

Effective Exercising

Once you begin your daily exercise routine, keep these points in mind to get the best results:

- Always drink water before, during, and after your exercise session.

- Make exercising a part of your daily routine. You may want to set a regular time to exercise each day and invite a friend to join you.

- Start gradually, about 5 to 10 minutes at first.

- Increase the amount of exercise each day, up to about 30 to 60 minutes.

- Breathe deeply and evenly during and between exercises. Don't hold your breath.

- Rest whenever it is necessary.

- Keep a daily written record of your progress.

- Exercise to lively music, TV, or with friends for added enjoyment.

Cool Down

If you have been participating in vigorous physical activity, it is extremely important not to stop suddenly. Abrupt stopping interferes with the return of the blood to the heart and may result in dizziness or fainting. Simply reduce the intensity of the exercise gradually and end with a few slow stretches from the section on stretching.

Exercise: The Key To The Good Life

Exercise can help you take charge of your health and maintain the level of fitness necessary for an active, independent lifestyle. Many health problems can be helped or even reversed by improving lifestyle behaviors. One of the major benefits of regular physical activity is protection against coronary heart disease. Physical activity also provides some protection against other chronic diseases such as adult-onset diabetes, arthritis, hypertension, certain cancers, osteoporosis, and depression. In addition, research has proven that exercise can ease tension and reduce the amount of stress you feel.

To put it simply—exercise is one of the best things you can do for your health.

Source: President's Council on Fitness, Sports, and Nutrition (www.fitness.gov), 1998. Reviewed by David A. Cooke, MD, FACP, April 2012.

Flexibility

Exercises in this category will help you maintain your range of motion. In addition to performing flexibility exercises, you should try to bend, move, and stretch every day to keep joints flexible and muscles elastic. Avoid reliance on push buttons and conveniences that take away the need for personal motion. And, compliment this program with such recreational activities as dancing, yoga, swimming, golfing, gardening, and housework.

Be sure to begin each workout with deep breathing and continue deep breathing at intervals throughout the session. You should work up to a total of 50 deep breaths per workout.

Flexibility Level I

1. **Finger Stretching:** To maintain finger dexterity. With the palm of the hand facing down and using other hand for leverage, gently press fingers up and back toward the forearm; then push fingers down. Suggested repetitions: 5 each hand.

2. **Hand Rotation:** To maintain wrist flexibility and range of motion. Grasp one wrist with the other hand. Keep palm facing down. Slowly rotate hand 5 times each clockwise and counter-clockwise. Suggested repetitions: 5 each hand.

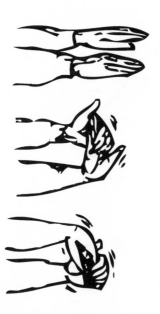

Figure 18.1. Finger Stretching.

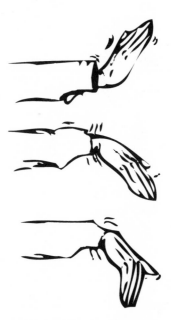

Figure 18.2. Hand Rotation.

3. **Ankle And Foot Circling:** To improve flexibility and range of motion of ankles. Cross leg over opposite knee, rotate foot slowly, making large complete circles. 10 rotations to the right, 10 to the left, each leg.

4. **Neck Extension:** To improve flexibility and range motion of neck. Sit up comfortably. Bend head forward until chin touches chest. You may want to stretch forward by simply jutting your chin out. Return to starting position and slowly rotate head to left. Return to starting position and slowly rotate head to right. Return to starting position. Suggested repetitions: 5.

5. **Single Knee Pull:** To stretch lower back and back of leg. Lie on back, hands at sides. Pull one leg to chest, grasp with both arms and hold for five counts. Repeat with opposite leg. Suggested repetitions: 3–5.

6. **Simulated Crawl Stroke/Back Stroke/Breast Stroke:** To stretch shoulder girdle. Stand with feet shoulder-width apart, arms at sides, relaxed. Bend knees and alternately swing right and left arms backwards, upward, and forward as if swimming. Suggested repetitions: 6–8 movements on each stroke.

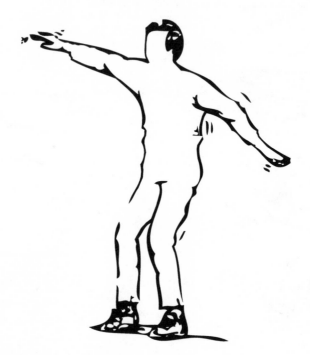

Figure 18.3. Simulated Crawl Stroke.

7. **Reach:** To stretch shoulder girdle and rib cage. While standing, take a deep breath, extend arms overhead. Rise on toes while reaching. Exhale slowly, lowering arms (can also be done in a seated position). Suggested repetitions: 6–8.

8. **Backstretch:** To improve the flexibility of the lower back. Sit up straight. Bend far forward and straighten up. Repeat, clasping hands on left knee. Repeat clasping hands on right knee. Exhale while bending forward. Suggested repetitions: 4–6 over each knee.

9. **Chain Breaker:** To stretch chest muscles. Stand erect, feet about six inches apart. Tighten leg muscles, tighten stomach by drawing it in, with hips forward, extend chest, bring arms up with clenched fists chest high, take deep breath, let it out slowly. Slowly pull arms back as far as possible keeping elbows chest high. Suggested repetitions: 8–10.

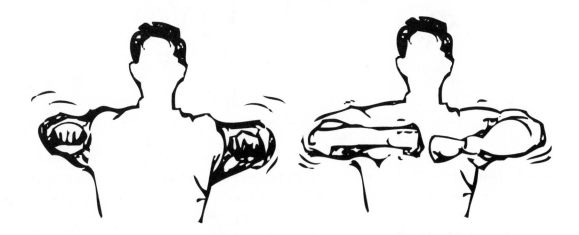

Figure 18.4. Chain Breaker.

Flexibility: Level II

1. **Double Knee Pull:** To stretch lower back and buttocks. Lie on back, hands at sides. Pull legs to chest, lock arms around legs, pull buttocks slightly off ground. Hold for 10 to 15 counts. Suggested repetitions: 3–5.

2. **Seated Pike Stretch:** To stretch lower back and hamstrings. Sit on floor, with legs forward, knees together. Exhale and stretch forward, slowly sliding hands down to ankles. Stretch only as far as is comfortable and use your hands for support. Hold for 5 to 8 counts. Don't bounce. Inhale deeply. Repetitions: 3–4.

3. **Chest Stretch:** To stretch muscles in chest and shoulders. Stand arm-length distant from a doorway opening. Raise one arm shoulder height with slight bend in elbow. Place hand against door jamb and turn upper body away so that the muscles in chest and shoulders are stretched. Suggested repetitions: 3–4 each arm.

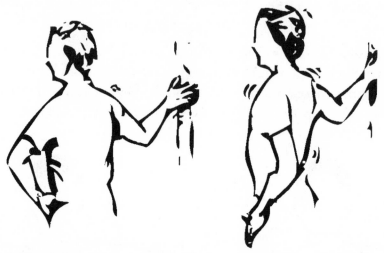

Figure 18.5. Chest Stretch.

4. **Seated Stretch:** To stretch lower back and hamstrings. Sit on floor one leg extended to your side and one leg bent comfortably in front of your body. Supporting your body weight with your hands and keeping your back straight, lean forward until you feel a comfortable leg and hamstring. Hold the stretch for a few seconds, exhaling. Switch sides. Suggested repetitions: 3–5 each side.

Flexibility Level III

1. **Sitting Stretch:** To increase flexibility of lower back and hamstrings. Sit on floor with legs extended as far apart as is comfortable. Exhale and stretch forward slowly, sliding your hands down your legs. Reach as far as is comfortable and hold for 5–8 counts. Suggested repetitions: 3–4.

2. **Achilles Stretch:** To stretch calf muscles on back leg and Achilles tendon. Stand facing a wall, two to three feet away. Extend arms, lean into wall. Move left leg forward a half step and right leg backward a half step or more. Lower right heel to floor. Press hips forward, stretching the calf muscles in the right leg. Hold 5 to 10 counts. Breathe normally. Reverse leg position and repeat. Suggested repetitions: 3–6 each leg.

3. **Modified Seal:** To stretch abdominal wall, chest, and front of neck. Lie on the floor with arms extended, stomach down, feet extended, with toes pointed. While exhaling, slowly lift head and push up until arms are bent at right angles, with back arching gently. Keep hips on the floor. Keeping arms bent, hold for 5–10 counts, Return to starting position, inhaling deeply. Suggested repetitions: 4–6.

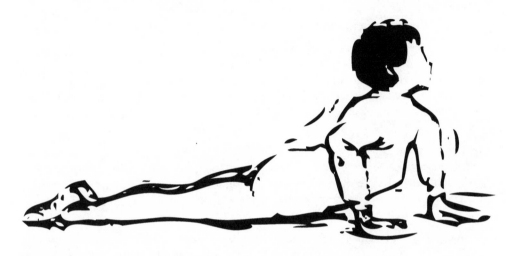

Figure 18.6. Modified Seal.

4. **Half Bow:** To stretch the top of the thigh and groin area. Lie on your side. Bend top leg so foot is near buttocks. Hold ankle of top foot with top hand just above toes. Slightly arch back. Hold 5 to 10 counts. Switch sides. Suggested repetitions: 3–5.

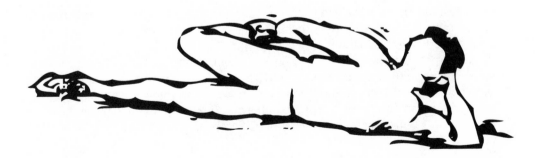

Figure 18.7. Half Bow.

Types Of Stretches

There are several types of stretches one may incorporate into their fitness training. The following information provides an overview of stretching variations:

- Static stretching is probably the most commonly used flexibility technique and is very safe and effective. A muscle or muscle group is gradually stretched to the point of limitation (a mild, even tension) and then typically held in that position for 15–30 seconds.

- Dynamic stretching incorporates active range-of-motion (ROM) movements that tend to resemble sport or movement-specific actions. For instance, a volleyball player might do some shoulder flexion and extension actions prior to a game. The rhythmic nature of a controlled dynamic stretch has a functional application owing to its similarity to the primary movement task. Dynamic stretching is often incorporated in the active phase of warm-ups.

- Ballistic stretching involves a bouncy approach to reach the target muscle's motion endpoint. A concern, however, with ballistic stretching is that it is often performed in a jerky, bobbing fashion that may produce undesirable tension or trauma to the stretched muscle and associated connective tissues. It may produce a potent stretch reflex that will oppose the muscle lengthening.

- Passive stretching is usually performed with a partner who applies a sustained stretch to another person's relaxed joint. The person who is stretching their muscles is not actively involved in the stretch, but is manipulated into the stretch by his or her partner. Passive stretching, therefore, requires close communication between the two individuals, along with a slow application of the stretch in order to prevent a forceful manipulation of the body segment and possible injury.

- Contract-relax and proprioceptive neuromuscular facilitation (PNF) stretching involves initially contracting the target muscle, then relaxing and stretching it with an assist from a partner or an applied force (such as a towel or rope). A variation (contract-relax agonist-contract method) involves performing a contraction of the opposing muscle during the stretching phase to take the target muscle to a new, farther motion endpoint.

- Resistance stretching has gained much attention and interest. It focuses on contracting the target muscles as they are lengthened. Some of these stretching moves can be done alone and others with a partner. In the first phase, the target muscles are placed in the shortened position. Then the person who is stretching his or her muscles contracts the target muscle(s). While contracted, the muscles are taken through a full range of motion (lengthened), either by the person alone or with assistance from his or her partner. So, resistance stretching incorporates a strengthening component through the entire range of motion. In essence, it is a carefully performed eccentric contraction.

Source: Excerpted from "Stretching," by LCDR Scott McGrew, U.S. Public Health Service, 2011. The complete text of this document, including references, is available online at http://dcp.psc.gov/ccbulletin/articles/stretching_03_2011.aspx.

Strength

The benefits of strength exercises include improving reaction time, reducing the rate of muscle atrophy, increasing work capacity, and helping prevent back problems and injury. Calisthenics work muscles against resistance, enabling them to grow and maintain muscle tone. In addition to the suggested strength exercises, other physical activities that are essentially recreational can provide benefits to help maintain muscle integrity. Such activities include bicycling and swimming,

Strength: Level I

1. **Finger Squeeze:** To strengthen the hands. Extend arms in front at shoulder height, palms down. Squeeze fingers slowly, then release. Turn palms up, squeeze fingers, release. Extend arms in front, shake fingers. Suggested repetitions: 5 in each position.

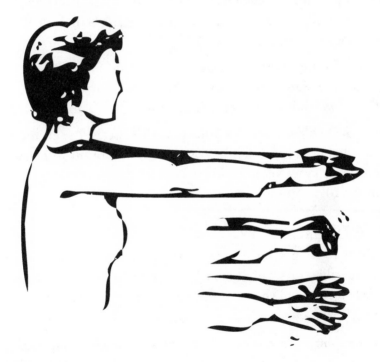

Figure 18.8. Finger Squeeze.

2. **Touch Shoulders:** To increase flexibility of the shoulders and elbows and tone the upper arm (can be done in a seated position). Touch shoulders with hands, extend arms out straight. Bring arms back to starting position. Suggested repetitions: 10–15.

3. **Leg Extensions:** To tone the upper leg muscles. Sit upright in a chair. Lift 1eft leg off the floor and extend it fully. Lower it very slowly. Suggested repetitions: 10–15 each leg.

4. **Back Leg Swing:** To firm the buttocks and strengthen the lower back. Stand up, holding on to the back of a chair. Keep your back and hips in line with the chair as you do the exercise. Extend one leg back, foot pointed towards the floor. Keeping the knee straight, lift the leg backwards approximately four inches and concentrate on squeezing the muscles in the buttocks with each lift. Make sure you keep your back straight as you raise your legs. Return to starting position. Suggested repetitions: 10 each leg.

5. **Quarter Squat:** To tone and strengthen lower leg muscles. Stand erect behind a chair, hands on chair back for balance. Bend knees, then rise to an upright position. Be careful not to let knees go beyond the line of your toes. Suggested repetitions: 8–12.

6. **Heel Raises:** To strengthen the calf muscles and ankles. Stand erect, holding a chair for balance if needed, hands on hips, feet together. Raise body on toes. Return to starting position. Suggested repetitions: 10.

7. **Knee Lift:** To strengthen hip flexors and lower abdomen. Stand erect. Raise knee to chest or as far upward as possible while back remains straight. Return to starting position. Repeat with other leg. Suggested repetitions: 5 each leg.

8. **Head And Shoulder Curl:** To firm stomach muscles. Lie on the floor, knees bent, arms at sides, head bent slightly forward. Reach forward with arms extended, until finger tips touch your knees. Hold for 5 counts. Return to starting position. Suggested repetitions: 10.

Strength: Level II

1. **Arm Curl:** To strengthen arm muscles. Use a weighted object such as a book or a can of vegetables or small dumbbell. Stand or sit erect with arms at side, holding weighted object. Bend your arm, raising the weight. Lower it. Suggested repetitions: 10–15 each arm.

2. **Arm Extension:** To tone muscles in the back of the arm. Sit or stand erect. Holding a weighted object of less than five pounds, raise your arm overhead. Slowly bend arm behind head. Slowly extend arm up. Suggested repetitions: 10–15 each arm.

3. **Modified Knee Push-up:** To strengthen upper back, chest, and back of arms. Start on bent knees, hands on floor and slightly forward of shoulders. Lower body until chin touches floor. Return to start. Suggested repetitions: 5–10.

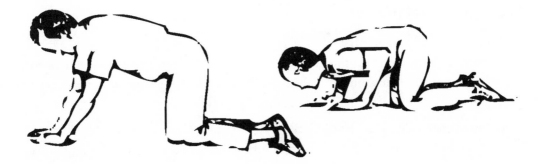

Figure 18.9. Modified Knee Push-up.

4. **Calf Raise:** To strengthen lower leg and ankle. Stand erect, hands on hip or on back of chair for balance. Spread feet 6" to 12". Slowly raise body up to toes, lifting heels. Return to starting position. Breathe normally. Suggested repetitions: 10–15

5. **Alternate Leg Lunges:** To strengthen upper thighs and inside legs. Also stretches back of leg. Take a comfortable stance with hands on hips. Step forward 18" to 24" with right leg. Keep left heel on floor. Shove off right leg and resume standing position. Suggested repetitions: 5–10 each leg.

6. **Modified Sit-up:** To improve abdominal strength. Lie on back, feet on the floor with finger tips behind your ears. Look straight up at the ceiling and lift head and shoulders off floor. Suggested repetitions: 10.

7. **Side Lying Leg Lift:** To strengthen and tone outside of thigh and hip muscles. Lie on side, legs extended. Raise leg four to five inches. Lower to starting position. Suggested repetitions: 10 on each side.

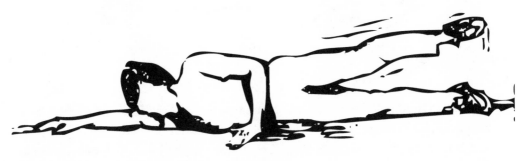

Figure 18.10. Side Lying Leg Lift.

Strength: Level III

Note: In Level III strength exercise, lightweight resistance equipment, such as the dumbbell, is introduced to overload the muscles. While equipment of this kind is low in cost and desirable, a number of substitutes can be used. These include a bucket of soil, a heavy household item such as an iron, a can of food, a stone, or a brick.

1. **Seated Alternate Dumbbell Curls:** To strengthen biceps of upper arms. Sit comfortably on a flat bench with arms at side. Hold a pair of dumbbells with an underhand grip, so that palms face up. Bending left elbow, raise dumbbell until left arm is fully flexed. Lower left dumbbell while raising right dumbbell from the elbow until right arm is fully flexed. Breathe normally. Suggested repetitions: 2 sets of 8–10 each arm.

2. **Dumbbell Fly:** To strengthen chest muscles and improve lateral range of motion in shoulder girdle. Lie on your back on a flat bench or floor if bench is not available. Grasp dumbbells in each hand and lift toward each other over chest. Inhale and lower dumbbell to side with elbow slightly bent. Raise dumbbell in an arc to the starting position, exhaling in the process. Suggested repetitions: 8–12.

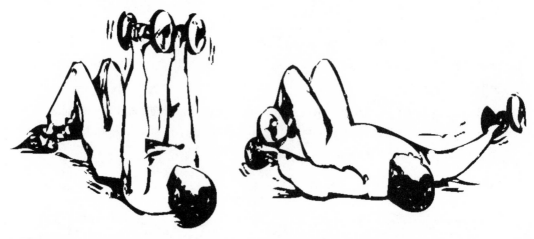

Figure 18.11. Dumbbell Fly

3. **Alternate Dumbbell Shrug:** To strengthen muscles in shoulders, upper back, and neck. Stand comfortably with dumbbells in each hand. Elevate shoulders as high as possible, rolling them first backward and then down to the starting position. Exhale as you lower the shoulders. Suggested repetitions: 10 forward, 5 backward.

4. **One Arm Dumbbell Extension:** To strengthen triceps (back of arm) and improve range of motion. Bring weight up to shoulder and lift overhead. Slowly lower it behind the back as far as is comfortable. Extend arm to original position. Inhale on the way down, exhale on the way up. Suggested repetitions: 8–12 on each arm.

5. **Dumbbell Calf Raise:** To strengthen calf muscle and improve range of motion of ankle joint. Stand with feet shoulder-width apart, weights in each hand, toes on a 2" x 4" block (preferred but not necessary). Raise up on toes lifting heels as high as possible. Slowly lower heels to starting position. Breathe normally. Suggested repetitions: 5 with heels straight back, 5 with heels turned out, 5 with heels turned in.

6. **Dumbbell Half Squats:** To strengthen thigh muscles in front. Stand with feet shoulder-width apart and heels on a 2" x 4" block (not necessary, but preferred). Holding weights in each hand, slowly descend to a comfortable position where the tops of the thighs are about at a 45 degree angle to the floor. There is no benefit to a deeper squat. Inhale on the way down. Stand up slowly, keeping knees slightly bent. Exhale on the way up. Suggested repetitions: 10–12.

7. **Modified Sit-up:** To improve abdominal strength. Lie on back, feet on the floor, with finger tips behind your ears. Look straight up at ceiling and lift head and shoulders off floor. Suggested repetitions: 12–15.

Endurance

Endurance-building or aerobic exercises improve the functions of the heart, lungs, and blood vessels. Vital to fitness are a strong heart to pump blood to nourish billions of body cells, healthy lungs where the gases of cell metabolism are exchanged for oxygen and elastic blood vessels free of obstructions. Without a healthy level of endurance, you may feel tired, lack zest. You may also experience shortness of breath, rapid heartbeat or even nausea.

Activities to improve endurance include brisk walking, cycling, swimming, dancing and jogging. Walking is actually one of the best all-round exercises. The massaging action the leg muscles exert on the veins as you walk improves the flow of blood back to the heart and also strengthens the leg muscles.

Walking For Fitness

Walking offers several advantages over other forms of exercise; it requires no previous instructions, it can be done almost anywhere, it can be done almost anytime, it costs nothing, and it has the lowest rate of injury of any form of exercise.

It takes a little longer to achieve conditioning results through walking than through more strenuous activities, but not much. One study showed, for example, that jogging a mile in 8½ minutes burns only 26 more calories than walking a mile in 12 minutes. Conditioning benefits from walking improve dramatically if you increase the pace to faster than three miles per hour (20-minute mile). In another study, participants burned an average of 66 calories per mile walking three miles per hour, but 124 calories per mile when they increased the pace to five miles per hour.

Choose a comfortable time of day to exercise, not too soon after eating and when the air temperature is not too high. Many people find it more enjoyable to exercise with others. Be careful not to overexert. Stop if you find yourself panting or feeling nauseous, if your breathing does not return to normal within ten minutes after exercising or if sleeping is affected

How To Walk

A good walking workout is a matter of stepping up your pace, increasing your distance, and walking more often. Here are some tips to help you get the most out of walking:

- Move at a steady clip, brisk enough to make your heart beat faster and cause you to breathe more deeply.

- Hold your head erect, back straight, and abdomen flat. Toes should point straight ahead and arms swing at your sides.

- Land on your heel and roll forward to drive off the ball of your foot. Walking only on the ball of the foot or walking flat-footed may cause soreness.

- Take long, easy strides, but don't strain. When walking up hills rapidly, lean forward slightly.

- Breathe deeply, with your mouth open if that's more comfortable.

What To Wear

Shoes that are comfortable, provide good support, and don't cause blisters or calluses are the only special equipment necessary. They should have arch supports and should elevate the heel one-half to three-quarters of an inch above the sole. They should also have uppers made of materials that breathe such as leather or nylon mesh. Some examples are: training models of running shoes with thick soles, light trail or hiking boots, or casual shoes with thick rubber or crepe rubber soles.

Wear lighter clothing than the temperature would ordinarily dictate because brisk walking generates a lot of body heat. In cold weather, wear several layers of light clothing. They trap body heat and are easy to shed if you get too warm. A woolen cap and mittens are important in very cold temperatures.

Chapter 19

Facts About Protective Equipment

The Facts

- Protective equipment should be worn at all times (training and games).

- It should fit correctly.

- It is important to regularly check and maintain protective equipment.

- Try out equipment prior to using it in competition.

- Equipment should be specific and appropriate for the sport, size, and age of the athlete.

- Equipment should always be used according to the manufacturer's guidelines and the recommendations of the sporting body concerned.

- Remember injuries usually mean time on the sideline—prevention is the key.

Wrist, Elbow And Knee Guards

- Protective wrist guards are useful to protect from impact when falling onto an out-stretched hand.

- Padded knee protectors absorb impact forces from falls onto concrete and skating surfaces, and collisions with racing poles.

- Elbows are at risk when falling and padding will reduce grazing and protect the joint from impact.

About This Chapter: "Gear Up: Your Guide to Protective Equipment," © 2012 Smartplay. All rights reserved. For additional information, visit http://www.smartplay.com.au.

Shin Pads

- Shin injuries are common in sports where there is a fast moving object, for example hockey, softball, cricket, lacrosse.

- Properly fitting shin pads will prevent a large number of these injuries.

- You should ensure that the shin pads are appropriate for the sport, that is different shin pads for hockey and soccer.

Shoulder Padding And Body Protectors

- In tackling sports such as rugby league and union, shoulder protectors are recommended to protect the top of the shoulder joint from impact injury

- Padded body protectors help to protect the trunk, particularly the chest area, from impact injury in sports such as fencing or softball and baseball (catcher and referee).

- "Boxes" (athletic cups) for boys in sports such as cricket and hockey are essential to protect the genitals.

Helmets

- In sports where high-speed collisions are likely (for example, motorcycling, cycling) hard-shell helmets are of proven value.

- In sports that have the potential for missile injuries (for example baseball, lacrosse) or for falls onto hard surfaces (for example, gridiron [American football], ice-hockey) specific helmets can reduce head injuries.

- Helmets should be approved by the sporting association concerned.

Ankle Taping And Braces

- Ankle taping and braces can protect the ankle from injury when an athlete lands awkwardly.

- They can be used to protect a previously injured ankle when a player returns to sport.

- Ankle braces and tape can be purchased from your local pharmacy or sports store.

- For advice about what type of braces to buy and how to tape effectively, contact your local sports physiotherapist, sports doctor, or sports trainer.

Gloves

- Protective gloves help to prevent bruising and fractures of the fingers, thumbs and hand in sports such as cricket, baseball, and softball.

- Gloves can also protect the hands from blisters in equestrian sports.

Mouthguards

- If participants are involved in sports where they are at risk of a blow to the head or face from either opponents or equipment, they should wear a properly fitted mouthguard.

- A mouthguard correctly fitted by a dentist will protect teeth, stop biting into the lips, and act as a cushioned layer between teeth to reduce the risk of concussion and jaw fracture.

- Mouthguards should fit the mouth accurately, allow normal breathing and speech, and be custom designed and fitted by a qualified professional.

Footwear

- Footwear that fits correctly and is designed for the sport or activity is essential to prevent many injuries. Important features of correct footwear include fit, cushioning and stability.

- See a sports podiatrist for more advice on specific foot problems and the correct footwear for you.

Chapter 20

Helmets

Which Helmet For Which Activity?

Why are helmets so important?

For many recreational activities, wearing a helmet can reduce the risk of a serious head injury and even save your life. During a fall or collision, most of the impact energy is absorbed by the helmet, rather than your head and brain.

Are all helmets the same?

No. There are different helmets for different activities. Each type of helmet is made to protect your head from the impacts common to a particular activity or sport. Be sure to wear a helmet that is appropriate for the particular activity you're involved in (see Table 20.1 for guidance). Other helmets may not protect your head as effectively.

How can I tell which helmet is the right one to use?

Bicycle and motorcycle helmets must comply with mandatory federal safety standards. Many other recreational helmets are subject to voluntary safety standards.

Helmets certified to a safety standard are designed and tested to protect the user from serious head injury while wearing the helmet. For example, all bicycle helmets manufactured

About This Chapter: The main text in this chapter begins with "Which Helmet for Which Activity," U.S. Consumer Product Safety Commission, 2006. It continues with information from "Hard Facts about Helmets," BAM! Body and Mind, Centers for Disease Control and Prevention, 2003. Reviewed by David A. Cooke, MD, FACP, April 2012.

after 1999 must meet the U.S. Consumer Product Safety Commission (CPSC) bicycle helmet standard. Helmets meeting this standard provide substantial head protection when the helmet is used properly. The standard requires that chin straps be strong enough to keep the helmet on the head and in the proper position during a fall or collision.

Helmets specifically marketed for exclusive use in an activity other than bicycling (for example, go-karting, horseback riding, lacrosse, and skiing) do not have to meet the requirements of the CPSC bicycle helmet standard. However, these helmets should meet other federal and/or voluntary safety standards.

Don't rely on the helmet's name or claims made on the packaging (unless the packaging specifies compliance with an appropriate standard) to determine if the helmet meets the appropriate requirements for your activity. Most helmets that meet a particular standard will contain a special label that indicates compliance (usually found on the liner inside of the helmet). See Table 20.1 for more information on what to look for.

Questions About Winter Sports Helmets

Are skiers and snowboarders at risk of head injury?

An international review, which included Canada, concluded that head injuries are the most common cause of death among skiers and snowboarders. Traumatic brain injuries account for 50–88 percent of the fatalities at ski resorts and 67 percent of skier deaths in children. Head injuries comprise 3–15 percent of all injuries suffered by skiers and snowboarders.

Novice skiers and snowboarders are most susceptible to injury; however novice snowboarders in particular are more likely to suffer severe head injuries. Children and adolescents experience more head and neck injuries than adults, which may be due to a number of factors unique to children. Children have immature muscles and bones that could result in more falls and they tire more quickly from physical activity. In addition they often wear ill-fitting ski equipment due to their continued growth from one ski season to the next.

Does wearing a helmet effectively protect a skier or snowboarder?

Several studies have demonstrated that ski and snow board helmets are effective at preventing head injuries. It is estimated that for every 10 people who wear a helmet, up to five may avoid head injuries. Studies also show that even at a speed of 19km/h, a ski helmet can minimize brain damage. Helmets may prove to offer even greater protection, as many individuals wear them incorrectly. Current evidence is limited on the relationship between helmet use and neck injury.

Are there helmets that I can wear for more than one activity?

Yes, but only a few. You can wear a CPSC-compliant bicycle helmet while bicycling, recreational roller or in-line skating, and riding a nonpowered scooter. Look at Table 20.1 for other activities that may share a common helmet.

Take off your helmet before playing on playgrounds or climbing trees. If a person wears a helmet during these activities, the helmet's chin strap can get caught on the equipment or tree and pose a risk of strangulation. The helmet itself may present an entrapment hazard.

How can I tell if my helmet fits properly?

A helmet should be both comfortable and snug. Be sure that it is level on your head—not tilted back on the top of the head or pulled too low over your forehead. It should not move in any direction, back-to-front or side-to-side. The chin strap should be securely buckled so that the helmet doesn't move or fall off during a fall or collision.

Is helmet fit important?

In order for helmets to protect adults and children properly, they must be correctly fitted and secured. Ski and snowboard helmets should rest two fingers width above the eyebrow and the helmet should be snug and comfortable, with only one finger width under the chinstrap. The helmet pads should touch the cheeks and the forehead, and the helmet back should not touch the nape of the neck. If wearing goggles, there should be little or no gap between the top of the goggles and the helmet. Most helmets come with fitting instructions.

When should a ski or snowboard helmet be replaced?

If a helmet has been dropped or the wearer has been in a fall or collision while wearing the helmet, a new one should be purchased, even if it appears undamaged.

Which helmets are recommended for tobogganing?

Experts recommend a ski/snowboarding helmet for tobogganing. Since the activity of going downhill is a similar mechanism of injury for tobogganing, a ski/snowboarding helmet is an appropriate choice. Certification from CSA, CE, Snell or ASTM is important when selecting a helmet.

Source: Excerpted and reprinted with permission from "Frequently asked questions ski/snowboard helmets," © 2010 Safe Kids Canada. All rights reserved. The complete text, including references, can be found online at http://www.safe kidscanada.ca/Professionals/Safety-Information/Winter-Helmets/Ski-Helmets-Winter/Ski-Helmets.aspx.

Facts About Equestrian Helmets

Proper Helmet Fit Is Important

In the past, helmets have been uncomfortable, hot, and ill fitting, leading many riders to forego the use of helmets. Recent advances, such as ventilation, lighter weight, and adjustable chin straps, have made helmets safer and more comfortable. More western looking helmets are being developed for those riders that want safety with a western look.

Each rider should have a helmet that is properly fitted to his/her head for maximum safety. Therefore, equestrian helmets should not be shared among riders. Helmets should also be replaced after a maximum of five years or after each major impact to ensure the rider's continued protection.

Helmet Certification

When purchasing an equestrian helmet, riders should look for American Society for Testing Materials (ASTM) and Safety Equipment Institute (SEI) certification. These certifications insure that the helmet complies with the basic helmet safety regulations. Helmets not certified by ASTM and SEI do not comply with industry standard and may offer sub-standard protection.

Equestrian helmets are constructed differently from other safety helmets (bicycle and motorcycle) as they are designed to protect more of the rider's head while not interfering with sight or balance. They are specifically made to reduce penetration by blunt objects (such as a horse's hoof) and to absorb some of the impact from a fall. Bicycle and motorcycle helmets do not provide the flexibility and safety offered by equestrian helmets.

Helmet Fitting

Equestrian helmets come in many sizes and styles. Finding a proper fitting helmet for your riding discipline can save money, time, and effort. Helmet sizes are based on the circumference at the widest part of the rider's head, approximately one inch above the eyebrows (Figure 20.1). This measurement is then matched to the proper helmet size (each style of helmet should have an appropriate sizing chart).

Figure 20.1. Helmet sizes are based on the circumference at the widest part of the rider's head.

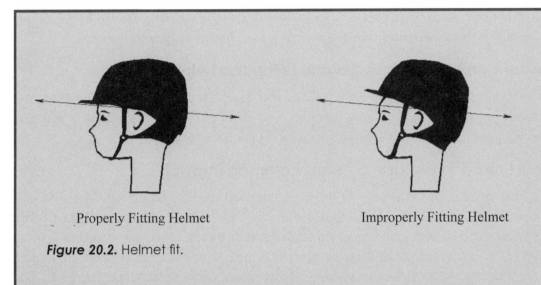

Properly Fitting Helmet   Improperly Fitting Helmet

Figure 20.2. Helmet fit.

Helmets may vary with style and brand so trying on helmets before purchase is highly recommended. The helmet should fit around the rider's entire head with the visor level just above the eyebrows (should not be above 1.5 inches, Figure 20.2). The chin strap should be attached so the strap is touching the skin under the rider's chin, not hanging loose. The suspension and chin straps should not pinch the rider's ears.

The rider should be able to move his/her head vigorously with minimal helmet movement. If the helmet slides, a smaller size may be needed while a larger size is warranted if the helmet is too tight, causing discomfort. Long hair should not be placed under the helmet in a bun, in a high pony tail, or flipped underneath, but rather should be pulled back into a low enough pony tail so that it does not interfere with fitting. Most helmet retailers can assist in the helmet fitting process if the rider remains unsure as to proper fit.

Summary

Injuries are a part of working with or riding horses. The use of safety equipment is important to equestrians' well-being. The use of helmets is a simple and effective means of decreasing the number of head injuries associated with falls from horses. All youth should use this simple solution to potentially devastating injuries. An ASTM or SEI approved helmet, worn and properly fitted can decrease the incidence of serious head injuries that result from horse activities. Overall, the helmet should be certified, snug, and comfortable to encourage maximum wear and protection.

Source: Excerpted from "Helmets, Heads, and Health for Horse Enthusiasts," by Colette Floyd-Tebeau, 4-H Equine Program Coordinator, and Dr. Patricia Evans, Extension Equine Specialist, Utah State University Cooperative Extension, August 2009. For additional information, including the complete text of this publication, visit http://utah4horse.org.

When buying a helmet, be sure to try it on so that the helmet can be tested for a good fit. Carefully examine the helmet and accompanying instructions and safety literature.

What can I do if I have trouble fitting the helmet?

You may have to apply the foam padding that comes with the helmet and/or adjust the straps. If this doesn't work, consult with the store where you bought the helmet or with the helmet manufacturer. Don't wear a helmet that doesn't fit correctly.

Will I need to replace a helmet after an impact?

That depends on the severity of the impact and whether the helmet can withstand one impact (a single-impact helmet) or more than one impact (a multiple-impact helmet). For example, bicycle helmets are designed to protect against a single severe impact, such as a bicyclist's fall onto the pavement. The foam material in the helmet will crush to absorb the impact energy during a fall or collision and can't protect you again from an additional impact. Even if there are no visible signs of damage to the helmet, you must replace it.

Other helmets are designed to protect against multiple moderate impacts. Two examples are football and ice hockey helmets. These helmets are designed to withstand multiple impacts of the type associated with the respective activities. However, you may still have to replace the helmet after one severe impact, or if it has visible signs of damage, such as a cracked shell or permanent dent in the shell or liner. Consult the manufacturer's instructions for guidance on when the helmet should be replaced.

Where can I find specific information about which helmet to use?

Look at the information in Table 20.1 and follow these easy steps:

- Find the activity of interest in the first column (Activity).
- Read across the row to find the appropriate helmet type for that activity listed in the second column (Helmet Type).
- Once you've found the right helmet, look for a label or other marking stating that it complies with an applicable standard listed in the third column (Applicable Standard(s)).

Hard Facts About Helmets

Your helmet should sit flat on your head—make sure it is level and is not tilted back or forward. The front of the helmet should sit low—about two finger widths above your eyebrows to protect your forehead. The straps on each side of your head should form a "Y" over your ears,

Table 20.1. Helmet types for common activities.

❶ Activity	❷ Helmet Type	❸ Applicable Standard(s)
Individual Activities — Wheeled		
Bicycling (including low speed, motor assisted) Roller & In-line Skating — Recreational Scooter Riding (including low speed, motor assisted)	Bicycle	**CPSC**, ASTM F1447, Snell B-90/95, Snell N-94†
BMX Cycling	BMX	**CPSC**, ASTM F2032
Downhill Mountain Bike Racing	Downhill	**CPSC**, ASTM F1952
Roller & In-line Skating — Aggressive/Trick Skateboarding	Skateboard	ASTM F1492†, Snell N-94†
Individual Activities — Wheeled Large Motor		
ATV Riding Dirt- & Mini-Bike Riding Motocrossing	Motocross or Motorcycle	DOT FMVSS 218, Snell M-2005
Karting/Go-Karting	Karting or Motorcycle	DOT FMVSS 218, Snell K-98, Snell M-2005
Moped Riding Powered Scooter Riding	Moped or Motorcycle	DOT FMVSS 218, Snell L-98, Snell M-2005
Individual Activities — Non-Wheeled		
Horseback Riding	Equestrian	ASTM F1163, Snell E-2001
Rock- & Wall-Climbing	Mountaineering	EN 12492†, Snell N-94†
Team Sport Activities ‡		
Baseball, Softball & T-Ball	Baseball Batter's	NOCSAE ND022
	Baseball Catcher's	NOCSAE ND024
Football	Football	NOCSAE ND002, ASTM F717
Ice Hockey	Hockey	NOCSAE ND030, ASTM F1045
Lacrosse	Lacrosse	NOCSAE ND041
Winter Activities		
Skiing Snowboarding	Ski	ASTM F2040, CEN 1077, Snell RS-98 or S-98
Snowmobiling	Snowmobile	DOT FMVSS 218, Snell M-2000
Although a helmet has not yet been designed for the following two activities, until such helmets exist, wearing one of the three listed types of helmets may be preferable to wearing no helmet at all.		
Ice Skating Sledding	Bicycle	**CPSC**, ASTM F1447, Snell B-90/95 or N-94†
	Skateboard	ASTM F1492†, Snell N-94†
	Ski	ASTM F2040, CEN 1077, Snell RS-98 or S-98

The federal CPSC Safety Standard for Bicycle Helmets is mandatory for those helmets indicated by **CPSC**.

† This helmet is designed to withstand more than one moderate impact, but protection is provided for only a limited number of impacts. Replace if visibly damaged (e.g., a cracked shell or crushed liner) and/or when directed by the manufacturer.

‡ Team sport helmets are designed to protect against multiple head impacts typically occurring in the sport (e.g., ball, puck, or stick impacts; player contact; etc.), and, generally, can continue to be used after such impacts. Follow manufacturer's recommendations for replacement or reconditioning.

Definitions: ASTM - ASTM International; CEN - European Committee for Standardization; DOT – Dept. of Transportation; EN - Euro-norm or European Standard; NOCSAE - National Operating Committee on Standards in Athletic Equipment; Snell - Snell Memorial Foundation.

with one part of the strap in front of your ear, and one behind — just below your earlobes. If the helmet leans forward, adjust the rear straps. If it tilts backward, tighten the front straps. Buckle the chinstrap securely at your throat so that the helmet feels snug on your head and does not move up and down or from side to side.

Helmets: Fact Or Fiction?

RIGHT

WRONG

Figure 20.3. The right way and the wrong way to wear a bicycle helmet.

Fiction: Helmets aren't cool.

Fact: Who says helmets can't be cool? If you're shopping for a helmet, there are lots of options, so you can pick out your favorite color. Or decorate your helmet with stickers and reflectors to show your personal style. Helmets are designed to help prevent injuries to your head, because a serious fall or crash can cause permanent brain damage or death. And that's definitely not cool.

Fiction: Helmets just aren't comfortable.

Fact: Today's helmets are lightweight, well ventilated, and have lots of padding. Try on your helmet to make sure it fits properly and comfortably on your head before you buy it.

Fiction: Really good riders don't need to wear helmets.

Fact: Crashes or collisions can happen at any time. Even professional bike racers get in serious wrecks. In three out of four bike crashes, bikers usually get some sort of injury to their head.

Helmet Program For Skaters

Helmet for a Promise™ is an opt-in free helmet program for skaters who do not own a helmet and cannot afford to buy one. The Helmet for a Promise™ approach is simple and direct. If a skater will promise to wear a helmet whenever skating, he or she will receive a custom-ordered helmet for FREE. Helmets offered include top skate brands such as S-ONE, Bern, ProTec, and Triple 8 in a wide range of styles and colors. Each skater gets to choose a helmet style, color, and size to fit properly. Helmet for a Promise™ requires that a registration form be filled in with required information and a signed Promise. The Registrations for Free Helmets are released as funds become available. Skaters are asked to OTP-IN to the e-mail registry that forms Helmet Nation™. Once skaters join Helmet Nation™ and receive helmets, the Ian Tilmann Foundation continues to ride, rap, and grow with them and their crews to pay it forward and spread word on the streets and skate parks about the Helmet for a Promise program.

Source: Reprinted with permission from The Ian Tilmann Foundation, © 2012. For additional information, visit www.theiantilmannfoundation.org.

Chapter 21

Eye Protection

Sports Eye Safety

More than 40,000 people a year suffer eye injuries while playing sports.

For all age groups, sports-related eye injuries occur most frequently in baseball, basketball and racquet sports.

Almost all sports-related eye injuries can be prevented. Whatever your game, whatever your age, you need to protect your eyes.

Take the following steps to avoid sports eye injuries:

- Wear proper safety goggles (lensed polycarbonate protectors) for racquet sports or basketball.
- Use batting helmets with polycarbonate face shields for youth baseball.
- Use helmets and face shields approved by the U.S. Amateur Hockey Association when playing hockey.
- Know that regular glasses don't provide enough protection

Recommended Sports Eye Protectors

Prevent Blindness America recommends that athletes wear sports eyeguards when participating in sports. Prescription glasses, sunglasses, and even occupational safety glasses do not provide adequate protection.

About This Chapter: This chapter includes "Sports Eye Safety," "Recommended Sports Eye Protectors," and "Tips for Buying Sports Eye Protectors," © 2011 Prevent Blindness America (www.preventblindness.org). Reprinted with permission.

Eye injuries are common in the following sports, so it's important to know what kind of protective eyewear is appropriate for each activity.

Baseball

Recommended protection:

- Faceguard (attached to helmet) made of polycarbonate material
- Sports eyeguards

Injuries prevented:

- Scratches on the cornea
- Inflamed iris
- Blood spilling into the eye's anterior chamber
- Traumatic cataract
- Swollen retina

Basketball

Recommended protection:

- Sports eyeguards

Injuries prevented:

- Fracture of the eye socket
- Scratches on the cornea
- Inflamed iris
- Blood spilling into the eye's anterior chamber
- Swollen retina

Soccer

Recommended protection:

- Sports eyeguards

Injuries prevented:

- Inflamed iris
- Blood spilling into the eye's anterior chamber
- Swollen retina

Football

Recommended protection:

- Polycarbonate shield attached to a faceguard
- Sports eyeguards

Injuries prevented:

- Scratches on the cornea
- Inflamed iris
- Blood spilling into the eye's anterior chamber
- Swollen retina

Hockey

Recommended protection:

- Wire or polycarbonate mask
- Sports eyeguards

Facts About Sports And Eye Injuries

- Eye injuries are the leading cause of blindness in children.
- Every 13 minutes, an emergency department in the United States treats a sports-related eye injury.
- Most eye injuries among kids aged 11 to 14 occur while playing sports.
- Baseball is a leading cause of eye injuries in children 14 and under.
- Basketball is a leading cause of eye injuries among 15-to 24-year-olds.
- Sports-related eye injuries represent a significant eye health hazard worldwide.
- Sports-related eye injuries cost $175 to $200 million a year.
- Hockey face protectors have saved society $10 million a year.
- Protective eyewear may prevent 90 percent of sports-related eye injuries.
- Experts agree that protective eyewear must meet ASTM standards.
- Many sports-related eye injuries result in permanent vision loss.
- Protective eyewear will keep you in the game rather than on the bench with an eye injury.

Source: Excerpted from "Sports-Related Eye Injuries: What You Need to Know and Tips for Prevention," National Eye Institute and the National Eye Health Education Program, 2008.

Injuries prevented:

- Scratches on the cornea
- Inflamed iris
- Blood spilling into the eye's anterior chamber
- Traumatic cataract
- Swollen retina

Tips For Buying Sports Eye Protectors

Eyeguards designed for use in racquet sports are now commonly used for basketball and soccer and in combination with helmets in football, hockey, and baseball. The eyeguards you choose should fit securely and comfortably and allow the use of a helmet if necessary. Expect to spend between $20 and $40 for a pair of regular eyeguards and $60 or more for eyeguards with prescription lenses.

The following guidelines can help you find a pair of eyeguards right for you:

- If you wear prescription glasses, ask your eye doctor to fit you for prescription eyeguards. If you're a monocular athlete (a person with only one eye that sees well), ask your eye doctor what sports you can safely participate in. Monocular athletes should always wear sports eyeguards.

- Don't buy sports eyeguards without lenses. Only "lensed" protectors are recommended for sports use. Make sure the lenses either stay in place or pop outward in the event of an accident. Lenses that pop in against your eyes can be very dangerous.

- Fogging of the lenses can be a problem when you're active. Some eyeguards are available with anti-fog coating. Others have side vents for additional ventilation. Try on different types to determine which is most comfortable for you.

- Check the packaging to see if the eye protector you select has been tested for sports use. Also check to see that the eye protector is made of polycarbonate material. Polycarbonate eyeguards are the most impact resistant.

- Sports eyeguards should be padded or cushioned along the brow and bridge of the nose. Padding will prevent the eyeguards from cutting your skin.

- Try on the eye protector to determine if it's the right size. Adjust the strap and make sure it's not too tight or too loose. If you purchased your eyeguards at an optical store, an optical representative can help you adjust the eye protector for a comfortable fit.

Until you get used to wearing a pair of eyeguards, it may feel strange, but bear with it. It's a lot more comfortable than an eye injury.

Chapter 22

Mouthguards

Mouthguards In Sports

Youth and adolescent sports participation has grown steadily over the years. It is estimated that 20 to 25 million youths participate in competitive sports. As a result of this growth in participation levels, incidence of injury has also increased. Some reports show sports account for approximately 36% of all unintentional injuries to children and adolescents. Of those injuries, 10–20% of all sports related injuries are maxillofacial injuries according to the American Dental Association.

The National Youth Sports Foundation for Safety reports dental injuries as the most common type of orofacial injury sustained during sports participation. They contend that an athlete is 60 times more likely to sustain damage to the teeth when not wearing a protective mouthguard. Often times these injuries will result in permanent damage to oral structures which require medical intervention.

Many dental injuries are easily prevented. Experts recommend that mouthguards be worn by athletes in competitive and recreational sports in which impact, contact, and collision are likely to occur. The American Dental Association (ADA) recommends wearing mouthguards for the following sports: acrobats, basketball, boxing, field hockey, football, gymnastics, handball, ice hockey, lacrosse, martial arts, racquetball, roller hockey, rugby, shot putting, skateboarding, skiing, skydiving, soccer, squash, surfing, volleyball, water polo, weightlifting, and wrestling. Other experts include baseball and softball infielders on that list. They further recommend the mouthguard to be worn during all practices and competition.

About This Chapter: "Mouthguards in Sports" © 2012 Nationwide Children's Hospital. All rights reserved. Reprinted with permission. For additional information from the Nationwide Children's Hospital Sports Medicine Program, visit http://www.nationwidechildrens.org/sports-medicine.

Position Statement And Recommendations For Mouthguard Use In Sports

Prior to implementation of the National Federation of State High Schools Associations (NFHS) mouthguard rule an athlete participating in contact sports had a better than 50% chance of sustaining a significant oral-facial injury during his or her secondary school career. Multiple studies by the American Dental Association, the American Academy of Pediatric Dentistry, and the American Academy of Sports Dentistry convincingly show the reduction of oral-facial injuries with the use of a properly fitted mouthguard. Prior to the use of properly fitted mouthguards and facemasks, over 50% of football players' injuries were oral-facial. They now represent less than 1% of all injuries.

The NFHS currently mandates the use of mouthguards in football, field hockey, ice hockey, lacrosse and wrestling (for wrestlers wearing braces). The Sports Medicine Advisory Committee (SMAC) of the NFHS recommends that athletes consider the use of a properly fitted, unaltered mouthguard for participation in any sport that has the potential for oral-facial injury from body or playing apparatus (stick, bat, ball, etc) contact. Current research does not support the theory that mouthguard use minimizes the risk or severity of concussion. The SMAC encourages further study in this important area.

Mouthguards should include occlusal (protecting and separating the biting surfaces) and labial (protecting the teeth and supporting structures) components covering all of the upper teeth. Mouthguards which cover the lower, rather than the upper, teeth may be used if recommended by a dentist. It is strongly recommended that mouthguards be properly fitted and not be altered in any manner which decreases the effective protection. Proper fit is insured by: (1) being constructed from a model made from an impression of the individual's teeth or (2) being constructed and fitted to the individual by impressing the teeth into the mouthguard itself. Mouthguards used in wrestling must be designed to cover both upper and lower orthodontic appliances (braces). Mouthguards cannot be clear and must be of any visible color other than white to allow for easier rule enforcement by officials in all sports in which their use is mandated (except wrestling).

Source: Excerpted from "Position Statement and Recommendations for Mouthguard Use in Sports," October 2011. © National Federation of State High School Associations. Reprinted with permission. To view the complete text of this position statement and additional information, visit www.nfhs.org.

There are three types of mouthguards:

- Ready-made or stock mouthguard

- Mouth-formed "boil and bite" mouthguard

- Custom-made mouthguard made by a dentist

These mouthguards vary in price and comfort, yet all provide some protection. According to the ADA, the most effective mouthguard should be comfortable, resistant to tearing, and resilient. A mouthguard should fit properly, be durable, easily cleaned, and not restrict speech or breathing.

It has been suggested that a properly fitted custom mouthguard may also reduce the risk of concussion, however there is currently no evidence to support this assertion.

It is important to remember damaged teeth do not grow back. Protect that perfect smile—wear a mouthguard.

Consult your primary care physician for more serious injuries that do not respond to basic first aid. As an added resource, the staff at Nationwide Children's Sports Medicine is available to diagnose and treat sports-related injuries for youth or adolescent athletes. To make an appointment, call 614-355-6000.

Chapter 23

Braces And Taping

To Tape Or Brace

To tape or to brace... is that the question?

Millions of children and adolescents participate in sports across the country. Injuries can occur as a result of being active in sports. One of the most common injuries is a sprain. A sprain is a stretch injury to a ligament, which attaches two bones together. One of the most common injuries in sports is an ankle sprain. Since these injuries can require several weeks to return to athletics, trying to prevent these injuries in the first place is important. Additionally, once an athlete sprains his/her ankle, it is common to experience recurrent ankle sprains as the ankle can be weaker following an injury. This is why many athletes tape their ankles or use ankle braces during their sports.

There are two explanations for how bracing or taping can help prevent injuries. One theory is that these devices provide mechanical support for the ankle—that is, they give extra support to the ankle ligaments. Several studies have shown that ankle tape stretches after 30 minutes of activity and may not really support the ankle joint. Ankle braces can get loose too, but can be easily tightened by the athlete. Another explanation for how taping or bracing can prevent injuries is that they improve proprioception. This is the body's ability to know where the foot and ankle are in space and to be able to balance and control motion at these joints. Taping and bracing may be more important after an ankle sprain to prevent further injuries—several studies have shown these are effective ways to decrease recurrent ankle sprains. Another great way to prevent initial and recurrent ankle sprains is balance training. This also improves proprioception and can help strengthen the muscles around the ankle joint which can decrease not only the number of ankle sprains but their severity as well.

Many athletes worry that using an ankle brace or tape can cause the ankle to become weakened over time and actually cause more injuries, however this has never been proven to be true. Although long term brace or tape wear has not been studied extensively, one study showed that eight weeks of using an ankle brace did not affect the ability of the peroneus longus muscle to prevent an ankle sprain. The peroneus longus muscle is one of the most important muscles that helps prevent inversion, which is the most common cause of ankle sprains.

So which is better, ankle tape or an ankle brace? Several studies have tried to determine which one is better at preventing injuries. Most of them show that braces may be slightly better, but that taping is better than no support. Often this comes down to user preference. Some athletes prefer tape because is less bulky than many of the braces. Some athletes prefer braces because they can tighten the braces themselves if they start getting loose.

Key Tips On Athletic Taping Of The Foot And Ankle

Excerpted from "Key Tips on Athletic Taping of the Foot and Ankle," by Tim Durta, DPM, MS, Podiatry Today, April 2006. Copyright 2006 HMP Communications. Reproduced with permission via Copyright Clearance Center. Reviewed by David A. Cooke, MD, FACP, April 2012.

Taping is a critical art as well as a science when it comes to the treatment and prevention of athletic injuries. Taping takes practice, creativity, and adaptability. It is a very important part of a sports medicine practice. Not only is taping therapeutic, it can also be diagnostic in the evaluation and treatment of injuries in athletes since the athlete's response to taping can indicate the effectiveness of orthotics in controlling biomechanical issues.

While taping is not a substitute for a comprehensive rehabilitation program, it is a key element in allowing an athlete to return to activity and prevent further injury.

We utilize taping for injury care and protection. It allows functional movement while limiting excessive motion. Taping stabilizes and supports the injured area and prevents additional injury. Taping also provides proprioceptive feedback. Improper application of tape can lead to blisters, skin irritation, and abnormal stress on the affected area as well as an increased risk of injury.

A Guide To The Different Types Of Tape

Athletic tape can be porous or nonporous. Porous tape allows for heat and moisture to pass through and help keep the skin cool and dry. Nonporous tape is more occlusive and increases the potential for skin damage and irritation from friction and heat. An added benefit of porous tape occurs if the tape has to be left on for an extended period of time. For example, a high school athlete who does not have access to an athletic trainer on a daily basis can shower and dry it off with a hair dryer.

Sometimes one may use elastic tape, which allows for muscles to contract without impeding circulation or neurological function. One should stretch the elastic tape one-third to one-half of its elastic capabilities before applying it. If it is too tight, the tape can restrict the function of the body part and lead to discomfort.

No matter what kind of tape one uses, always emphasize monitoring of the taped area for tingling, numbness, or impairment of circulation at all times.

Spray tape adherent helps the tape adhere better to the skin and also offers a layer of protection. Be sure to use the spray in a well-ventilated area. While areas such as the Achilles tendon or the dorsum of the foot and ankle may be sensitive to friction, one can protect these areas by adding a pad with lubricant such as petroleum jelly. Clinicians should cover any areas of blisters or open wounds prior to taping.

How To Safeguard Against Skin Irritation And Allergic Reactions

Remind patients that it is best to remove the tape immediately after the sport activity in order to minimize skin irritation. It is important for clinicians to inspect the skin regularly for any signs of irritation or allergic reaction when taping an athlete on a regular basis.

When dealing with an athlete who is sensitive to tape, is taped on a daily basis, or is allergic to tape, it is important to use a foam underwrap or prewrap. One should apply underwrap over the skin in a single layer as several layers will increase sweating and moisture retention under the tape. Always ask the athlete about any history of tape irritation or allergies and beware of the fair skinned athletes.

Nine Key Principles Of Taping

Here are some additional principles of taping that clinicians should keep in mind when working with athletes.

1. Place the area to be taped in the position it is to be stabilized. Any movement while taping will cause wrinkles and uneven application to the tape.

2. Select the appropriate type of tape for the area and overlap tape at least half the width of the tape below to help prevent irritating the skin from skin separation.

3. To prevent constriction of the area to be taped, be sure to avoid continuous taping whenever possible (or use elastic tape).

4. Always attempt to keep the roll of tape in hand while taping.

5. While applying the tape to the skin, smooth and mold it to avoid wrinkles or excessive pressure over prominent areas.

6. Apply the tape firmly and with a purpose. Don't just lay it on the skin but fit the contour of the skin with the pull in the desired direction in order to control the motion in that area.

7. Begin taping with an anchor piece, which will serve as a substrate to attach strips to, and finish with a lock strap to secure the tape job.

8. Tape directly to the skin in order to give the maximum amount of support and protection.

9. In order to minimize strain, one must be in the proper position for applying tape at a comfortable height. Otherwise, it can be tough on the back and wrists.

Chapter 24

How To Select The Right Athletic Shoes

Selecting Athletic Shoes

Proper-fitting sports shoes can enhance performance and prevent injuries. Follow these specially-designed fitting facts when purchasing a new pair of athletic shoes.

- Try on athletic shoes after a workout or run and at the end of the day. Your feet will be at their largest.

- Wear the same type of sock that you will wear for that sport.

- When the shoe is on your foot, you should be able to freely wiggle all of your toes.

- The shoes should be comfortable as soon as you try them on. There is no break-in period.

- Walk or run a few steps in your shoes. They should be comfortable.

- Always relace the shoes you are trying on. You should begin at the farthest eyelets and apply even pressure as you a crisscross lacing pattern to the top of the shoe.

- There should be a firm grip of the shoe to your heel. Your heel should not slip as you walk or run.

- If you participate in a sport three or more times a week, you need a sports specific shoe.

- It can be hard to choose from the many different types of athletic shoes available. There are differences in design and variations in material and weight. These differences have been developed to protect the areas of the feet that encounter the most stress in a particular athletic activity.

About This Chapter: "How to Select the Right Athletic Shoes," © 2011 American Orthopaedic Foot and Ankle Society. All rights reserved. Reprinted with permission. For additional information, visit www.aofas.org.

Know Your Sports Shoes

If you play a sport three or more times per week, a sport-specific shoe may be necessary. Remember that after 300–500 miles of running or 300 hours of aerobic activity, the cushioning material in the shoe is usually worn down and it's time to toss the shoes.

Types of Athletic Shoes

Athletic shoes are grouped into seven categories:

Running, Training, And Walking (includes shoes for hiking, jogging, and exercise walking): Look for a good walking shoe to have a comfortable soft upper, good shock absorption, smooth tread, and a rocker sole design that encourages the natural roll of the foot during the walking motion. The features of a good jogging shoe include cushioning, flexibility, control and stability in the heel counter area, lightness, and good traction.

Court Sports: Includes shoes for tennis, basketball, and volleyball. Most court sports require the body to move forward, backward, and side-to-side. As a result, most athletic shoes used for court sports are subjected to heavy abuse. The key to finding a good court shoe is its sole. Ask a coach or shoes salesman to help you select the best type of sole for the sport you plan on participating in.

Field Sports: Includes shoes for soccer, football, and baseball. These shoes are cleated, studded, or spiked. The spike and stud formations vary from sport to sport, but generally are replaceable or detachable cleats, spikes, or studs affixed into nylon soles.

Winter Sports: Includes footwear for figure skating, ice hockey, alpine skiing, and cross-country skiing. The key to a good winter sports shoe is its ability to provide ample ankle support.

Track And Field Sport Shoes: Because of the specific needs of individual runners, athletic shoe companies produce many models for various foot types, gait patterns, and training styles. It is always best to ask your coach about the type of shoe that should be selected for the event you are participating in.

Specialty Sports: Includes shoes for golf, aerobic dancing, and bicycling.

Outdoor Sports: Includes shoes used for recreational activities such as hunting, fishing, and boating.

Choices, Choices

The fitness boom of the last 25 years led to an explosion in the manufacture of sports shoes. The sports shoe consumer of the 1960s only had to make one choice—the all-purpose sneaker. Today's consumer must choose from among hundreds of brands and styles of athletic shoes designed for every sport and activity.

You may feel overwhelmed by the choices available to you, particularly since the athletic footwear industry introduces more technologically sophisticated shoes with new designs and features every year. Slick ads and television commercials tout these features, but offer little in the way of advice in selecting the shoes that match your feet. One brand does not meet the needs of everyone and the latest innovation or most expensive shoe with all the features may not be your best choice.

The below information will help you determine the right shoe for you, the one that will help you enjoy sports and lessen your chance of injury. The information includes: what you should look for in sports specific shoes, features in construction that provide comfort and prevent injuries, how to obtain a proper shoe fit, and shoe adjustments that can be made to treat foot problems.

Running Shoes

Joggers should wear a shoe with more cushioning impact. Running shoes are designed to provide maximum overall shock absorption for the foot. Such a shoe should also have good heel control. Although not a cure-all, these qualities in a running/sports shoe help to prevent shin splints, tendinitis, heel pain, stress fractures, and other overuse syndromes.

Walking Shoes

If walking is your sport or your doctor's recommendation for cardiovascular conditioning, wear a lightweight shoe. Look for extra shock absorption in the heel of the shoe and especially under the ball of the foot (the metatarsal area). This will help reduce heel pain (plantar fasciitis and pump bumps) as well as burning and tenderness in the ball of the foot (metatarsalgia). A shoe with a slightly rounded sole or "rocker bottom" also helps to smoothly shift weight from the heel to the toes while decreasing the forces across the foot. Walking shoes have more rigidity in the front so you can roll off your toes rather than bend through them as you do with running shoes.

Aerobic Shoes

Shoes for aerobic conditioning should be lightweight to prevent foot fatigue and have extra shock absorption in the sole beneath the ball of the foot (metatarsal area) where the most stress occurs. If possible, work out on a carpet.

Tennis Shoes

Tennis players need a shoe that supports the foot during quick side to side movements or shifts in weight. A shoe that provides stability on the inside and outside of the foot is an important choice. Flexibility in the sole beneath the ball of the foot allows repeated quick forward movements for a fast reaction at the net. You need slightly less shock absorption in the shoe if you're playing tennis or other racquet sports. On soft courts, wear a softer soled shoe that allows better traction. On hard courts, you want a sole with greater tread.

Basketball Shoes

If basketball is your sport, choose a shoe with a thick, stiff sole. This gives extra stability when running on the court. A high-top shoe provides support when landing from a jump and may help prevent ankle sprains.

Cross Trainers

Cross-training shoes, or cross trainers, combine several of the above features so that you can participate in more than one sport. A good cross trainer should have the flexibility in the forefoot you need for running combined with the lateral control necessary for aerobics or tennis.

You do not necessarily need a different pair of shoes for every sport in which you participate. Generally, you should wear sport-specific shoes for sports you play more than three times a week. If you have worked out for some time injury-free, then stick with the particular shoe you have been wearing. There is really no reason to change.

For special problems, you may need a special shoe. A well-cushioned shoe may not be a good shoe for someone who overpronates. If your ankles turn easily, you may need to wear a shoe with a wide heel. If you have trouble with shin splints, you may need a shoe with better shock absorption.

Design Features

Sport shoes vary in materials, design, and how they are made. Look inside the shoe before you decide which to buy. This will help you select a shoe that fits both your foot and your sport.

Special features in construction give comfort to the wearer as well as help prevent injury.

A slip-lasted shoe is made by sewing together the upper like a moccasin and then gluing it to the sole. This lasting method makes for a lightweight and flexible shoe with no torsional rigidity.

A board-lasted shoe has the "upper" leather or canvas sewn to a cardboard-like material. A person with flat feet (pes planus) feels more support and finds improved control in this type of shoe.

A combination-lasted shoe combines advantages of both other shoes. It is slip-lasted in the front, and board-lasted in the back. These shoes give good heel control but remain flexible in the front under the ball of the foot. They are good for a wide variety of foot types.

Shoe Fit

The best-designed shoes in the world will not do their job if they do not fit properly. You can avoid foot problems by finding a shoe store that employs a pedorthist or professional shoe fitter who knows about the different shapes and styles of shoes. Or, you can become an informed consumer by following these guidelines:

- Don't go just by size—have your feet measured.
- Visit the shoe store at the end of a workout when your feet are largest.
- Wear the sock you normally wear when working out.
- Fit the shoe to the largest foot.
- Make sure the shoe provides at least one thumb's breadth of space from the longest toe to the end of the toe box.
- If you have bunions or hammertoes, find a shoe with a wide toe box. You should be able to fully extend your toes when you're standing and shoes should be comfortable from the moment you put them on. They will not stretch out. Women who have big or wide feet should consider buying men's or boys' shoes which are cut wider for the same length.

When Foot Problems Develop

If you begin to develop foot or ankle problems, simple adjustments in the shoes sometimes can relieve the symptoms. Many of these simple devices are available without prescription.

A heel cup provides an effective way to alleviate pain beneath the heel (plantar fasciitis). Made of plastic or rubber, the heel cup is designed to give support around the heel while providing relief of pressure beneath the tender spot.

An arch support (orthosis) can help treat pain in the arch of the foot. Made of many types of materials, arch supports can be placed in a shoe after removing the insole that comes with the shoe.

A metatarsal pad can help relieve pain beneath the ball of the great toe (sesamoiditis) or beneath the ball of the other toes (metatarsalgia). Made of a felt material or firm rubber, the pad has adhesive on its flat side. Fixed to the insole behind the tender area, the pad shares pressure normally placed on the ball of the foot. This relieves pressure beneath the tender spot.

Custom Arch Supports

Many problems in the feet respond to stretching and conditioning, choosing a different shoe, and simple over-the-counter shoe modifications. However, long term (chronic) and complicated problems of the feet may require specially designed inserts (orthoses) made of materials that concentrate relief on a particular area while supporting other areas. Severe flat foot, high arched feet, shin splints, Achilles tendinitis, and turf toe are but a few of these conditions. To obtain the best relief for such problems, see an orthopedic surgeon, a doctor specializing in diseases of the bones and joints. The orthopedic surgeon is trained to treat problems of the foot and ankle. Pedorthists and orthotists are trained to make and modify arch supports (orthoses) and fulfill the surgeon's prescription. Working with these professionals ensures you will get the right shoe for the best possible treatment.

Chapter 25

Safety Tips For Popular Sports

Weather

- The weather can affect athletes' safe participation in sports activities. Young people are highly susceptible to extremes in temperature. Fluid replacement is important during any sporting activity, particularly in hot and humid environments. Athletes should hydrate themselves regularly before partaking in trainings and/or competitions. The weather (heat, humidity, wind, and rain) should be assessed before beginning an activity to determine if training/competition should commence.

- If athletes are exercising in the heat, do acclimatize them to the warm and humid weather conditions. Start activities slowly and build endurance. If an athlete does not feel well, stop the activity, rest, and assess fitness status before returning to play.

- Ensure adequate shade and sunscreens are available. All participants, officials, and spectators should have appropriate clothing, hats, and sunglasses to prevent overexposure to the sun.

- Do not train outdoors during a thunderstorm to minimize lightning risks.

Hydration

- Everyone should establish a hydration plan that allows drinking of water or sports drinks throughout sports sessions, whether you are a participating athlete, official, and/or

About This Chapter: Excerpts from *Sports Safety Tips for Popular Competitive Sports*, a publication by the Singapore Sports Council (www.ssc.gov.sg) Reprinted with permission. All rights reserved. The information in this publication is regularly updated. To view the complete text in its current form, and additional sports safety information, visit http://sportssafety.ssc.gov.sg/publish/sports_safety/home/resources.html. This version was accessed September 12, 2011.

spectator. Hydrate BEFORE, DURING, and AFTER training, sports activity, and/or competition. Without proper hydration, the risk of developing exertional heat related illnesses is higher.

- Adequate hydration is essential to avoid dehydration and overheating. It is best to drink 500 ml of water half an hour before exercise, 250–500 ml every half an hour during exercise and 1000 ml after exercise. Isotonic drinks are recommended for any activities that last more than an hour.

- It is important to note that although isotonic drinks provide some replacement of salt and sugar lost during vigorous activity, they also may be high in sugar content which can sometimes cause cramps, nausea and diarrhea. Water is usually the best choice of fluid intake.

- Always bring along a drinking bottle when training and exercising.

- Preferable to have cold fluid available during training and competition.

- Always drink enough (a gauge is based on the color of urine; clear or pale yellow).

Heat Illness

Heat illness is a serious matter and can be life-threatening if not taken seriously. Vigorous exercise under hot and humid weather may cause internal body heat to build up and result in heat illness. Athletes who still exercise at their cool climate intensity while lacking acclimatization will also be at increased risk of heat illness.

The risk of heat illness increases when a person can't produce enough sweat to release heat and cool down, and when high humidity hinders the effective evaporation of sweat.

Symptoms of heat illness include:

- Excessive thirst
- Nausea or vomiting
- Headaches
- Light headedness or dizziness
- Fatigue or weakness
- Profuse perspiration, often accompanied by cold, clammy skin
- Obvious loss of skill and coordination/clumsiness or unsteadiness

- Anxiety or confusion

- Aggressive or irrational behavior

- Collapse

- Paleness

- Muscle aches and cramps

General Sports Safety Tips

- Acclimation is the body's adaptation to a higher heat tolerance. Gradually increase practice intensity and duration over at least five days of training in hot or humid conditions.

- Rest frequently to help stay hydrated and cool, seek shade when possible.

- If you feel unusually fatigued, or if your exercise performance is suffering, stop activity and try to cool off.

- Assist the cooling process with the use of fans or by wetting the skin.

- Under hot conditions, adjust duration and intensity of warm-up to minimize increase in body heat and temperature before competition.

- Avoid intense exercise during the hottest time of day; train closer to sunrise or sunset.

- Wear fewer and loose-fitting, lightweight clothing in hot weather so sweat can evaporate.

Injury Prevention

Warming up prepares the mind, heart, muscles and joints for the upcoming activity. It also improves performance and prevents injuries. Any sporting activity should start with warming up. It is advised to start with some cardiovascular exercises like jogging, brisk walking, or jumping jacks to get the muscles warmed up. Stretching exercises should follow after the above initial warm up routine. It is important because the tissue is more elastic (flexible) due to the increase in heat and blood flow to the muscles.

Cooling down after each session helps the body recover and return to its normal temperature. It also releases the lactic acid in the muscles. This would reduce the likelihood of sore muscles and allows the heart rate to return to its resting state.

Physical Activity Readiness Questionnaire—PAR-Q

Regular physical activity is fun and healthy, and increasingly more people are starting to become more active every day. Being more active is very safe for most people. However, some people should check with their doctor before they start becoming much more physically active.

If you are planning to become much more physically active than you are now, start by answering the seven questions below. If you are between the ages of 15 and 69, the PAR-Q will tell you if you should check with your doctor before you start.

Common sense is your best guide when you answer these questions. Please read the questions carefully and answer each one honestly: Yes or No.

1. Has your doctor ever said that you have a heart condition <u>and</u> that you should only do physical activity recommended by a doctor?
2. Do you feel pain in your chest when you do physical activity?
3. In the past month, have you had chest pain when you were not doing physical activity?
4. Do you lose your balance because of dizziness or do you ever lose consciousness?
5. Do you have a bone or joint problem (for example, back, knee, or hip) that could be made worse by a change in your physical activity?
6. Is your doctor currently prescribing drugs (for example, water pills) for your blood pressure or heart condition?
7. Do you know of <u>any other reason</u> why you should not do physically activity?

If You Answered YES To One Or More Questions

Talk with your doctor by phone or in person before you start becoming much more physically active or before you have a fitness appraisal. Tell your doctor about the PAR-Q and which questions you answered "Yes."

- You may be able to do any activity you want—as long as you start slowly and build up

Archery

Archery is a sport involving the use of a bow and arrows, with the aim of scoring the most points by accurately shooting the arrow to the center of the target.

General Safety Tips

- Set up a distinct single shooting line for archers to shoot from.
- Archers should leave an arm's length distance from other archers.
- Heed instructions on when to commence shooting, cease shooting, and retrieve arrows.

gradually. Or, you may need to restrict your activities to those which are safe for you. Talk with your doctor about the kinds of activities you wish to participate in and follow his/her advice.

- Find out which community programs are safe and helpful for you.

IF You Answered NO To All Questions

If you answered "No" honestly to all PAR-Q questions, you can be reasonably sure that you can:

- Start becoming much more physically active—begin slowly and build up gradually. This is the safest and easiest way to go.
- Take part in a fitness appraisal—this is an excellent way to determine your basic fitness so that you can plan the best way for you to live actively. It is also highly recommended that you have your blood pressure evaluated. If your reading is over 144/94, talk with your doctor before you start becoming much more physically active.

Delay Becoming Much More Active

- If you are not feeling well because of a temporary illness such as a cold or fever—wait until you feel better; or
- If you are or may be pregnant—talk to your doctor before you start becoming more active.

Please Note

If your health changes so that you then answer "Yes" to any of the above questions, tell your fitness or health professional. Ask whether you should change your physical activity plan.

Source: *Physical Activity Readiness Questionnaire (PAR-Q)*, © 2002, reviewed 2012. Used with permission from the Canadian Society for Exercise Physiology, www.csep.ca. Informed Use of the PAR-Q: The Canadian Society for Exercise Physiology, Health Canada, and their agents assume no liability for persons who undertake physical activity, and if in doubt after completing this questionnaire, consult your doctor prior to physical activity.

- Ensure appropriate protective gears are worn (for example, finger tabs, arm guards, and chest guards).
- Store archery equipment safely.

Track And Field

Athletics, or track and field, is about running faster, jumping higher, and throwing further than competitors and enduring long distances.

General Safety Tips

- Ensure proper footwear is worn (for example, sports shoes, running, throwing, or jumping spikes).

- Equipment should be used with an adult's supervision.

- Stay in the demarcated areas for your own sport.

- Survey the field for others during field event practices.

Badminton

Badminton is a racquet sport played by two opposing players/pairs. The objective is to score points by hitting the shuttlecock over the net into the opponent's half of the court so that it hits the ground before the opponent is able to return it.

General Safety Tips

- Ensure that the court is dry.

- Wear appropriate footwear.

- Play within demarcated areas.

Basketball

Basketball is a ball sport played by two opposing teams consisting of five people each. Players score by shooting the ball into the opposing team's basket.

General Safety Tips

- Wear appropriate footwear with good ankle support.

- Ensure the boundaries of the court are clear of spectators and belongings.

- Trim or tape long fingernails.

- Ensure that the court is dry.

Boxing

Amateur boxing is a sport where points are scored through punches to an opponent above his waistline.

General Safety Tips

- Ensure appropriate protective gear is worn (for example, hand wraps, mouth guards, helmets, soft sole shoes, etc).

- Ensure boxing ring is free from hazards.

- Ensure training equipment is in working condition.

Canoe/Kayak

The kayak is a covered deck canoe propelled with a double-bladed paddle with the paddler seated in the boat. The canoe is an open canoe propelled with a single-bladed paddle with the paddler kneeling in the boat.

General Safety Tips

- Equip yourself with necessary swimming and survival skills.

- Be familiar with capsize drills.

- A well-fitting personal flotation device (PFD) should be worn at all times when out in the water.

Cycling

Cycling can be divided into four main events: BMX, mountain bike, road race, and time trial, testing the speed and endurance of athletes as they speed through the course.

General Safety Tips

- Ensure that bicycles and accessories (for example, brakes, tires, chains, and gears) are in good working condition.

- Wear a well-fitting helmet with the chin strap securely fastened.

- Wear lightweight, breathable clothing.

Diving

Diving combines artistry and athleticism with undeniable courage—divers hit the water at about 55 km/h.

General Safety Tips

- Equip yourself with necessary swimming and survival skills.

- Attempt advance jumps progressively.

- Be careful of wet and slippery floors.

- Only one swimmer is allowed on the diving board or platform at any one time.

- Wait for the previous diver to leave the water before diving.

- Do not swim under the boards to exit the water.

Equestrian Sports

In equestrian sports, the horse and rider work together to demonstrate feats of grace, agility, and speed. There are seven equestrian disciplines recognized by the International Equestrian Federation which includes dressage, jumping, eventing, reining, vaulting, endurance, and driving.

General Safety Tips

- Ensure appropriate protective gear is worn (for example, riding helmet, body protectors, and riding boots).

- Saddles and harnesses should be undamaged and properly secured.

- Adjust the horse bit correctly to make sure that it is not worn at the joints.

- Undergo proper training in riding style and horse safety (for example, mounting and dismounting from horse).

Fencing

Fencing is a traditional sport developed based on ancient sword fighting, involving two competitors contesting bouts using light weapons: épée, foil, or sabre.

General Safety Tips

- Ensure appropriate protective gear is worn (for example, padded white jacket, underarm protector, gloves, wire mesh mask, flat soled shoes).

- Refrain from using the weapons when off training mats.

- Only engage in fencing activities in the presence of an instructor.

- Check your weapon regularly to ensure it is safe and usable. Use a new blade if you are in doubt about the safety of your weapon.

Soccer

Soccer is played between two teams of 11 players on the field of play at any one time. The ball may be passed, tapped, rolled, or dribbled in any direction using the feet, as well as thrown from the sideline in the case of a throw-in.

General Safety Tips

- Ensure shin pads and soccer boots are worn during play.

- Goal keepers should wear gloves.

- Ensure the boundaries of the field/court are clear of spectators and belongings.

- Wear lightweight, breathable clothing.

Gymnastics

Gymnastics is a sport involving the performance of sequences of movements. It requires competitors to perform set moves either on the floor, apparatus, or in the air, requiring a high level of flexibility, agility, and strength.

General Safety Tips

- Ensure gymnastic equipment is in proper condition.

- Acquire basic skills and have someone to help when attempting more advanced moves.

- Perform a skill only if you are confident on executing it.

- Wear well-fitting clothing.

Handball

Handball is a fast-paced, contact sport involving two teams of seven players on the field of play at any one time. Amid intense physical contact, players pass, throw, roll, catch, and dribble the ball with their hands while trying to score goals. The team which has scored more goals than the opponent is the winner.

General Safety Tips

- Ensure the boundaries of the court are clear of spectators and belongings.
- Trim or tape long fingernails.
- Ensure that the court is dry.
- Ensure proper footwear is worn.
- Wear lightweight, breathable clothing.

Field Hockey

Field hockey is an exciting sport played on artificial turf with two teams of 11 players. Players use their hockey stick to control, dribble, and hit the ball. The team that scores the most goals wins the match.

General Safety Tips

- Goalkeepers are advised to remove their protective gear, including helmet, during the break to prevent the body from overheating.
- Ensure goalkeepers wear appropriate protective gear (for example, helmet with face guard, chest protector, gloves, protective pads, and kickers).
- Wear face masks when defending a penalty corner.
- All players are to use well fitted shin-guards and mouth guards.
- Check goal posts and structures for stability.
- Ensure proper footwear is worn.

Judo

Judo, a traditional Japanese martial art sport, means *gentle way*. Governed by the philosophy "minimum strength, maximum efficiency," Judo involves two individuals who, by gripping the Judo uniform (or Judo gi), use the forces of balance, power, and movement to throw the opponent over. There is no kicking, punching, or weapons involved.

General Safety Tips

- Put on proper footwear when off the mat. Do not exit and return to the mat barefoot.
- Spar with an opponent with a level of skill similar to you.
- The instructor must be notified when an individual enters or exits the mat during practice.

- Wear undamaged Judo gi and/or appropriate athletic clothing.
- Hard metal objects (for example, jewelry, ear studs, rings, etc) are not to be worn.

Rowing

Rowing is an Olympic sport where athletes (one or more depending on the event) sit in a rowing boat, facing backwards, and use oars or sculls to propel the boat forward over a straight course of 1,000 m.

General Safety Tips

- Equip yourself with necessary swimming and survival skills.
- Be familiar with capsize drills.
- Personal flotation device (PFD) should be worn at all times when out in the water.
- Apply ample sun block to all areas of exposed skin to prevent sunburn caused by the reflection of the sun on water. Reapply regularly.

Sailing

Sailing is a sport involving the maneuvering of a boat using wind as the only source of power to navigate a specially marked course in a race.

General Safety Tips

- Check your equipment before casting off.
- Always protect your head, hands, and feet when sailing.
- Equip yourself with necessary swimming and survival skills.
- Be familiar with capsize drills.
- Wear light and thin clothing to prevent heat stroke and dehydration.

Shooting

General Safety Tips

- Treat every gun as if it were loaded and ready to fire.
- Never load a gun until you are sure that it is safe to shoot.

- Always keep the gun pointed in a safe direction.

- Always keep your fingers off the trigger until ready to shoot.

- Ensure appropriate protective gears are worn (for example, ear muffs, shooting glasses, and vest).

Swimming

Swimming events include freestyle, breaststroke, backstroke, butterfly, and medley, testing the speed and endurance of participants in individual and team competitions.

General Safety Tips

- Equip yourself with swimming and survival skills.

- Take note of depth markers.

- Be careful of wet and slippery floors.

Table Tennis

Table tennis, also known as ping pong, is a sport in which two or four players hit a lightweight, hollow ball back and forth with paddles. A game is won by the player or pair who first scores 11 points.

General Safety Tips

- Ensure no table tennis balls are near your feet where you might easily trip over them.

- Avoid hitting or running into your partner while playing doubles.

- Check equipment for cracks.

- Ensure that courts are dry.

- Avoid jumping across barriers between courts.

Taekwondo

Taekwondo, a martial art sport, involves the use of both hands and legs to score points by hitting the legal scoring areas. The sport prohibits the use of dangerous techniques. The trademark of the sport is its fast and flamboyant kicks delivered to permitted regions of the body and head.

General Safety Tips

- Spar with an opponent with a level of skill similar to you.
- Observe the rules and regulation of the sport.
- Ensure appropriate protective gear is worn (for example, head gear, groin guard, body protector).
- Hard metal objects (for example, jewelry, ear studs, rings, etc) are not to be worn.

Tennis

A tennis match is a game of endurance, quick-wittedness, and precise execution. It consists of a predetermined number of sets, which in turn consists of games. Each game is made up of a sequence of points played with the same player serving.

General Safety Tips

- Clear the court of all tennis balls at all times.
- Ensure that the court is dry.
- Wear appropriate footwear with good support.
- Avoid jumping or climbing over the net.

Triathlon

The triathlon competition format for individual competitions includes a 750 m swim in open water, a 20 km cycle ride (three-lap course), and a 5 km run (two-lap course). The 4 x mixed team relay competition includes a 250 m swim in open water, a 7 km cycle ride (one-lap course), and a 1.7 km run (one-lap course)

General Safety Tips

Swimming

- Acclimatize to the open sea factors such as water temperature, waves, and currents.
- Use the buddy system during training sessions regardless of how good a swimmer you are.

Cycling

- Be prepared for unfamiliar terrain (for example, uneven/slippery surfaces, speed bumps, etc).

- Wear a well-fitting helmet with straps secured in place.

- Ensure that bicycles and accessories are in good working condition (gears, brakes, lights, etc).

Running

- Wear appropriate footwear with good support.

Volleyball

Volleyball is played by two teams of six players on court at any one time. Players try to score points by grounding the ball on the opponent's court under specific rules.

General Safety Tips

- Wear well-fitting protective gear such as elbow and knee pads to prevent injuries.

- Wear appropriate shoes with good support to prevent injuries.

- Ensure the boundaries of the court are clear of spectators and belongings.

Tips For Safe Physical Activity

When To Stop Or Slow Down

Stop your activity right away if you experience these symptoms:

- Have pain, tightness, or pressure in your chest or neck, shoulder, or arm
- Feel dizzy or sick
- Break out in a cold sweat
- Have muscle cramps
- Are extremely short of breath
- Feel pain in your joints, feet, ankles, or legs. You could hurt yourself if you ignore the pain.

Ask your health care provider what to do if you have any of these symptoms.

Slow down if you feel out of breath. The "talk test" is an easy way to monitor your physical activity intensity:

- You should be able to talk during your activity without gasping for breath.
- When talking becomes difficult, your activity may be too hard.
- If talking becomes difficult for you while exercising, slow down until you are able to talk comfortably again.

- Ensure that the courts are dry.

- Trim or tape long fingernails.

Weightlifting

In weightlifting, competitors compete to lift a weighted bar above their head and hold it under control until signaled by the referee to replace it on the platform.

General Safety Tips

- Put the weights back to their respective places after use.

- Ensure pins are firmly in place in weight stack machines.

- Ensure proper footwear is worn.

- Bring a towel and wipe down gym benches before and after use.

- Adopt a proper weight advancement training program.

Wear Suitable Clothes

- Wear lightweight, loose-fitting tops so you can move easily.
- Wear clothes made of fabrics that absorb sweat and remove it from your skin.
- Never wear rubber or plastic suits. Plastic suits could hold the sweat on your skin and make your body overheat.
- Women should wear a good support bra.
- Wear supportive athletic shoes for weight-bearing activities.
- Wear a knit hat to keep you warm when you are physically active outdoors in cold weather. Wear a tightly woven, wide-brimmed hat in hot weather to help keep you cool and protect you from the sun.
- Wear sunscreen when you are physically active outdoors.
- Wear garments that prevent inner-thigh chafing, such as tights or spandex shorts.

Drink Fluids

Drink fluids regularly while you are being physically active. Water or other fluids will help keep you hydrated when you are sweating.

Source: Excerpted from "Active at Any Size," National Institute of Diabetes and Digestive and Kidney Diseases (www .niddk.nih.gov), February 2010.

- Engage spotters when trying major lifts.

- Maintain good lifting position, back management techniques, and correct breathing techniques while lifting weights.

Wrestling

Wrestling is an ancient individual combat sport fought between two wrestlers. Each competitor attempts to throw the other to the mat, and *pin* their shoulders to the ground to register a *fall*. There are several distinctions in rules between the two major international styles of wrestling: Greco-Roman and freestyle.

General Safety Tips

- Spar with an opponent with a level of skill similar to you.

- Ensure appropriate protective gear is worn (for example, proper fitting clothing, padded and protective safety gear).

- Wrestle within a safe distance from hazards.

- Hard metal objects (for example, jewelry, ear studs, rings, etc) are not to be worn.

Chapter 26

Bike Safety

The Basics

Riding bikes is a great way for you to get active and have fun. Riding a bike can help you get in shape, lose weight, lower your risk of health conditions like heart disease, spend time with your family, and save money on gas.

Follow these safety tips every time you ride: use the right size bike; check the brakes before you ride; always wear a bike helmet; wear bright colors and reflective tape; and ride in the same direction as cars.

A bike crash could send you to the emergency room. The good news is that many bike injuries can be prevented.

Take Action

Riders of any age should be able to put one leg on each side of the top tube (or bar) of their bike with both feet flat on the ground. If your feet can't reach the ground, the bike isn't safe for you to ride.

Check The Brakes

Make sure the brakes are working before you ride. Bikes that brake when you pedal backwards are best for kids. Young children's hands aren't big enough or strong enough to use hand brakes.

About This Chapter: From "Ride Your Bike Safely," National Health Information Center (www.healthfinder.org), U.S. Department of Health and Human Services, December 30, 2011.

Always Wear A Bike Helmet

Get in the "helmet habit." Wear helmets every time and everywhere you ride bikes. A bike helmet is the best way to prevent injury or death from a bike crash.

Make sure your helmet is certified. Look for a sticker on the inside that says "CPSC." This means it's been tested for safety.

Bike helmets only protect you if you wear them the right way. Every time you put your helmet on, make sure that the helmet is flat on the top of your head, the helmet is covering the top of your forehead, and the strap is buckled snugly under your chin.

Replace your helmet if you crash. Even if your helmet doesn't look cracked or damaged, it might not protect you in another crash.

Make Sure People Can See You Easily

Drivers can have a hard time seeing bike riders, even during the day. Wear neon, fluorescent, or other bright colors, and put something on your clothes or bike that reflects light, like reflective tape.

Try to plan ahead so your bike rides are over before it gets dark. If you are going to ride at night, make sure your bike has reflectors on the front, back, and tires, and put battery powered lights on your bike. A red light is for the back, and a white light is for the front—just like with cars.

Follow The "Rules Of The Road"

Look both ways before entering the street, and ride in the same direction as the cars. Remember to stop at all stop signs and intersections. Use hand signals to show others what you plan to do next. For a left turn, look behind you, hold your left arm straight out to the side, and turn carefully. For a right turn, hold your left arm out and up in an "L" shape. To signal that you are stopping, hold your left arm out and down in an upside-down "L" shape.

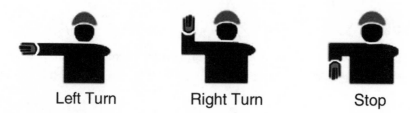

Left Turn   Right Turn   Stop

Figure 26.1. Hand signals for left turn, right turn, and stop.

Chapter 27

Skateboard Safety

An estimated 90% of skateboard injuries are among those ages 15 and younger. Injuries from skateboarding vary from minor to fatal. The most common are sprains and fractures to the wrist and elbow followed by legs and ankles. However the most dangerous is head injury which can lead to brain damage or death. By wearing a properly fitted skateboard helmet can reduce your risk head injury by 85% and the risk of brain injury by 90%. Follow the safety tips below. Remember, wearing a properly fitted and fastened helmet when riding It will not only keep you safe, but riding like a pro.

Helmets

- Protect your head. Always wear a helmet.
- Helmets need to be worn by all skaters, at all ability levels, at all times to prevent head injuries.
- The helmet must fit securely and be buckled or fastened.
- Do not buy a helmet that moves on the head when the head moves.
- The front of the helmet should come down to just a finger's width above the eyebrows.

Knee Pads

- All skaters, and especially beginners, should wear knee pads to prevent knee injuries and scrapes.

About This Chapter: "Skateboard Safety Tips," April 2012, reprinted with permission from the Los Angeles Department of Public Health, Injury and Violence Prevention Program (http://publichealth.lacounty.gov/ivpp), © 2012. All rights reserved.

- Pads need to be fastened securely around the leg.

- Pads are usually sized small, medium, and large according to body size.

Elbow Pads

- Elbow pads are also highly recommended for beginners as well as all aggressive skaters.

- Elbow pads are sized small, medium, and large according to body size.

Wrist Guards

- Hand protection is recommended to be worn at all times.

- Some guards and gloves are manufactured with a hard plastic splint. These offer the maximum protection against injury.

- They are sized small, medium, and large according to body size

Riding Safely

- Always keep your board maintained (check with a local shop for maintenance).

- Always ride during daylight hours.

- Wear bright-colored clothes that make you more visible.

- Stay alert! Watch for potholes, dogs, water, rocks, and people.

- Look both ways before crossing alleyways and driveways.

- Children younger than five years of age should not use skateboards. Their center of gravity is higher, their neuromuscular system is not well developed, their judgment is poor, and they are not sufficiently able to protect themselves from injury. More developmentally appropriate activities need to be encouraged.

- Children ages six to ten must have close adult supervision.

- Skateboards must never be ridden near traffic. Their use should be prohibited on streets and highways.

- Activities that bring skateboards and motor vehicles together ("catching a ride") are especially dangerous.

- It is safest to ride in a community skateboard park.

- Obey city laws and observe areas where you cannot skate.

- Do not skate in crowds of pedestrians or bicyclists.

- Do not take chances. Complicated tricks require careful practice and specially designed areas.

- Do not use headphones while skating—pay attention to your surroundings.

Learning To Fall

- Learn the basic skills of skateboarding along with knowing how to stop safely.

- Learning how to fall will help reduce your chances of being seriously injures.

- If you lose your balance, crouch down on the skateboard so you will not have as far to fall.

- If you fall:
  - Try to roll rather than have your body absorb the force with your arms.
  - Relax your body, rather than stiffening your body and arms.

If You Fall

- If you fall and are taken to the hospital, bring the helmet with you.

- Any impact can crush the protective foam of the helmet. Even if it doesn't look damaged, it will still be less able to absorb future impacts. Replace a helmet on a regular basis because of wear and tear to the protective foam.

- If a helmet is damaged, either during an actual crash or in some other way, it should be replaced immediately.

Chapter 28

Football Safety

It's hard to overstate football's popularity in the United States. The Super Bowl is the biggest sports event of the year. College football and the NFL dominate headlines in the fall—and even in the spring as the NFL draft takes center stage. And high school football is a revered institution in big cities and small towns from sea to shining sea. In short, football has supplanted baseball as America's game.

But football is an inherently violent sport, with large bodies colliding with one another with tremendous force. The name of the game is to hit somebody, and as a result, injuries in football are very common and often serious enough to require a trip to the emergency room.

To learn how to keep things as safe as possible on the football field, follow these tips.

Why Is Football Safety Important?

Because of its violent nature and the sheer numbers of people who play, football is the leading cause of school sports injuries. Aside from minor aches and pains, common football injuries include ankle sprains, pulled muscles, broken bones, torn ligaments, and concussions.

Fortunately, many football injuries can be prevented by wearing the right equipment, playing within the rules, and using proper technique.

About This Chapter: "Football Safety," August 2010, reprinted with permission from www.kidshealth.org. Copyright © 2010 The Nemours Foundation. This information was provided by KidsHealth, one of the largest resources online for medically reviewed health information written for parents, kids, and teens. For more articles like this one, visit www.KidsHealth.org or www.TeensHealth.org.

Gear Guidelines

You'll need a lot of protective gear to play football, and you'll need to remember to wear all of it each time you play. If you show up for a practice or game without a necessary piece of equipment, tell your coach, and don't try to play until you fix the situation.

At a minimum, you should never take the field without the following gear.

Helmet

All football helmets should have a hard plastic outer shell and a thick layer of padding. Helmets should meet the safety standards developed by the National Operating Committee on Standards for Athletic Equipment (NOCSAE). Ask for help from your coach or a trained professional at a sporting goods store to make sure you get a helmet that meets these standards and fits well.

Helmets also should have a rigid facemask made from coated carbon steel. Check your facemask to make sure it is properly secured to the helmet. There are different face masks for different positions and purposes. Ask your coach which one would be appropriate for you.

Finally, all helmets should have a chin strap with a protective chin cup. Always keep your chin strap fastened and snug whenever you play.

Pants With Leg Pads

Some football pants include pads that snap into place or fit into pockets within the pants. Other pants are shells that you pull over your pads. Regardless of which style you choose, you should have pads for your hips, thighs, knees, and tailbone.

Shoulder Pads

Football shoulder pads should have a hard plastic shell with thick padding.

Shoes

Different leagues have different rules dictating the type of shoes and cleats (non-detachable or detachable) you can use. Check with your coach and consult your league's guidelines regarding which types of shoes are allowed.

Mouthguard

All football leagues will require you to use a mouthguard. Be sure to get one with a keeper strap that attaches it securely to your facemask.

Athletic Supporter With Cup

Worn properly, this essential piece of equipment helps male athletes avoid testicular injuries.

Additional Gear

Other items that you might want to consider using for protection include: padded neck rolls; forearm pads; padded or non-padded gloves; "flak jackets" that protect the ribcage and abdomen.

If you need to wear glasses on the field, be sure they're made of shatterproof glass or plastic.

Before Kickoff

Get yourself in shape before the season starts. Ideally, you should eat a healthy diet and get regular exercise year-round, but if you can't, be sure to start preparing for the football season by working out and eating right during the summer. This will help you be a better player and help prevent injuries.

Have a pre-season physical exam. Many schools won't let athletes play unless they've had a sports physical. If your school doesn't require or schedule an exam for you, have your parents take you to your own doc. He or she will make sure you're physically able to play.

Warm up and stretch before every game or practice. Start by doing jumping jacks or jogging in place for a few minutes, and then slowly and gently stretch your muscles, holding each stretch for at least 30 seconds. This is particularly important if you will be playing in cold weather.

Drink plenty of water before, during, and after games and practices. This helps you avoid dehydration and overheating, especially when it's hot out.

Work with your coach and teammates to learn proper techniques. You'll want to know how to avoid unsafe play before you participate in a game or full-speed practice. Once play begins, things will happen quickly. If you aren't knowledgeable about what's going on, you'll be more susceptible to getting hurt.

During Games And Practices

Know and obey the rules of football. There's a reason why things like tripping, clipping, grabbing the facemask, blocking below the knees, and helmet-to-helmet contact are illegal. They can be dangerous to both you and others. The point of the game is to hit opposing players, but if you don't do it in a legal manner, you will cost your team on the field and greatly increase your risk of injury.

When making a tackle, keep your head up and never lead with the top of your helmet. Known as "spearing," this is not only illegal, it also greatly increases your chances of a traumatic head or neck injury. Practice tackling with correct form until you are sure you can do it safely in a game.

Know your vulnerabilities. If you will be playing an offensive "skill position" such as wide receiver, running back, or quarterback, you'll find yourself in a vulnerable position as defenders try to tackle you. Learn how to absorb contact and protect yourself when you have the ball or are making a throw or catch.

Be aware of where you are on the field and what is going on around you at all times. Football can seem a little chaotic, but if you pay attention to what you're doing, you can usually avoid accidental collisions that might otherwise lead to injuries.

If you have any pain or discomfort, take yourself out of the game. Never try to play through pain. It only increases the severity of an injury and keeps you out of action longer. Don't start playing again until the pain goes away or you get cleared to play by a doctor.

If you feel like an opposing player is deliberately trying to injure you, don't start a fight or try to retaliate. Let your coach and the referee know, and let them handle the situation.

Stop at the whistle. Give it your all when a play is in progress, but be sure to stop as soon as you hear the whistle. It's not uncommon for a player to get hurt when one player keeps going after everyone else relaxes at the whistle.

A Few Other Reminders

Make sure there is first aid available at the fields where you play and practice, as well as someone who knows how to administer it. This can be a coach or other responsible adult. Have a plan for emergency situations, and be sure there is someone available to take injured players to the emergency room or contact medical personnel to quickly treat serious injuries.

When you are on the sidelines waiting to go into a game, stand well back from the playing field so you don't find yourself in the way if a play spills out of bounds.

Study the playbook and know what you are supposed to be doing on every play. Then practice, practice, practice until you have your responsibilities down pat. The more confident you are in what you're doing on the field, the less likely you are to get hurt.

Lastly, don't forget to have fun out there. Football can be a very demanding sport, and between all the repetition of practice and the hype and glitz of college and pro football, it can be easy to forget what attracted you to the game in the first place.

Football is tons of fun to play. Wear the right gear and use a little common sense, and you can help keep yourself injury free and out on the field having a great time.

Chapter 29

Water Sports Safety

Health Benefits Of Water-Based Exercise

Swimming is the second most popular sports activity in the United States and a good way to get regular aerobic physical activity. Just two and a half hours per week of aerobic physical activity, such as swimming, bicycling, or running can decrease the risk of chronic illnesses. This can also lead to improved health for people with diabetes and heart disease. Swimmers have about half the risk of death compared with inactive people. People report enjoying water-based exercise more than exercising on land. They can also exercise longer in water than on land without increased effort or joint or muscle pain.

Water-based exercise can help people with chronic diseases. For people with arthritis, it improves use of affected joints without worsening symptoms. Water-based exercise also improves mental health. Swimming can improve mood in both men and women. For people with fibromyalgia, it can decrease anxiety and exercise therapy in warm water can decrease depression and improve mood.

Because exercising in water offers many physical and mental health benefits and is a good choice for people who want to be more active. When in the water, remember to protect yourself and others from illness and injury by practicing healthy and safe swimming behaviors.

About This Chapter: This chapter includes excerpts from the following documents produced by the Centers for Disease Control and Prevention: "Health Benefits of Water-Based Exercise," February 24, 2012; "Unintentional Drowning: Fact Sheet," May 16, 2011; "White-Water Rafting Activity Card," BAM! Body and Mind, undated (accessed 4/4/2012); and "Frequently Asked Questions" [about Recreational Water Illnesses], November 18, 2011.

Unintentional Drowning

Every day, about ten people die from unintentional drowning. Of these, two are children aged 14 or younger. Drowning is the sixth leading cause of unintentional injury death for people of all ages, and the second leading cause of death for children ages one to 14 years.

Healthy Swimming Fast Facts

- There are 8.8 million residential and public-use swimming pools in the United States.
- In the United States during 2007, there were approximately 339 million pool visits each year by persons over the age of six.
- Forty-one percent of children aged 7–17 years, and 17.4% of adults in the United States, swim at least six times per year.
- There are over 6.6 million hot tubs in operation in the United States.
- Sunburn is a risk factor for both basal cell carcinoma and melanoma (types of skin cancer). In 2003, a total of 45,625 new cases of melanoma were diagnosed in the United States, and 7,818 persons died from the disease.
- Over 12 percent (13,532 of 111,487) of pool inspections conducted during 2008 resulted in an immediate closure, pending the correction of the violations.
- A total of 78 recreational water-associated outbreaks affecting 4,412 persons were reported to CDC for 2005–2006, the largest number of outbreaks ever reported in a 2-year period.
- Because of its resistance to chlorine, *Cryptosporidium* has become the leading cause of gastroenteritis outbreaks associated with swimming pool venues. Reporting of cryptosporidiosis cases increased 208 percent from 2004 (3,411) to 2008 (10,500).
- Drowning is the second leading cause of all unintentional injury deaths in children aged 1–14 years.
- Among 0–4 year olds, 69% of drownings for which the location was known occurred in swimming pools.
- In the United States in 2007, almost 32 million individuals participated in motor or power boat activities.
- In 2006, 3,474 persons were injured and 710 died while boating.
- The U.S. Coast Guard's 2006 statistics stated that approximately 87 percent of boaters who drowned were not wearing life jackets.

Source: Excerpted from "Healthy Swimming Fast Facts," Centers for Disease Control and Prevention, July 29, 2010. The complete text of this document, including references, can be found online at http://www.cdc.gov/healthywater/swimming/fast_facts.html.

How big is the problem?

In 2007, there were 3,443 fatal unintentional drownings (non-boating related) in the United States, averaging ten deaths per day. An additional 496 people died from drowning in boating-related incidents.

More than one in five people who die from drowning are children 14 and younger. For every child who dies from drowning, another four received emergency department care for nonfatal submersion injuries.

More than 55% of drowning victims treated in emergency departments require hospitalization or transfer for higher levels of care (compared to a hospitalization rate of 3-5% for all unintentional injuries). These injuries can be severe.

Nonfatal drownings can cause brain damage that may result in long-term disabilities including memory problems, learning disabilities, and permanent loss of basic functioning (for example, permanent vegetative state).

Who is most at risk?

Males: Nearly 80% of people who die from drowning are male.

Children: Children ages one to four have the highest drowning rates. In 2007, among children one to four years old who died from an unintentional injury, almost 30% died from drowning. Fatal drowning remains the second-leading cause of unintentional injury-related death for children ages one to 14 years.

Minorities: Between 2000 and 2007, the fatal unintentional drowning rate for African Americans across all ages was 1.3 times that of whites. For American Indians and Alaskan Natives, this rate was 1.7 times that of whites.

Rates of fatal drowning are notably higher among these populations in certain age groups. The fatal drowning rate of African American children ages 5 to 14 is 3.1 times that of white children in the same age range. For American Indian and Alaskan Native children, the fatal drowning rate is 2.3 times higher than for white children.

Factors such as the physical environment (for example, access to swimming pools) and a combination of social and cultural issues (for example, wanting to learn how to swim, and choosing recreational water-related activities) may contribute to the racial differences in drowning rates. Current rates are based on population, and not on participation. If rates could be determined by actual participation in water-related activities, disparity in minorities drowning rates compared to whites would be much greater.

What factors influence drowning risk?

Lack of Supervision And Barriers: Supervision by a lifeguard or designated water-watcher is important to protect young children when they are in the water, whether a pool or bathtub. But when children are not supposed to be in the water, supervision alone isn't enough to keep them safe. Barriers such as pool fencing should be used to help prevent young children from gaining access to the pool area without caregivers' awareness. There is an 83% reduction in the risk of childhood drowning with a four-sided isolation pool fence, compared to three-sided property-line fencing.

Among children ages one to four years, most drownings occur in residential swimming pools. Most young children who drowned in pools were last seen in the home, had been out of sight less than five minutes, and were in the care of one or both parents at the time.

Natural Water Settings (such as lakes, rivers, or the ocean): The percent of drownings in natural water settings increases with age. When a location was known, 65% of drownings among those 15 years and older occurred in natural water settings.

Lack Of Life Jacket Use In Recreational Boating: In 2009, the U.S. Coast Guard received reports for 4,730 boating incidents; 3,358 boaters were reported injured, and 736 died. Among those who drowned, nine out of ten were not wearing life jackets. Most boating fatalities that occurred during 2008 (72%) were caused by drowning with 90% of victims not wearing life jackets; the remainder were due to trauma, hypothermia, carbon monoxide poisoning, or other causes.

Alcohol Use: Alcohol use is involved in up to half of adolescent and adult deaths associated with water recreation and about one in five reported boating fatalities. Alcohol influences balance, coordination, and judgment, and its effects are heightened by sun exposure and heat.

Seizure Disorders: For persons with seizure disorders, drowning is the most common cause of unintentional injury death, with the bathtub as the site of highest drowning risk.

What has research found?

Participation in formal swimming lessons can reduce the risk of drowning by 88% among children aged one to four years.

Seconds count. CPR performed by bystanders has been shown to improve outcomes in drowning victims. The more quickly intervention occurs, the better change of improved outcomes.

A CDC study about self-reported swimming ability found that younger adults reported greater swimming ability than older adults. Self-reported ability increased with level of education. Among racial groups, African Americans reported the most limited swimming ability.

Men of all ages, races, and educational levels consistently reported greater swimming ability than women.

How can drowning be prevented?

The following guidelines can help prevent water-related injuries:

- **Supervision In Or Around The Water:** Designate a responsible adult to watch young children while in the bath and all children swimming or playing in or around water. Supervisors of preschool children should provide "touch supervision"—be close enough to reach the child at all times. Adults should not be involved in any other distracting activity (such as reading, playing cards, talking on the phone, or mowing the lawn) while supervising children.

- **Buddy System:** Always swim with a buddy. Select swimming sites that have lifeguards whenever possible.

- **Seizure Disorder Safety:** If you or a family member has a seizure disorder, provide one-on-one supervision around water, including swimming pools. Consider taking showers rather than using a bath tub for bathing.

- **Learn To Swim:** Formal swimming lessons can protect young children from drowning. However, even when children have had formal swimming lessons, constant, careful supervision when children are in the water, and barriers, such as pool fencing, to prevent unsupervised access are necessary.

- **Learn Cardiopulmonary Resuscitation (CPR):** In the time it might take for paramedics to arrive, your CPR skills could make a difference in someone's life.

- **Do Not Use Air-Filled Or Foam Toys:** Do not use air-filled or foam toys, such as "water wings," "noodles," or inner-tubes in place of life jackets (personal flotation devices). These toys are not designed to keep swimmers safe.

- **Avoid Alcohol:** Teens should not drink alcohol, and all people should avoid drinking alcohol before or during swimming, boating, or water skiing. Do not drink alcohol while supervising children.

If you have a swimming pool at home, follow these guidelines:

- **Four-Sided Fencing:** Install a four-sided pool fence that completely separates the house and play area of the yard from the pool area. The fence should be at least four feet high. Use self-closing and self-latching gates that open outward with latches that are out of reach of children. Also, consider additional barriers such as automatic door locks or alarms to prevent access or notify you if someone enters the pool area.

- **Clear The Pool And Deck Of Toys:** Remove floats, balls, and other toys from the pool and surrounding area immediately after use so children are not tempted to enter the pool area unsupervised.

If you are in or around natural bodies of water:

- Know the local weather conditions and forecast before swimming or boating. Strong winds and thunderstorms with lightning strikes are dangerous.

- Use U.S. Coast Guard approved life jackets when boating, regardless of distance to be traveled, size of boat, or swimming ability of boaters.

- Know the meaning of and obey warnings represented by colored beach flags, which may vary from one beach to another.

Safety Tips For Open Water Swimming

Open-water swimming is, as we say, a whole different animal. While training in a pool is often times more convenient and is necessary for interval training, those training for an open water swim should attempt at least a few open-water training swims before a race. Here is what you need to know to stay safe and get the most out of your open water swims.

Never Swim Alone: While it may be difficult to find like-minded individuals to spend a Saturday morning braving the algae levels in the local lake with you, the presence of a swim buddy will keep you accountable. Additionally, the added visibility will keep you safer from boat traffic. Even better yet is either a powered boat or a kayak to act as a support craft. The crafts, which sit higher in the water, reduce the danger of boat traffic. An added bonus of a support craft is that it can carry bottled water and some sort of food (for example, gel packet) to keep you hydrated and fueled.

Always Swim Parallel To And Near The Shoreline: If you swim parallel to the shoreline you will never be far from land in the event that you tire or have a panic attack (not uncommon among beginning open water swimmers). Also, boat traffic is generally limited close to shore. If there is a "No Wake Zone" where boats are required to keep speeds to a minimum, stick to this area. Keep in mind that swimmers can disappear from a boat operator's view behind a wave or swell.

Beat The Morning Traffic: With the exception of fishermen and water skiers; most boaters will wait until early afternoon to push off the dock. Try to swim early in the morning so that you can finish up before their boats are even loaded. While swimming in the dark is almost never

- Watch for dangerous waves and signs of rip currents (for example, water that is discolored and choppy, foamy, or filled with debris and moving in a channel away from shore). If you are caught in a rip current, swim parallel to shore; once free of the current, swim toward shore.

White-Water Safety

White-water rafting is an exciting way to see the great outdoors while testing your strength and ability to think on your feet. It's also a great way to meet new people, and learn how to work as part of a team. If everyone pulls together, the accomplishments are greater—so get out and conquer that river.

White-water rafting takes place on a river, but not just any river will do—it has to have rapids. Rapids occur where the water moves very quickly downhill over rocks or boulders. To the experts, rapids are classified on a scale of 1–6. Class 1 rapids are small with low waves, a slow current, and no obstructions in the water, while Class 6 rapids can have large, frequent

---

recommended, there are circumstances when it can be beneficial to a swimmer that might have a night-swimming portion of his or her race (think ultra-marathon swims). If this is the case, training in the dark is highly recommended to acclimate the swimmer to the anxiety that may accompany the situation. Glow sticks should be attached to the swimmer's swimsuit and goggle straps for added visibility.

Be Prepared: The unique qualities of open-water call for some slight gear changes. A mirrored goggle will protect eyes from the sun, and sunscreen is a must. The swimmer should wear a bright colored (yellow or orange are great choices) swim cap to increase visibility. Thinner straps on swimsuits are preferable to thicker ones for chaffing reasons. For use with a regular swimsuit, Vaseline or an anti-chaffing product should be applied under the straps of the suit, the underarms, and even the back of the next. If a wetsuit is necessary, take care to apply the anti-chaffing product liberally and make sure the wetsuit fits properly. An ill-fitting wetsuit worn for even a short period of time can leave a swimmer bloodied.

Whenever swimming in open water, safety is the number one priority. Do not hesitate to abort a swim if you feel it is not safe. Weather conditions can change in an instant and careless boat operators make the waters unsafe for everyone. Always be alert and look around as you look for and listen for watercraft. Use caution, but don't forget to take in all the beautiful and meditative qualities of open water.

waves that are often unavoidable, and in some cases, you may even have to navigate a waterfall. Class 6 rapids are extremely difficult and almost impossible to pass. Beginners should stick to Class 1 and 2 rapids—they're exciting, extreme, and safe. If you have other questions about rapid classifications, river guides are always glad to explain the rating system.

Gear Up

You'll need a raft and paddles (usually eight people per raft) to navigate the rapids, as well as a good life jacket and helmet. If you're heading out into cooler temperatures, wear warm, waterproof clothing and wool socks—these will keep you warm and dry while splashing down the river. If it's warm outside, nylon shorts, a bathing suit or swim trunks, a t-shirt, or a tank top are all good choices—just make sure to lather on that sunscreen to protect yourself from the sun. As for shoes, your best bet is to wear a pair with rubber soles or slip-on water shoes that you don't mind getting wet—because even during a good run, you're sure to get wet.

Some rafting trips can take a few hours (or even an entire day), so pack plenty of drinking water and food—just make sure to pack it up tight to keep the water out.

Play It Safe

Before jumping into that raft, it's important to know how to swim. Even if you're a strong swimmer, always wear a life jacket. It should fit snugly and have back and shoulder protection as well as floatation to help you swim safely in white water. Also, don't forget to wear your helmet—it should be designed for water sports, fit properly and snugly on your head, and allow for water to drain from the helmet. It should also cover your ears, temples, and the back of your neck. Once you have the proper gear and are sure it's all in working order, you're ready to run the river.

It's also really helpful if you've done a little exploring first. Make sure you know the river you are rafting on—check out the rating of the rapids and what the current is like. It's best to a have a trained, experienced guide on your team and in your raft. The guide will know the best course and the safest passage. Don't enter a rapid unless you're sure you can run it safely or swim it without getting hurt. If you fall out of the raft, position your body so that you are on your back with your feet facing down river—try to keep your feet and legs up.

Usually a group of three boats is the minimum on a river—but only one boat should run the rapids at a time. Safe rafting is all about teamwork, so pick a captain to call out directions so everyone can work together.

Most importantly, be prepared. Get a first aid and survival kit, and include extra ropes, a raft repair kit, and extra life vests. Better safe than stranded.

Recreational Water Illnesses: Frequently Asked Questions

What's an "RWI"?

RWI stands for "recreational water illness," which is an illness caused by germs spread by swallowing, breathing in mists or aerosols of, or having contact with contaminated water in swimming pools, hot tubs, water parks, water play areas, interactive fountains, lakes, rivers, or oceans. RWIs can also be caused by chemicals in the water or chemicals that evaporate from the water and cause indoor air quality problems.

Can I get diarrhea from swimming?

Yes. You share the water—and the germs in it—with every person who enters the pool. Infectious diarrhea can contain anywhere from hundreds of millions to one billion germs in each bowel movement. This means that a single diarrheal incident from one person could contaminate water throughout a large pool system or waterpark. Swallowing even a small amount of water that has been contaminated with these germs can make you sick. That is why it is so important to stay out of the pool if you are sick with diarrhea, shower before swimming, and avoid swallowing pool water.

Can I get head lice from a swimming pool?

Head lice are unlikely to be spread through the use of swimming pools. Head lice survive by holding onto hair and, although pool chlorine levels do not kill lice, the lice are not likely to let go when a person's head goes under water.

Can I get pinworm from a swimming pool?

Pinworm infections are rarely spread through the use of swimming pools. Pinworm infections occur when a person swallows pinworm eggs picked up from contaminated surfaces or fingers. Although chlorine levels found in pools are not high enough to kill pinworm eggs, the presence of a small number of pinworm eggs in thousands of gallons of water (the amount typically found in pools) makes the chance of infection unlikely.

What is hot tub rash?

Hot tub rash is an infection of the skin that occurs from extended exposure to contaminated water. Hot tub rash is caused by the germ *Pseudomonas*, which is common in the environment (water, soil). Symptoms of hot tub rash include itchy spots on the skin that become a bumpy red rash, rash worse in areas previously covered by swimsuit, and pus-filled blisters around hair follicles.

Hot tub rash can occur if disinfectant levels in the hot tub water are low, allowing the *Pseudomonas* to multiply. To protect yourself from hot tub rash, ask your pool manager about the disinfectant and pH testing program at your hot tub, ensuring frequent testing. Appropriate disinfectant (usually chlorine or bromine) levels, and pH control are key. Check the disinfection levels with test strips. Remove swimsuits and shower with soap after leaving the hot tub., and clean swimsuits after leaving the hot tub.

Three Steps For All Swimmers

Keep germs from causing recreational water illnesses (RWIs):

- Don't swim when you have diarrhea. You can spread germs in the water and make other people sick.
- Don't swallow the pool water. Avoid getting water in your mouth.
- Practice good hygiene. Shower with soap before swimming and wash your hands after using the toilet or changing diapers. Germs on your body end up in the water.

Source: Excerpted from "Six Steps for Healthy Swimming: Protection Against Recreational Water Illnesses (RWIs)," Centers for Disease Control and Prevention, April 6, 2010.

What causes stinging eyes, nose irritation and/or breathing difficulty at the pool and what can I do about it?

Many people experience stinging eyes, nasal irritation, or difficulty breathing after being in the water or breathing in the air at swimming pools, particularly indoor pools. These symptoms are typically caused by a build-up of irritants, known as chloramines, in the water and air. This build-up is usually caused by poor air circulation and lack of fresh air in the pool area.

To avoid this problem at home, you can open doors or windows to increase the amount of fresh air coming through the room. You can also turn on a fan to help boost the air flow over the pool surface. Good hygiene practices, such as showering before entering the pool and using the bathroom regularly (to avoid urinating in the pool), will also help reduce the amount of irritants in the air and water.

In a public setting, ask your pool operator to open any doors or windows and suggest that they use a fan to increase air flow.

Chapter 30

Winter Sports Safety

Winter sports are lots of fun—just ask any kid who's just scored the winning goal during an ice-hockey game or finished sledding to the bottom of a giant hill.

But when you're sitting on that sled, getting ready to ski, or doing a figure-eight on the pond in your skates, you have to know how to be safe. Otherwise, you could get injured and be stuck inside while everyone else is enjoying the snow.

Stay Warm

No matter which winter sport you choose, staying warm is important. The right clothing and equipment will help you do that. Dress in layers, people often say. This is true, but some of the newer fabrics for cold weather give you the warmth of layers without all the bulk. Ask an adult if you're not sure what to wear outside.

Sometimes kids say, "I don't mind being cold." The tough guy (or girl) approach isn't a good idea. Staying warm isn't just about feeling comfortable. Your body needs to stay warm to work properly. And when your body is at the right temperature, it won't need to spend as much energy getting warm. That will give you maximum energy for winter fun. Also, if you're dressed properly, it means you can stay outside longer without worrying about frostbite.

About This Chapter: "Winter Sports: Sledding, Skiing, Snowboarding, Skating," July 2009 reprinted with permission from www.kidshealth.org. Copyright © 2009 The Nemours Foundation. This information was provided by KidsHealth, one of the largest resources online for medically reviewed health information written for parents, kids, and teens. For more articles like this one, visit www.KidsHealth.org or www .TeensHealth.org.

Fun In The Sun

Even though it might seem odd in winter, don't forget to put on sunscreen (with a minimum SPF of 15) when you're skiing, sledding, skating, or snowboarding. Sunlight reflects off all that bright white snow and ice and back onto your face—so cover up with sunscreen, and put some lip balm that contains sunscreen on your lips (even when it's cloudy outside).

Sledding

Zipping down a hill at what feels like a million miles an hour can be a great time—as long as you're sledding safely. When you grab your sled, make sure it's sturdy and that it's one you can really steer. The handholds should be easy to grab, and the seat of the sled should be padded. Never use homemade sleds like garbage-can lids, plastic bags, or pool floats—these are dangerous and you may lose control while you're sledding. Also, never use a sled that has any sharp, jagged edges or broken parts (this might happen if you're using an old sled).

It's especially important to wear gloves or mittens and boots while you're on the sled because in addition to keeping you warm, they can help prevent you from injuring your hands and feet. Wearing a bike helmet is also a good habit to get into—doctors say it's a great way to protect your head while you're sledding.

When you're picking your sledding spot, it's best to have an adult check it first to make sure it's OK. Hills designated for sledding are always a good bet—they can be safer than private areas like backyards. (Having an adult around while everyone is sledding is a good idea, too.)

Make sure the hill isn't too steep and that it's covered with packed snow, not ice. The hill must not end anywhere near cars on the road. This is important. If it's a new hill you're trying out and you've never been to the bottom, you might want to walk it first just to be sure. Also, look for obstacles like trees, bushes, and rocks that are covered in snow. Sled only in daylight or in well-lit areas.

If you're sledding with a friend, make sure that you don't go over the weight limit—look at the label on the sled for the number of pounds it will hold. If everybody has his or her own sled and is taking turns sledding down the hill, make sure the person sledding before you is well out of the way before you take off.

And whether you're on the sled by yourself or with pals, you always want to be sitting up, not lying down. Lying flat puts your body at greater risk for injuries if you lose control and flip out. Finally, there is only one kind of energy that's right for moving a sled: kid power. Never ride on a sled that's being pulled by a car, truck, or snowmobile.

Do you really need a hat?

Yep. Mom is right. You lose a lot of heat through your head and neck. Wear a hat and you'll put a lid on the head your body needs.

Source: Nemours Foundation, July 2009. Reprinted with permission.

Skating

Whether you're tending goal or going for a triple-spin in the air, it's cool to glide across the ice. Whichever ice sport you like, one rule is always the same: only skate on approved ice. In places where it gets really cold, you might be able to skate outdoors on frozen ponds and lakes. But these spots must be approved for skating. You'll know because they'll be marked by one or more signs from the police or recreation department saying that skating is OK. If the safe area is blocked off, be sure to stay within that area.

Never try skating on ice that hasn't been approved, even for a second. Ice that looks and seems strong may not be able to hold a kid's weight. And just like with swimming, never skate alone.

Once you have a safe skating spot, you need safe skates. Ice skates need to fit you properly. Don't try to fit into skates that are too small, or put on lots of socks to fit into an older brother's or sister's pair. Skates should be snug but not too tight, laced up to the top.

If you play ice hockey, take a tip from the pros: don't step out onto the ice without all the proper gear. This means padding, and most important, the right helmet. An ice-hockey helmet is the only kind you can wear—not a football helmet or a bike helmet. If you're ever in doubt about what makes up the right ice-hockey gear, ask an ice-hockey coach or a professional at a sporting-goods store.

When you're out skating around for fun, skate in the same direction as the rest of the crowd. Don't dart across the ice—you might smack into someone who doesn't have time to get out of the way. The same goes for trying out new skating moves—be sure to watch where you're going and make sure that you have lots of room.

Finally, throw out any gum or candy you have in your mouth before going onto the ice—you don't want to choke on it or have it fall out of your mouth onto the ice and cause someone to trip.

Skiing And Snowboarding

Before you hit the slopes to ski or snowboard, make sure you have the right equipment—and that it fits you correctly. Many kids have problems because the equipment they use is too big for them. It may have belonged to an older brother or sister and they're hoping that they can "grow into it." Equipment that is too big will make it hard for you to keep control.

The same goes for boots and bindings—make sure these are the right size for your feet before getting on the slopes. Ski boots that are designed just for kids are a good bet because they're more flexible than boots for adults, and they have buckles that are easier to manage, too—making it quicker for you to get skiing.

Helmets are a must for skiing and snowboarding. Goggles will protect your eyes from bright sunlight and objects that could get in the way and poke you in the eye (like tree branches). Just like with inline skating, snowboarders need kneepads and elbow pads. Some snowboarders who are just learning wear specially padded pants to cushion their falls.

Top Winter Safety Tips

- Always wear sport-specific, properly fitting safety gear when participating in winter sports.

- Kids should always wear helmets when they ski, sled, snowboard and play ice hockey. There are different helmets for different activities.

- Dress in layers and wear warm, close-fitting clothes. Make sure that long scarves are tucked in so they don't get entangled in lifts, ski poles or other equipment.

- Stay hydrated. Drink fluids before, during and after winter play.

- Kids—or caregivers—who become distracted or irritable, or begin to hyperventilate, may be suffering from hypothermia or altitude sickness, or they may be too tired to participate safely in winter sports. They need to go indoors to warm up and rest.

- Children under six should not ride a snowmobile, and nobody under 16 should drive one. All snowmobile drivers and passengers should wear helmets designed for high-speed motor sports. A bike helmet isn't sufficient for a four-wheeled motorcycle that can go up to 90 miles per hour.

Source: Excerpted from "Winter Sports Safety," © 2012 Safe Kids Worldwide (www.safekids.org). All rights reserved. Reprinted with permission.

Speaking of learning, it's a good idea to take at least one skiing or snowboarding lesson before you take off. This can keep you from getting frustrated or getting hurt before you have a chance to enjoy this new sport. For instance, your instructor can teach you how to stop. Even after a lesson, it's good to have an adult nearby in case you need help. Grownups can help you choose the right trails and hills. If you're in doubt, it's always safer to start with easier slopes and move on to harder ones later.

Skiing and snowboarding can be a little like driving a car. You have to learn to share the road or, in this case, the trail. It also means watching out for others to avoid collisions, so keep your eye on the other snowboarders and skiers.

Anything else you need to know? Yep—go out and enjoy the snow.

Part Three
Diagnosing And Treating Common Sports Injuries

Chapter 31

What Are Sports Injuries?

Sports injuries are injuries that happen when playing sports or exercising. Some are from accidents. Others can result from poor training practices or improper gear. Some people get injured when they are not in proper condition. Not warming up or stretching enough before you play or exercise can also lead to injuries. The most common sports injuries are the following:

- Sprains and strains
- Knee injuries
- Swollen muscles
- Achilles tendon injuries
- Pain along the shin bone
- Fractures
- Dislocations

What's the difference between an acute and a chronic injury?

There are two kinds of sports injuries: acute and chronic. Acute injuries occur suddenly when playing or exercising. Sprained ankles, strained backs, and fractured hands are acute injuries. Signs of an acute injury include the following:

- Sudden, severe pain
- Swelling
- Not being able to place weight on a leg, knee, ankle, or foot

About This Chapter: From "What Are Sports Injuries?" Fast Facts: An Easy-to-Read Series of Publications for the Public, National Institute of Arthritis and Musculoskeletal and Skin Diseases (www.niams.nih.gov), June 2009.

- An arm, elbow, wrist, hand, or finger that is very tender

- Not being able to move a joint as normal

- Extreme leg or arm weakness

- A bone or joint that is visibly out of place

Common Sports Injuries

The following are some of the most common sports injuries.

Sprains And Strains

A sprain is a stretch or tear of a ligament and can be caused by a trauma such as a fall or blow to the body that knock a joint out of position. Areas of the body most vulnerable to sprains are ankles, knees, and wrists. Signs of a sprain include the following:

- Varying degrees of tenderness or pain
- Bruising
- Inflammation
- Swelling
- Inability to move a limb or joint or
- Joint looseness, laxity, or instability

A strain is a twist, pull, or tear of a muscle or tendon. It is an acute, noncontact injury that results from overstretching or overcontraction. These are common symptoms of a strain:

- Pain
- Muscle spasm
- Loss of strength

Knee Injuries

The knee is the most commonly injured joint. Some of the less severe knee problems are runner's knee and tendonitis. More severe injuries include bone bruises or damage to the cartilage or ligaments. Knee injuries can result from a blow to or twist of the knee, from improper landing after a jump, or from running too hard, too much, or without proper warm-up.

Shin Splints

Shin splints are primarily seen in runners and refer to pain along the tibia or shin bone. Risk factors for shin splints include overuse or incorrect use of the lower leg; improper stretching,

Chronic injuries happen after you play a sport or exercise for a long time. Signs of a chronic injury include the following:

- Pain when you play

- Pain when you exercise

---

warm-up, or exercise technique; overtraining; running or jumping on hard surfaces; and running in shoes that don't have enough support.

Achilles Tendon Injuries

This injury refers to a stretch, tear, or irritation to the tendon connecting the calf muscle to the back of the heel. The most common cause of Achilles tendon tears is a problem called tendonitis (a degenerative condition caused by aging or overuse). When a tendon is weakened, trauma can cause it to rupture. These injuries are common in middle-aged "weekend warriors" who may not exercise regularly or take time to stretch properly before an activity, or in professional athletes involved in quick-acceleration, jumping sports like football and basketball.

Fractures

A fracture is a break in the bone that can occur from either a quick, one-time injury to the bone (acute fracture) or from repeated stress to the bone over time (stress fracture).

- **Acute Fractures:** These fractures can be a simple (a clean break with little damage to the surrounding tissue) or compound (a break in which the bone pierces the skin). Most acute fractures are emergencies.

- **Stress Fractures:** These occur largely in the feet and legs and are common in sports that require repetitive impact (running/jumping sports such as gymnastics or track and field). The most common symptom of a stress fracture is pain at the site that worsens with weight-bearing activity—tenderness and swelling often accompany the pain.

Dislocations

The injury occurs when the two bones that come together to form a joint become separated. The majority of dislocations occur in contact sports such as football and basketball, as well as high-impact sports and sports that can result in excessive stretching or falling. The joints most likely to be dislocated are the hand and shoulder. A dislocated joint is an emergency situation that requires medical treatment.

Source: Excerpted from "Sports Health and Safety," Federal Citizen Information Center, April 30, 2010.

- A dull ache when you rest

- Swelling

What should I do if I get injured?

Never try to "work through" the pain of a sports injury. Stop playing or exercising when you feel pain. Playing or exercising more only causes more harm. Some injuries should be seen by a doctor right away. Others you can treat yourself.

Call a doctor in these circumstances:

- The injury causes severe pain, swelling, or numbness

- You can't put any weight on the area

- An old injury hurts or aches

- An old injury swells

- The joint doesn't feel normal or feels unstable

If you don't have any of these signs, it may be safe to treat the injury at home. If the pain or other symptoms get worse, you should call your doctor.

RICE (Rest, Ice, Compression, And Elevation)

The RICE method is used to relieve pain, reduce swelling, and speed healing. Follow these four steps right after the injury occurs and do so for at least 48 hours:

- **Rest:** Reduce your regular activities. If you've injured your foot, ankle, or knee, take weight off of it. A crutch can help. If your right foot or ankle is injured, use the crutch on the left side. If your left foot or ankle is injured, use the crutch on the right side.

- **Ice:** Put an ice pack to the injured area for 20 minutes, four to eight times a day. You can use a cold pack or ice bag. You can also use a plastic bag filled with crushed ice and wrapped in a towel. Take the ice off after 20 minutes to avoid cold injury.

- **Compression:** Put even pressure (compression) on the injured area to help reduce swelling. You can use an elastic wrap, special boot, air cast, or splint. Ask your doctor which one is best for your injury.

- **Elevation:** Put the injured area on a pillow, at a level above your heart, to help reduce swelling.

Source: National Institute of Arthritis and Musculoskeletal and Skin Diseases (www.niams.nih.gov), June 2009.

How are sports injuries treated?

Treatment often begins with the RICE method [see box]. Here are some other things your doctor may do to treat your sports injury.

Nonsteroidal Anti-Inflammatory Drugs (NSAIDs): Your doctor will suggest that you take a NSAID such as aspirin, ibuprofen, ketoprofen, or naproxen sodium. These drugs reduce swelling and pain. You can buy them at a drug store. Another common drug is acetaminophen. It may relieve pain, but it will not reduce swelling.

Immobilization: Immobilization is a common treatment for sports injuries. It keeps the injured area from moving and prevents more damage. Slings, splints, casts, and leg immobilizers are used to immobilize sports injuries.

Surgery: In some cases, surgery is needed to fix sports injuries. Surgery can fix torn tendons and ligaments or put broken bones back in place. Most sports injuries don't need surgery.

Rehabilitation (Exercise): Rehabilitation is a key part of treatment. It involves exercises that step by step get the injured area back to normal. Moving the injured area helps it to heal. The sooner this is done, the better. Exercises start by gently moving the injured body part through a range of motions. The next step is to stretch. After a while, weights may be used to strengthen the injured area.

As injury heals, scar tissue forms. After a while, the scar tissue shrinks. This shrinking brings the injured tissues back together. When this happens, the injured area becomes tight or stiff. This is when you are at greatest risk of injuring the area again. You should stretch the muscles every day. You should always stretch as a warm-up before you play or exercise.

Don't play your sport until you are sure you can stretch the injured area without pain, swelling, or stiffness. When you start playing again, start slowly. Build up step by step to full speed.

Rest: Although it is good to start moving the injured area as soon as possible, you must also take time to rest after an injury. All injuries need time to heal; proper rest helps the process. Your doctor can guide you on the proper balance between rest and rehabilitation.

Other Therapies: Other common therapies that help with the healing process include mild electrical currents (electrostimulation), cold packs (cryotherapy), heat packs (thermotherapy), sound waves (ultrasound), and massage.

What can people do to prevent sports injuries?

These tips can help you avoid sports injuries.

- Don't bend your knees more than half way when doing knee bends.

- Don't twist your knees when you stretch and keep your feet as flat as you can.

- When jumping, land with your knees bent.

- Do warm-up exercises before you play any sport.

- Always stretch before you play or exercise.

- Don't overdo it.

- Cool down after hard sports or workouts.

- Wear shoes that fit properly, are stable, and absorb shock.

- Use the softest exercise surface you can find; don't run on asphalt or concrete.

- Run on flat surfaces.

- Don't be a "weekend warrior" and don't try to do a week's worth of activity in a day or two.

- Learn to do your sport right. Use proper form to reduce your risk of overuse injuries.

- Use safety gear.

- Know your body's limits.

- Build up your exercise level gradually.

- Strive for a total body workout of cardiovascular, strength-training, and flexibility exercises.

- Be in proper condition to play the sport.

- Get a physical exam before you start playing sports.

- Follow the rules of the game.

- Wear gear that protects, fits well, and is right for the sport.

- Know how to use athletic gear.

- Don't play when you are very tired or in pain.

- Always warm up before you play.

- Always cool down after you play.

Chapter 32

Overuse Injuries

What is an overuse injury?

There are basically two types of injuries: acute injuries and overuse injuries. Acute injuries are usually the result of a single, traumatic event (macro-trauma). Common examples include wrist fractures, ankle sprains, shoulder dislocations, and hamstring muscle strain.

Overuse injuries are more subtle and usually occur over time. They are the result of repetitive micro-trauma to the tendons, bones and joints. Common examples include tennis elbow (lateral epicondylitis), swimmer's shoulder (rotator cuff tendinitis and impingement), Little League elbow, runner's knee, jumper's knee (infrapatellar tendinitis), Achilles tendinitis, and shin splints.

In most sports and activities, overuse injuries are the most common and the most challenging to diagnose and treat.

Why do overuse injuries occur?

The human body has a tremendous capacity to adapt to physical stress. In fact, many positive changes occur as a result of this. With exercise and activity, bones, muscles, tendons, and ligaments get stronger and more functional. This happens because of an internal process called remodeling. The remodeling process involves both the break down and buildup of tissue. There is a fine balance between the two and if break down occurs more rapidly than build up, injury occurs.

This can happen when you first begin a sport or activity and try to do too much too soon. If you begin playing tennis and play for several hours in an attempt to improve rapidly you are setting yourself up for an overuse injury. This is because you are trying to do too much and do not allow your body adequate time to recover. As a beginner, you may also have poor technique, which may predispose you to tennis elbow. With overuse injuries, it often takes detective-like work to understand why the injury occurred.

Acute Versus Chronic Injuries

Acute Injuries

Acute injuries such as a sprained ankle, strained back, or fractured hand, occur suddenly during activity. Signs of an acute injury include the following:

- Sudden, severe pain
- Swelling
- Extreme limb weakness
- Inability to place weight on a lower limb
- Extreme tenderness in an upper limb
- Inability to move a joint through its full range of motion
- A bone or a joint that is visibly out of place

Chronic Injuries

Chronic injuries are those that happen over a period of time and are usually the result of re-petitive training, such as running, or overhand throwing. If left untreated, a chronic injury will probably get worse over time. Signs of a chronic injury include the following:

- Pain when you play
- A dull ache when at rest
- Swelling

Source: Excerpted from "Sports Health and Safety, Federal Citizen Information Center, April 30, 2010.

What factors are usually responsible for overuse injuries?

Training errors are the most common cause of overuse injuries. These errors involve a too rapid acceleration of the intensity, duration or frequency of your activity. A typical example is a runner who has run several miles three times a week without any problem. That runner then begins advanced training for running in a marathon, running a longer distance every day at a faster pace. Injury or break down is inevitable. Overuse injuries also happen in people who are returning to a sport or activity after injury and try to make up for lost time.

There are also technical, biomechanical and individual factors. Proper technique is critical in avoiding overuse injuries. Slight changes in form may be the culprit. For this reason, coaches, athletic trainers and teachers can play a role in preventing recurrent overuse injuries.

Some people are more prone to overuse injuries and this is usually related to anatomic or biomechanical factors. Imbalances between strength and flexibility around certain joints predispose to injury. Body alignment, like knock-knees, bowlegs, unequal leg lengths and flat or high arched feet, is also important. Many people also have weak links due to old injuries, incompletely rehabilitated injuries or other anatomic factors.

Other factors include equipment, like the type of running shoe or ballet shoe, and terrain, hard versus soft surface in aerobic dance or running.

How are overuse injuries usually diagnosed?

The diagnosis can usually be made after a thorough history and physical examination. This is best done by a sports medicine specialist with specific interest and knowledge of your sport or activity. In some instances, X-rays are needed and occasionally additional tests like a bone scan or MRI are needed.

What is the treatment?

Treatment depends on the specific diagnosis. In general, for minor symptoms, cutting back the intensity, duration or frequency of the offending activity brings relief. Adopt a hard/easy workout schedule and cross train with other activities that allow you to maintain overall fitness levels while your injured part recovers. This is very important for treating the early symptoms of overuse injuries.

Working with a coach or teacher or taking lessons can assure proper training and technique. Paying particular attention to proper warm up before activity and using ice after activity may also help. Aspirin or other over the counter anti-inflammatory medications can also be taken to relieve symptoms.

If symptoms persist, a sports medicine specialist will be able to create a more detailed treatment plan for your specific condition. This may include a thorough review of your training program and an evaluation for any predisposing anatomic or biomechanical factors. Physical therapy and athletic training services may also be helpful.

Can overuse injuries be prevented?

Most overuse injuries can be prevented with proper training and common sense. Learn to listen to your body. Remember that "no pain, no gain" does not apply here.

The 10 percent rule is very helpful. In general, you should not increase your training program or activity more than 10 percent per week. This allows your body adequate time for recovery and response. The 10 percent rule also applies to increasing pace or mileage for walkers and runners, as well as to the amount of weight added in strength training programs.

Seek the advice of a sports medicine specialist when beginning an exercise program or sport to prevent chronic or recurrent problems. Your program can also be modified to maintain overall fitness levels in a safe manner while you recover from your injury.

Chapter 33

Heat Illness

Heat illness is a term which refers to a group of conditions which occur when the body is heated at a high rate and cannot cool itself fast enough. When young athletes who have a mild heat illness do not stop exercising and move to a cooler environment, they are at high risk for developing severe heat illness.

The types of heat illness include:

- **Heat Stress:** Body temperature is normal but an affected individual is uncomfortable and exercise performance is decreased.

- **Heat Exhaustion:** An individual experiences fatigue and cannot perform well because his or her body temperature is too high.

- **Heat Stroke:** This is the most severe form of heat illness. Heat stroke is a medical emergency resulting from a body temperature high enough to cause damage to cells in the body, including the brain, muscles, liver, kidney, and heart. Heat stroke can lead to permanent injury or death.

How It Occurs

As it becomes hotter and more humid, people are at increased risk for heat illness. In extremes high temperature and humidity, heat illness can occur even without activity. Heat illness most often occurs when athletes are exercising vigorously outdoors for too long in conditions that they are not used to. Other factors that predispose to heat illness include being dehydrated, attempting to play a sport at a high level without proper conditioning, and wearing heavy clothing that does not allow sweat to evaporate easily, such as the protective gear in football.

Signs And Symptoms

Heat exhaustion can cause muscle cramping, feeling faint, headache, dizziness, chills, thirst, nausea, vomiting, and profuse sweating due to elevated body temperature. Heat stroke occurs when body temperature has risen to above 104 degrees and the body is not able to cool fast enough. An individual with heat stroke is confused or delirious with flushed, dry, skin. Heat stroke causes severe dehydration. Some patients with heat stroke pass out or have a seizure.

Diagnosis

A medical professional can usually diagnose heat illness based on the patient's symptoms and physical exam. Taking a temperature at the time helps confirm the diagnosis. Laboratory tests often help guide treatment.

Treatment

Whenever there is a concern for heat illness, young athletes should immediately stop all activities and be taken to a cooler place in the shade or indoors. They should also be given cool liquids if they are able to drink. If there are any signs that the individuals are confused or "out of it," they need immediate medical attention. All unnecessary clothing should be removed. In more severe cases, intravenous fluids, immersion in ice water in order to bring the temperature down, and close monitoring in a hospital may be needed.

Preventing Heat Illness

Heat illness can be prevented by avoiding exposure to intense heat and with proper acclimatization. It can take two weeks for a body to adapt to heat and develop mechanisms to counteract it, so until then athletes should exercise daily at 50–70% of maximum effort in hotter weather, gradually increasing the time spent in the heat. Athletes should have frequent breaks (every 15–20 minutes) to drink water or sports drinks. Athletes should wear light, loose clothing and take frequent breaks in the shade. If possible during hot days, events should be scheduled for early morning or evening when it is cooler. Coaches and event organizers should be prepared to cancel sporting events in the event of extreme heat and/or humidity.

Chapter 34

Sprains And Strains

What is a sprain?

A sprain is an injury to a ligament (tissue that connects two or more bones at a joint). In a sprain, one or more ligaments is stretched or torn.

What causes a sprain?

Many things can cause a sprain. Falling, twisting, or getting hit can force a joint out of its normal position. This can cause ligaments around the joint to stretch or tear. Sprains can occur if people experience these situations:

- Fall and land on an arm

- Fall on the side of their foot

- Twist a knee

Where do sprains usually occur?

Sprains happen most often in the ankle. Sometimes when people fall and land on their hand, they sprain their wrist. A sprain to the thumb is common in skiing and other sports.

What are the signs and symptoms of sprains?

The usual signs and symptoms of a sprain are the following:

About This Chapter: From "What Are Sprains and Strains," Fast Facts: An Easy-to-Read Series of Publications for the Public, National Institute of Arthritis and Musculoskeletal and Skin Diseases (www.niams.nih.gov), June 2009.

- Pain
- Swelling
- Bruising
- Not being able to move or use the joint

Sometimes people feel a pop or tear when the injury happens. A sprain can be mild, moderate, or severe.

What is a strain?

A strain is an injury to a muscle or a tendon (tissue that connects muscle to bone). In a strain, a muscle or tendon is stretched or torn.

What causes strains?

A strain is caused by twisting or pulling a muscle or tendon. Strains can happen suddenly or develop over days or weeks. A sudden (acute) strain is caused by situations such as the following:

- A recent injury
- Lifting heavy objects the wrong way
- Overstressing the muscles

Chronic strains are usually caused by moving the muscles and tendons the same way over and over.

Where do strains usually occur?

Two common sites for a strain are the back and the hamstring muscle in the back of the thigh. Sports such as soccer, football, hockey, boxing, and wrestling put people at risk for strains in the back or legs. People who play some sports use their hands and arms a lot.

Examples are gymnastics, tennis, rowing, and golf. People who play these sports sometimes strain their hand or arm. Elbow strains can also happen when playing sports.

What are the signs and symptoms of strains?

A strain can cause the following symptoms:

- Pain

- Muscle spasms

- Muscle weakness

- Swelling

- Cramping

- Trouble moving the muscle

If a muscle or tendon is torn completely, it is often very painful and hard to move.

How are sprains and strains treated?

Treatments for sprains and strains are the same. To reduce swelling and pain in the first day or two, doctors usually say to do the following:

- Rest the injured area. If the ankle or knee is hurt, the doctor might tell you to use crutches or a cane.

- Put ice on the injury for 20 minutes at a time. The doctor might say to do this four to eight times a day.

- Compress (squeeze) the injury using special bandages, casts, boots, or splints. Your doctor will tell you which one is best for you and how tight it should be.

- Put the injured ankle, knee, elbow, or wrist up on a pillow.

- The doctor may recommend taking medicines, such as aspirin or ibuprofen.

After treating pain and swelling, doctors usually say to exercise the injured area. This helps to prevent stiffness and increase strength. Some people need physical therapy. You may need to exercise the injured area or go to physical therapy for several weeks. Your doctor or physical therapist will tell you when you can start to do normal activities, including sports. If you begin too soon, you can injure the area again.

It is important to see a doctor if you have a painful sprain or strain. This helps you get the right treatments.

Can sprains and strains be prevented?

To help prevent sprains and strains, you can do the following:

- Avoid exercising or playing sports when tired or in pain

- Eat a well-balanced diet to keep muscles strong

- Maintain a healthy weight

- Try to avoid falling (for example, put sand or salt on icy spots on your front steps or sidewalks)

- Wear shoes that fit well

- Get new shoes if the heel wears down on one side

- Exercise every day

- Be in proper physical condition to play a sport

- Warm up and stretch before playing a sport

- Wear protective equipment when playing

- Run on flat surfaces

Chapter 35

Broken Bones

Your bones are tough stuff—but even tough stuff can break. Like a wooden pencil, bones will bend under strain. But if the pressure is too much, or too sudden, bones can snap. You can break a bone by falling off a skateboard or crashing down from the monkey bars.

When a bone breaks it is called a fracture (say: frak-chur). There's more than one way to break or fracture a bone. A break can be anything from a hairline fracture (a thin break in the bone) to the bone that's snapped in two pieces like a broken tree branch.

Doctors describe fractures in the following ways:

- A complete fracture is when the bone has broken into two pieces.

- A greenstick fracture is when the bone cracks on one side only, not all the way through.

- A single fracture is when the bone is broken in one place.

- A comminuted (say: kah-muh-noot-ed) fracture is when the bone is broken into more than two pieces or crushed.

- A bowing fracture, which only happens in kids, is when the bone bends but doesn't break.

- An open fracture is when the bone is sticking through the skin.

What are bones made of?

Bones are made of bone cells, proteins, and minerals like calcium.

About This Chapter: "The Facts about Broken Bones," August 2009, reprinted with permission from www.kidshealth.org. Copyright © 2009 The Nemours Foundation. This information was provided by KidsHealth, one of the largest resources online for medically reviewed health information written for parents, kids, and teens. For more articles like this one, visit www.KidsHealth.org or www.TeensHealth.org.

What happens when you break a bone?

It hurts to break a bone. It's different for everyone, but the pain is often like the deep ache you get from a super bad stomachache or headache. Some people may experience sharper pain—especially with an open fracture. And if the fracture is small, a kid may not feel much pain at all. Sometimes, kids won't even be able to tell that they broke a bone

Breaking a bone is a big shock to your whole body. It's normal for you to receive strong messages from parts of your body that aren't anywhere close to the fracture. You may feel dizzy, woozy, or chilly from the shock. A lot of people cry for a while. Some people pass out until their bodies have time to adjust to all the signals they're getting. And other people don't feel any pain right away because of the shock of the injury (say: in-juh-ree).

If you think you or someone else has broken a bone, the most important things to do are to:

* stay calm

* make sure the person who is hurt is as comfortable as possible

Some Of Your Bones

Femur: The thigh bone.

Fibula: The long, thin outer bone of the lower leg.

Humerus: The bone of the upper arm.

Radius: The smaller of the two bones of the forearm. It is located on the thumb side of the arm.

Tibia: The larger of the two bones that make up the lower leg. It is also referred to as the shin bone.

Other Helpful Terms

Displaced Fracture: A fracture in which the two ends of the broken bone are separated from one another.

Ligaments: Tough bands of connective tissue that connect bones.

Orthopaedic Surgeon: A physician who specializes in treating (through surgery, casting, or other means) abnormalities of or injuries to the bones.

Tendons: Tough but flexible bands of tissue that connect muscles to bones.

Source: Excerpted from "Growth Plate Injuries," National Institute of Arthritis and Musculoskeletal and Skin Diseases (www.niams.nih.gov), August 2007. Reviewed by David A. Cooke, MD, FACP, April 2012.

- tell an adult

- if there are no adults around, call 911 or the emergency number in your area

The worst thing for a broken bone is to move it. This will hurt the person and it can make the injury worse. In the case of a broken arm or leg, a grown-up may be able to cushion or support the surrounding area with towels or pillows.

One super-important tip: If you're not sure what bone is broken or you think the neck or back is broken, do not try to move the injured person. Wait until a trained medical professional has arrived.

What does the doctor do?

To treat the broken bone, the doctor needs to know which kind of fracture it is. That's where x-rays come in handy. X-rays give doctors a map of fractures so that they can set the bones back in their normal position.

With breaks in larger bones or when a bone breaks in more than two pieces, the doctor may need to put in a metal pin—or pins—to help set it. For this operation, you'll get some medicine so you'll be asleep and unable to feel any pain. When your bone has healed, the doctor will remove the pin or pins.

After your bone has been set, the next step is usually putting on a cast, the special bandage that will keep the bone in place for the one to two months it will take for the break to mend. Casts are made of bandages soaked in plaster, which harden to a tough shell (that's why they last so long).

Sometimes casts are made of fiberglass or plastic—and some are even waterproof, which means you can still go swimming and get them wet. And sometimes they come in cool colors or patterns that you can choose.

How do broken bones heal?

Your bones are natural healers. At the location of the fracture, your bones will produce lots of new cells and tiny blood vessels that rebuild the bone. These cells cover both ends of the broken part of the bone and close up the break until it's as good as new.

What should you do when the cast comes off?

Can you believe they use a saw to remove your cast? The funny thing is this saw doesn't hurt your skin at all. It might even tickle. Once the cast is off, the injured area will probably look and feel pretty weird. The body part that was in a cast might look strange at first. The skin might be pale, dry, or flaky. Body hair might look darker and the body part itself might look smaller because you might have lost some muscle while it was healing.

Don't worry. This is all temporary. Kids are great healers, so you'll be back to normal soon. In some cases, your doctor might suggest you do special exercises to improve your strength and flexibility. You'll want to go slow and ask the doctor if there are any activities you should avoid, such as hanging from the monkey bars. If you want to return to a sport, ask the doctor how soon you'll be able to do it.

How can you be sure you don't break any more bones? Accidents happen, but you often can prevent injuries by wearing safety helmets, pads, and the right protective gear for your activity or sport.

It's also a smart idea to do what you can to build strong bones. How do you do that?

- Get a lot of physical activity, especially stuff like jumping and running.

- Feed your bones the calcium and vitamin D they need to stay strong. That means getting your share of milk and other calcium-rich foods and drinks, such as broccoli and calcium-fortified orange juice.

Chapter 36

Growth Plate Injuries

This chapter contains general information about growth plate injuries. It describes what the growth plate is, how injuries occur, and how they are treated. If you have further questions after reading this chapter, you may wish to discuss them with your doctor.

What is the growth plate?

The growth plate, also known as the epiphyseal plate or physis, is the area of growing tissue near the ends of the long bones in children and adolescents. Each long bone has at least two growth plates: one at each end. The growth plate determines the future length and shape of the mature bone. When growth is complete—sometime during adolescence—the growth plates close and are replaced by solid bone.

Because the growth plates are the weakest areas of the growing skeleton—even weaker than the nearby ligaments and tendons that connect bones to other bones and muscles—they are vulnerable to injury. Injuries to the growth plate are called fractures.

Who gets growth plate injuries?

Growth plate injuries can occur in growing children and adolescents. In a child, a serious injury to a joint is more likely to damage a growth plate than the ligaments that stabilize the joint. Trauma that would cause a sprain in an adult might cause a growth plate fracture in a child.

About This Chapter: Excerpted from "Growth Plate Injuries," National Institute of Arthritis and Musculoskeletal and Skin Diseases, August 2007. Reviewed by David A. Cooke, MD, FACP, April 2012. Brand names included in this chapter are provided as examples only, and their inclusion does not mean that these products are endorsed by the National Institutes of Health or any other Government agency. Also, if a particular brand name is not mentioned, this does not mean or imply that the product is unsatisfactory.

Growth plate fractures occur twice as often in boys as in girls, because girls' bodies mature at an earlier age than boys. As a result, their bones finish growing sooner, and their growth plates are replaced by stronger, solid bone.

One-third of all growth plate injuries occur in competitive sports such as football, basketball, or gymnastics, while about 20% of growth plate fractures occur as a result of recreational activities such as biking, sledding, skiing, or skateboarding.

Key Words

Computed (or computerized) Tomography (CT) Scan: An imaging technique that provides doctors with a three-dimensional picture of the bone. It also shows "slices" of the bone, making the picture much clearer than x-rays.

Epiphyseal Plate: The area of developing tissue near the end of the long bones in children and adolescents. It is also called the physis or growth plate.

Epiphysis: The end of a long bone, which is initially separated by cartilage from the shaft of the bone and develops separately. It eventually fuses with the shaft (diaphysis) of the bone to form a complete bone.

Growth Plate: The area of developing tissue near the end of the long bones in children and adolescents. Each long bone has at least two growth plates: one at each end. The growth plate determines the future length and shape of the mature bone. When growth is complete—sometime during adolescence—the growth plates are replaced by solid bone. The growth plate is also called the physis or epiphyseal plate.

Metaphysis: The growing portion of a long bone that lies between the ends of the bones (epiphyses) and the shaft (diaphysis).

Magnetic Resonance Imaging (MRI): A procedure in which a strong magnet is used to pass a force through the body, resulting in a clear, detailed, cross-sectional image. Unlike standard x-rays, it can show soft tissue as well as bone and thus is useful in diagnosing injuries to the growth plates.

Neurological: Having to do with the nervous system (made up of the brain, spinal cord and peripheral nerves), this system of tissues uses electrical and chemical means to record and distribute information within the body.

Physis: The area of developing tissue near the end of the long bones in children and adolescents. The physis is also called the growth plate.

Ultrasound: A technique that allows doctors to view the soft tissues of the body by bouncing sound waves off the tissue and then converting the echoes into a picture called a sonogram.

Fractures can result from a single traumatic event, such as a fall or automobile accident, or from chronic stress and overuse. Most growth plate fractures occur in the long bones of the fingers (phalanges) and the outer bone of the forearm (radius). They are also common in the lower bones of the leg (the tibia and fibula).

What causes growth plate injuries?

Growth plate injuries can be caused by an event such as a fall or blow to the limb, or they can result from overuse. For example, a gymnast who practices for hours on the uneven bars, a long-distance runner, and a baseball pitcher perfecting his curve ball can all have growth plate injuries.

Although many growth plate injuries are caused by accidents that occur during play or athletic activity, growth plates are also susceptible to other disorders, such as bone infection, that can alter their normal growth and development. Other possible causes of growth plate injuries include the following:

- **Child Abuse:** More than one million children each year are the victims of substantiated child abuse or neglect. The second most common injury among abused children is a fracture, and growth plate injuries are prevalent because the growth plate is the weakest part of the bone.

- **Injury From Extreme Cold (For Example, Frostbite):** Exposure to extreme cold can damage the growth plate in children and result in short, stubby fingers or premature degenerative arthritis (breakdown of the joint cartilage).

- **Radiation And Medications:** Research has suggested that chemotherapy given for childhood cancers may negatively affect bone growth. Prolonged use of steroids for inflammatory conditions such as juvenile idiopathic arthritis can also harm bone growth.

- **Neurological Disorders:** Children and teens with certain neurological disorders that result in sensory deficit or muscular imbalance are prone to growth plate fractures, especially at the ankle and knee. Children who are born with insensitivity to pain can have similar types of injuries.

- **Genetics:** The growth plates are where many inherited disorders that affect the musculoskeletal system appear. Scientists are just beginning to understand the genes and gene mutations involved in skeletal formation, growth, and development. This new information is raising hopes for improving treatment for children and teens who are born with poorly formed or improperly functioning growth plates.

- **Metabolic Disease:** Disease states such as kidney failure and hormone disorders can affect the growth plates and their function. The bone growth of children and teens with long-term conditions of this kind may be negatively affected.

Signs That Require A Visit To The Doctor

- Inability to continue play because of pain following an acute or sudden injury
- Decreased ability to play over the long term because of persistent pain following a previous injury
- Visible malformation of the arms or legs
- Severe pain from acute injuries that prevent the use of an arm or leg.

Adapted from *Play it Safe, a Guide to Safety for Young Athletes* with permission of the American Academy of Orthopaedic Surgeons.

How are growth plate fractures diagnosed?

A teen who has persistent pain, or pain that affects athletic performance or the ability to move and put pressure on a limb, should never be allowed or expected to "work through the pain." Whether an injury is acute or due to overuse, it should be evaluated by a doctor, because some injuries, if left untreated, can cause permanent damage and interfere with proper growth of the involved limb.

The doctor will begin the diagnostic process by asking about the injury and how it occurred and by examining the adolescent. The doctor will then use x-rays to determine if there is a fracture, and if so, the type of fracture. Often the doctor will x-ray not only the injured limb but the opposite limb as well. Because growth plates have not yet hardened into solid bone, neither the structures themselves nor injuries to them show up on x-rays. Instead, growth plates appear as gaps between the shaft of a long bone, called the metaphysis, and the end of the bone, called the epiphysis. By comparing x-rays of the injured limb to those of the noninjured limb, doctors can look for differences that indicate an injury.

Very often the x-ray is negative, because the growth plate line is already there, and the fracture is undisplaced (the two ends of the broken bone are not separated). The doctor can still diagnose a growth plate fracture on clinical grounds because of tenderness of the plate. Children do get ligament strains if their growth plates are open, and they often have undisplaced growth plate fractures.

Other tests doctors may use to diagnose a growth plate injury include magnetic resonance imaging (MRI), computed tomography (CT), and ultrasound.

Because these tests enable doctors to see the growth plate and areas of other soft tissue, they can be useful not only in detecting the presence of an injury, but also in determining the type and extent of the injury.

What are the different types of growth plate injuries?

Since the 1960s, the Salter-Harris classification, which divides most growth plate fractures into five categories based on the type of damage, has been the standard. The categories are as follows.

Type I—Fracture Through The Growth Plate: The epiphysis is completely separated from the end of the bone or the metaphysis, through the deep layer of the growth plate. The growth plate remains attached to the epiphysis. The doctor has to put the fracture back into place if it is significantly displaced. Type I injuries generally require a cast to protect the plate as it heals. Unless there is damage to the blood supply to the growth plate, the likelihood that the bone will grow normally is excellent.

Type II—Fracture Through The Growth Plate And Metaphysis: This is the most common type of growth plate fracture. It runs through the growth plate and the metaphysis, but the epiphysis is not involved in the injury. Like type I fractures, type II fractures may need to be put back into place and immobilized. However, the growth plate fracture heals a great deal, especially in younger children. If it is not too displaced, the doctor may not need to put it back into position. In this case, it will strengthen with time.

Type III—Fracture Through Growth Plate And Epiphysis: This fracture occurs only rarely, usually at the lower end of the tibia, one of the long bones of the lower leg. It happens when a fracture runs completely through the epiphysis and separates part of the epiphysis and growth plate from the metaphysis. Surgery is sometimes necessary to restore the joint surface to normal. The outlook or prognosis for growth is good if the blood supply to the separated portion of the epiphysis is still intact and if the joint surface heals in a normal position.

Type IV—Fracture Through Growth Plate, Metaphysis, And Epiphysis: This fracture runs through the epiphysis, across the growth plate, and into the metaphysis. Surgery is frequently needed to restore the joint surface to normal and to perfectly align the growth plate. Unless perfect alignment is achieved and maintained during healing, prognosis for growth is poor, and angulation (bending) of the bone may occur. This injury occurs most commonly at the end of the humerus (the upper arm bone) near the elbow.

Type V—Compression Fracture Through Growth Plate: This uncommon injury occurs when the end of the bone is crushed and the growth plate is compressed. It is most likely to occur at the knee or ankle. Prognosis is poor, since premature stunting of growth is almost inevitable.

Type VI: A newer classification, called the Peterson classification, adds a type VI fracture, in which a portion of the epiphysis, growth plate, and metaphysis is missing. This usually occurs with open wounds or compound fractures, and often involves lawnmowers, farm machinery, snowmobiles, or gunshot wounds. All type VI fractures require surgery, and most will require later reconstructive or corrective surgery. Bone growth is almost always stunted.

What kind of doctor treats growth plate injuries?

For all but the simplest injuries, a doctor will probably refer a teen to an orthopedic surgeon (a doctor who specializes in bone and joint problems in children and adults) for treatment. Some problems may require the services of a pediatric orthopedic surgeon, who specializes in injuries and musculoskeletal disorders in children and teens.

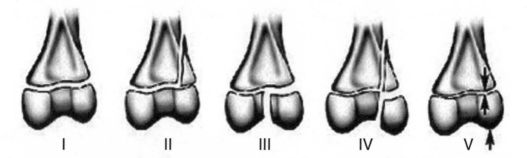

Figure 36.1. The Salter-Harris Classification of Growth Plate Injuries. Adapted from Disorders and Injuries of the Musculoskeletal System, 3rd Edition. Robert B. Salter. Baltimore. Williams and Wilkins, 1999. Used with the author's permission.

How are growth plate injuries treated?

Treatment for growth plate injuries depends on the type of injury. In all cases, treatment should be started as soon as possible after injury and will generally involve a mix of the following:

- **Immobilization:** The affected limb is often put in a cast or splint, and the teen is told to limit any activity that puts pressure on the injured area.

- **Manipulation Or Surgery:** If the fracture is displaced (meaning the ends of the injured bones no longer meet as they should), the doctor will have to put the bones or joints back in their correct positions, either by using his or her hands (called manipulation) or by performing surgery. Sometimes the doctor needs to fix the break and hold the growth plate in place with screws or wire. After the procedure, the bone will be set in place (immobilized) so it can heal without moving. This is usually done with a cast that encloses the injured growth plate and the joints on both sides of it. The cast is left in place until the injury heals, which can take anywhere from a few weeks to two or more months for serious injuries. The need for manipulation or surgery depends on the location and extent of the injury, its effect on nearby nerves and blood vessels, and the teen's age.

- **Strengthening And Range-Of-Motion Exercises:** These are exercises designed to strengthen the muscles that support the injured area of the bone and to improve or maintain the joint's ability to move in the way that it should. A doctor may recommend these after the fracture has healed. A physical therapist can work with a teen's doctor to design an appropriate exercise plan.

- **Long-Term Follow-Up:** Long-term follow-up is usually necessary to monitor the teen's recuperation and growth. Evaluation includes x-rays of matching limbs at three to six month intervals for at least two years. Some fractures require periodic evaluations until the teen's bones have finished growing. Sometimes a growth arrest line (a line on the x-ray where the bone stopped growing temporarily) may appear as a marker of the injury. Continued bone growth away from that line may mean there will not be a long-term problem, and the doctor may decide to stop following the patient.

Will the affected limb of a teen with a growth plate injury still grow?

About 85% of growth plate fractures heal without any lasting effect. Whether an arrest of growth occurs depends on the treatment provided, and the following factors, in descending order of importance.

- **Severity Of The Injury:** If the injury causes the blood supply to the epiphysis to be cut off, growth can be stunted. If the growth plate is shifted, shattered, or crushed, the growth plate may close prematurely, forming a bony bridge or "bar." The risk of growth arrest is higher in this setting. An open injury in which the skin is broken carries the risk of infection, which could destroy the growth plate.

- **Age Of The Child:** In a younger child, the bones have a great deal of growing to do; therefore, growth arrest can be more serious, and closer surveillance is needed. It is also true, however, that younger bones have a greater ability to heal.

- **Which Growth Plate Is Injured:** Some growth plates, such as those in the region of the knee, are more involved in extensive bone growth than others.

- **Type Of Fracture:** Of the six fracture types described earlier, types IV, V, and VI are the most serious.

The most frequent complication of a growth plate fracture is premature arrest of bone growth. The affected bone grows less than it would have without the injury, and the resulting limb could be shorter than the opposite, uninjured limb. If only part of the growth plate is injured, growth may be lopsided and the limb may become crooked.

Growth plate injuries at the knee have the greatest risk of complications. Nerve and blood vessel damage occurs most frequently there. Injuries to the knee have a much higher incidence of premature growth arrest and crooked growth.

Chapter 37

Concussions

Our brains help us do everything—walk, talk, think, breathe, eat, sleep, and lots more. Sometimes on TV or in cartoons people bang their heads and everybody laughs. But, hitting your head isn't silly or funny. Your brain is in there. We need to take good care of our heads to protect our brains. One way to do this is to always buckle up in cars. You should also always wear a helmet when riding a bike, rollerblading, or doing anything else where you might fall and hit your head.

What Is A Concussion?

A concussion is when you hit your head really hard and temporarily hurt your brain. Most of the time when we hit our heads we don't get concussions. This is because the brain is protected by our hard skulls and floats in a special protective fluid. But, if you hit your head hard enough, you may feel dizzy, get sick to your stomach, be confused, or have trouble remembering what happened. This could mean you've had a concussion.

What Happens After A Concussion?

After a concussion, most kids feel different for a little while. If you've had a concussion, you might feel extra tired or a bit slowed down, or you might have headaches or feel dizzy. Remembering stuff and doing homework might also be a little harder. Feeling different like this can be scary. Don't worry. Most kids feel normal again after a week or two.

About This Chapter: "Information about Concussions for Kids and Teens," © 2011 Children's Hospital Colorado (www.childrenscolorado.org). All rights reserved. Reprinted with permission.

Concussions Are Serious

A concussion is a brain injury:

- It is caused by a bump, blow, or jolt to the head or body
- Can change the way your brain normally works
- Can occur during practices or games in any sport or recreational activity
- Can happen even if you haven't been knocked out
- Can be serious even if you've just been "dinged" or "had your bell rung"

All concussions are serious. A concussion can affect your ability to do schoolwork and other activities (such as playing video games, working on a computer, studying, driving, or exercising). Most people with a concussion get better, but it is important to give your brain time to heal.

Concussion Symptoms

You can't see a concussion, but you might notice one or more of the symptoms listed below or that you "don't feel right" soon after, a few days after, or even weeks after the injury.

- Headache or "pressure" in head
- Nausea or vomiting
- Balance problems or dizziness
- Double or blurry vision
- Bothered by light or noise
- Feeling sluggish, hazy, foggy, or groggy
- Difficulty paying attention
- Memory problems
- Confusion

Source: Excerpted from "Heads Up Concussion in High School Sports A Fact Sheet for Athletes," Centers for Disease Control and Prevention (CDC), June 2010.

What Should I Do If I Think I've Had a Concussion?

The most important thing to do is to talk with an adult about what happened and how you feel. Make sure you tell your parents, doctor, and teachers if you've hit your head and you're feeling different than normal. They'll help figure out if you've had a concussion and how to get better.

If You Think You've Had A Concussion

- Tell your coaches and your parents. Never ignore a bump or blow to the head even if you feel fine. Also, tell your coach right away if you think you have a concussion or if one of your teammates might have a concussion.

- Get a medical check-up. A doctor or other healthcare professional can tell if you have a concussion and when it is OK to return to play.

- Give yourself time to get better. If you have a concussion, your brain needs time to heal. While your brain is still healing, you are much more likely to have another concussion. Repeat concussions can increase the time it takes for you to recover and may cause more damage to your brain. It is important to rest and not return to play until you get the OK from your health care professional that you are symptom-free.

Source: Excerpted from "Heads Up Concussion in High School Sports A Fact Sheet for Athletes," Centers for Disease Control and Prevention. June 2010.

Here Are Some Things You Can Do After A Concussion

Be Safe: Until you're all back to normal, don't do anything where you could hit your head again. Take it easy at recess. Take a break from doing things like riding your bike, skateboarding, and climbing trees. Your doctor will tell you when it's safe to do these types of things again.

Rest If You Need To: Right after a concussion, you might need to rest and sleep more than usual. If you feel tired, it's okay to rest or take a nap. But, don't stay in bed all day. To get better, your brain will need exercise too. Brains get exercise in lots of ways like by going to school, reading, and doing puzzles.

Tell An Adult If Your Head Hurts: If you get a headache, tell your parents or teacher. Try taking a break from what you were doing. If that doesn't work, lying down with the lights off usually helps headaches go away. For some headaches, your parents or doctor might need to give you medicine.

Take Breaks If You Have Trouble Paying Attention: For a little while after a concussion, concentrating on homework might be hard. If so, do your homework a bit at a time. Work for a while, take a short break, and then work some more. Take short breaks if you feel yourself losing focus or getting "spacey."

If You Can't Remember Something, Just Ask Again: Remembering things might be a little harder for a while too. Don't feel bad if you don't remember something. Just let your parents or teacher know you forgot. Writing things down or making lists can help if you have trouble remembering.

Watch Out For Crankiness: Some kids feel a little cranky after a concussion. They get mad or upset over small things. If this happens to you, take a deep breath. Then, take a break from what you were doing. Going to a quiet place to relax should help too.

Be Patient: After a concussion, you might feel a bit strange for a while. Don't worry. Be patient. Remember, your brain should get back to normal after it's had a little time to heal.

Preventing Concussions

Every sport is different, but there are steps you can take to protect yourself.

- Use the proper sports equipment, including personal protective equipment. In order for equipment to protect you, it must be the right equipment for the game, position, or activity; worn correctly and the correct size and fit; and used every time you play or practice.
- Follow your coach's rules for safety and the rules of the sport.
- Practice good sportsmanship at all times.

Source: Excerpted from "Heads Up Concussion in High School Sports A Fact Sheet for Athletes," Centers for Disease Control and Prevention (CDC), June 2010.

What Should I Do About School?

Most kids should stay home from school for a day or two after a concussion. The brain usually needs extra rest right after it's been hurt. But, getting back to school is important too. School is exercise for the brain and should help you get better. Make sure your teachers know you had a concussion. Tell them if you need a break during the day to rest. If you get worried or stressed about school, talk with your teachers and parents so they can figure out how best to help.

When Do I Get To Play Sports Again?

After a concussion, you'll need to take a break from sports and gym class for a little while. Your brain needs time to completely heal without getting hurt again. Your doctor will decide when it's safe for you to do these things. Most kids are allowed to play sports again a week or so after they're feeling all better.

Chapter 38

Muscle Contusion (Bruise)

A muscle contusion or muscle bruise is an injury to the soft tissue (muscle fibers, connective tissue, and/or blood vessels and nerves) of the upper leg. The most commonly involved muscle is the quadriceps. The muscle contusion may be accompanied by bone contusion (bruise) or even a fracture (broken bone). These contusions are graded 1, 2, or 3 depending on the severity.

- **Grade 1 (Mild):** A grade 1 muscle contusion produces mild bruising, little pain and no swelling at the site of impact. The knee moves normally or very close to normally. Athletes have some mild soreness when pressure is applied to the area of injury.

- **Grade 2 (Moderate):** This injury is slightly deep than a grade 1 contusion and produces mild pain and a little swelling. Athletes with a grade 2 quadriceps injury can only bend the knee part of the way and may walk with a slight limp. Pressure on the area of injury causes some pain.

- **Grade 3 (Severe):** Severe muscle contusions are very painful and are accompanied by noticeable swelling. Individuals with this type of injury usually develop obvious bruising at the sight of injury. A severe quadriceps contusion may result in a significant loss of motion in the knee and cause an obvious limp. Athletes have pain with pressure at the site of injury and the surrounding area.

How It Occurs

Muscle contusions occur when an individual receives one or more direct blows, to the body part, falls or jams of a body part against a hard surface. In essence, the muscles are compressed and crushed between the object or person delivering the blow and the underlying bone.

About This Chapter: "Muscle Contusion (Bruise)," reprinted with permission from Ann & Robert H. Lurie Children's Hospital of Chicago (www.luriechildrens.org). © 2012. All rights reserved.

Signs And Symptoms

Signs and symptoms of muscle contusions include swelling and bruising at the injury site, muscle tightness, pain with or without movement, and inability to move a joint fully.

Diagnosis

A complete physical examination will determine the exact location and extent of the injury. Your doctor can tell you if she feels a gap within the muscle indicating a possible tear. X-rays of the bone are often taken to rule a fracture (broken bone) or other conditions. Additional tests such as ultrasound, computed tomography (CT) scan or magnetic resonance imaging (MRI) may be required to determine the extent of the injury and to identify any additional injuries. The results of the physical exam and other diagnostic tests allow your doctor to determine how severe this injury is; this is very important for guiding the treatment plan and making decisions about when it is safe for you to return to athletics.

Treatment

Initial treatment includes rest and protecting the injury from further harm by stopping play or practice. Applying ice and elevating the injured area will help minimize injury to the muscle. For lower extremity injuries; if putting weight on the leg is painful, crutches may be needed to protect the injury site. Compressing the area with a soft bandage and keeping the muscle in a slightly stretched position may be beneficial as well. Anti-inflammatory medications such as ibuprofen (for example Motrin or Advil) can be used for pain relief. Once you are able to comfortably bend your knee to 90 degrees or more, your physician will prescribe a physical therapy or rehabilitation program. Massage and heat should be avoided for at least the first week after injury. If you notice numbness and weakness developing anywhere or rapidly increasing swelling in the injured area, you should seek immediate medical attention. Although this occurs very rarely, rapid bleeding into the muscle may cause a build-up of pressure in the thigh; this may require urgent surgery to drain blood from the thigh.

Returning To Activity And Sports

The time to return to activity and sports depends on the grade/severity of the injury and one's progress with stretching and strengthening exercises. Moderate-to-severe contusions take an average of four to six weeks to heal. Minor contusions take considerably less time. If you put too much stress on the injured area before it is healed, excessive scar tissue may develop.

Your physician will allow you to return to contact sports when you get back your full strength, motion, and endurance. You may need to wear a protective device or pad to prevent further injury to the area.

Chapter 39

Bursitis And Tendonitis

What is bursitis and what is tendonitis?

Bursitis and tendonitis are both common conditions that involve inflammation of the soft tissue around muscles and bones, most often in the shoulder, elbow, wrist, hip, knee, or ankle.

A bursa is a small, fluid-filled sac that acts as a cushion between a bone and other moving parts: muscles, tendons, or skin. Bursae are found throughout the body. Bursitis occurs when a bursa becomes inflamed (redness and increased fluid in the bursa).

A tendon is a flexible band of fibrous tissue that connects muscles to bones. Tendonitis is inflammation of a tendon. Tendons transmit the pull of the muscle to the bone to cause movement. They are found throughout the body, including the hands, wrists, elbows, shoulders, hips, knees, ankles, and feet. Tendons can be small, like those found in the hand, or large, like the Achilles tendon in the heel.

What causes these conditions?

Bursitis is commonly caused by overuse or direct trauma to a joint. Bursitis may occur at the knee or elbow, from kneeling or leaning on the elbows longer than usual on a hard surface, for example. Tendonitis is most often the result of a repetitive injury or motion in the affected area. These conditions occur more often with age. Tendons become less flexible with age, and therefore, more prone to injury.

People such as carpenters, gardeners, musicians, and athletes who perform activities that require repetitive motions or place stress on joints are at higher risk for tendonitis and bursitis.

About This Chapter: From "Questions and Answers about Bursitis and Tendinitis," National Institute of Arthritis and Musculoskeletal and Skin Diseases (www.niams.nih.gov), March 2011.

An infection, arthritis, gout, thyroid disease, and diabetes can also bring about inflammation of a bursa or tendon.

What parts of the body are affected?

Tendonitis causes pain and tenderness just outside a joint. Some common names for tendonitis identify with the sport or movement that typically increases risk for tendon inflammation. They include tennis elbow, golfer's elbow, pitcher's shoulder, swimmer's shoulder, and jumper's knee. Some common examples follow.

Tennis Elbow And Golfer's Elbow: Tennis elbow refers to an injury to the outer elbow tendon. Golfer's elbow is an injury to the inner tendon of the elbow. These conditions can also occur with any activity that involves repetitive wrist turning or hand gripping, such as tool use, hand shaking, or twisting movements. Carpenters, gardeners, painters, musicians, manicurists, and dentists are at higher risk for these forms of tendonitis. Pain occurs near the elbow, sometimes radiating into the upper arm or down to the forearm. Another name for tennis elbow is lateral epicondylitis. Golfer's elbow is also called medial epicondylitis.

What's It Mean?

Acromion: The outer part of the shoulder blade.

Arthroscopic Surgery: Repairing the interior of a joint by inserting a microscope-like device and surgical tools through small cuts rather than one, large surgical cut.

Biceps Muscle: The muscle in the front of the upper arm.

Bursa: A small sac of tissue located between a bone and other moving structures such as muscles, skin, or tendons. The bursa contains a lubricating fluid that allows these structures to glide smoothly.

Bursitis: Inflammation or irritation of a bursa.

Corticosteroids: Synthetic preparations of cortisol, which is a hormone produced by the body. Corticosteroids block the immune system's production of substances that trigger allergic and inflammatory responses. These drugs may be injected directly into the inflammation site. Generally, symptoms improve or disappear within several days. Frequent injections into the same site are not recommended.

Epicondylitis: A painful and sometimes disabling swelling of the tissues of the elbow.

Humerus: The upper arm bone.

Impingement Syndrome: When the rotator cuff becomes inflamed and thickened, it may get trapped under the acromion, resulting in pain or loss of motion.

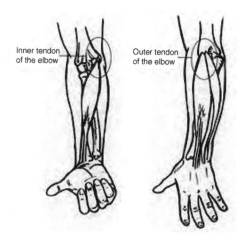

Inner tendon of the elbow

Outer tendon of the elbow

Figure 39.1. Structure of the Elbow.

Inflammation: The characteristic reaction of tissue to injury or disease. It is marked by swelling, redness, heat, and pain.

Joint: A junction where two bones meet. Most joints are composed of cartilage, joint space, the fibrous capsule, the synovium, and ligaments.

Muscle: A tissue that has the ability to contract, producing movement or force. There are three types of muscle: striated muscle, which is attached to the skeleton; smooth muscle, which is found in such tissues as the stomach and blood vessels; and cardiac muscle, which forms the walls of the heart. For striated muscle to function at its ideal level, the joint and surrounding structures must all be in good condition.

Patella: A flat triangular bone located at the front of the knee joint. Also called the kneecap.

Quadriceps Muscle: The large muscle at the front of the thigh.

Radius: The larger of the two bones in the forearm.

Range Of Motion: The extent to which a joint can move freely and easily.

Rheumatoid Arthritis: An autoimmune inflammatory disease that causes pain, swelling, stiffness, and loss of function in the joints.

Rotator Cuff: A set of muscles and tendons that secures the arm to the shoulder blade and permits rotation of the arm.

Tendonitis: Inflammation or irritation of a tendon.

Tendons: Fibrous cords that connect muscle to bone.

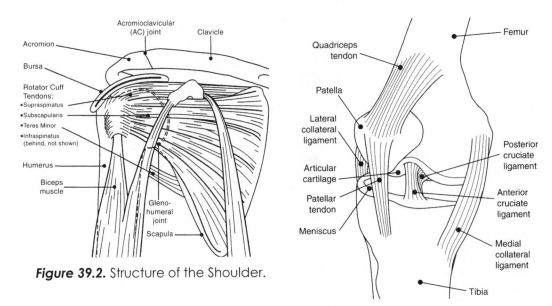

Figure 39.2. Structure of the Shoulder.

Figure 39.3. Lateral View of the Knee.

Shoulder Tendonitis, Bursitis, And Impingement Syndrome: Two types of tendonitis can affect the shoulder. Biceps tendonitis causes pain in the front or side of the shoulder and may travel down to the elbow and forearm. Pain may also occur when the arm is raised overhead. The biceps muscle, in the front of the upper arm, helps stabilize the upper arm bone (humerus) in the shoulder socket. It also helps accelerate and decelerate the arm during overhead movement in activities like tennis or pitching.

Rotator cuff tendonitis causes shoulder pain at the tip of the shoulder and the upper, outer arm. The pain can be aggravated by reaching, pushing, pulling, lifting, raising the arm above shoulder level, or lying on the affected side. The rotator cuff is primarily a group of four muscles that attach the arm to the shoulder joint and allow the arm to rotate and elevate. If the rotator cuff and bursa are irritated, inflamed, and swollen, they may become compressed between the head of the humerus and the acromion, the outer edge of the shoulder blade. Repeated motion involving the arms, or the aging process involving shoulder motion over many years, may also irritate and wear down the tendons, muscles, and surrounding structures. Squeezing of the rotator cuff is called shoulder impingement syndrome.

Inflammation caused by rheumatoid arthritis may cause rotator cuff tendonitis and bursitis. Sports involving overuse of the shoulder and occupations requiring frequent overhead reaching are other potential causes of irritation to the rotator cuff or bursa, and may lead to inflammation and impingement.

Knee Tendonitis Or Jumper's Knee: If a person overuses a tendon during activities such as dancing, cycling, or running, it may elongate or undergo microscopic tears and become inflamed. Trying to break a fall may also cause the quadriceps muscles to contract and tear the quadriceps tendon above the knee cap (patella) or the patellar tendon below it. This type of injury is most likely to happen in older people whose tendons tend to be weaker and less flexible. Tendonitis of the patellar tendon is sometimes called jumper's knee because in sports that require jumping, such as basketball, the muscle contraction and force of hitting the ground after a jump strain the tendon. After repeated stress, the tendon may become inflamed or tear.

People with tendonitis of the knee may feel pain during running, hurried walking, or jumping. Knee tendonitis can increase risk for ruptures or large tears to the tendon. A complete rupture of the quadriceps or patellar tendon is not only painful, but also makes it difficult for a person to bend, extend, or lift the leg, or to bear weight on the involved leg.

Achilles Tendonitis: Achilles tendon injuries involve an irritation, stretch, or tear to the tendon connecting the calf muscle to the back of the heel. Achilles tendonitis is a common overuse injury, but can also be caused by tight or weak calf muscles or any condition that causes the tendon to become less flexible and more rigid, such as reactive arthritis or normal aging.

Achilles tendon injuries can happen to anyone who regularly participates in an activity that causes the calf muscle to contract, like climbing stairs or using a stair-stepper, but are most common in middle-aged "weekend warriors" who may not exercise regularly or take time to warm up and stretch properly before an activity. Among professional athletes, most Achilles injuries seem to occur in quick-acceleration or jumping sports like football, tennis, and basketball, and almost always end the season's competition for the athlete.

Achilles tendonitis can be a chronic condition. It can also cause what appears to be a sudden injury. Tendonitis is the most common factor contributing to Achilles tendon tears. When a tendon is weakened by age or overuse, trauma can cause it to rupture. These injuries can be so sudden and agonizing that they have been known to bring down charging professional football players in shocking fashion.

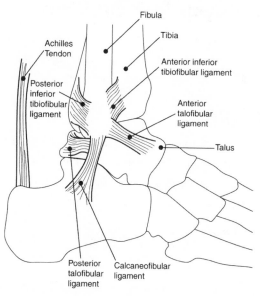

Figure 39.4. Lateral View of the Ankle.

How are these conditions diagnosed?

Diagnosis of tendonitis and bursitis begins with a medical history and physical examination. The patient will describe the pain and circumstances in which pain occurs. The location and onset of pain, whether it varies in severity throughout the day, and the factors that relieve or aggravate the pain are all important diagnostic clues. Therapists and physicians will use manual tests called selective tissue tension tests to determine which tendon is involved, and then will palpate (a form of touching the tendon) specific areas of the tendon to pinpoint the area of inflammation. X-rays do not show tendons or bursae, but may be helpful in ruling out problems in the bone or arthritis. In the case of a torn tendon, x-rays may help show which tendon is affected. In a knee injury, for example, an x-ray will show that the patella is lower than normal in a quadriceps tendon tear and higher than normal in a patellar tendon tear. The doctor may also use magnetic resonance imaging (MRI) to confirm a partial or total tear. MRIs detect both bone and soft tissues like muscles, tendons and their coverings (sheaths), and bursae.

An anesthetic-injection test is another way to confirm a diagnosis of tendonitis. A small amount of anesthetic (lidocaine hydrochloride) is injected into the affected area. If the pain is temporarily relieved, the diagnosis is confirmed.

To rule out infection, the doctor may remove and test fluid from the inflamed area.

What kind of health care professional treats these conditions?

A primary care physician or a physical therapist can treat the common causes of tendonitis and bursitis. Complicated cases or those resistant to conservative therapies may require referral to a specialist, such as an orthopedist or rheumatologist.

How are bursitis and tendonitis treated?

Treatment focuses on healing the injured bursa or tendon. The first step in treating both of these conditions is to reduce pain and inflammation with rest, compression, elevation, and anti-inflammatory medicines such as aspirin, naproxen, or ibuprofen. Ice may also be used in acute injuries, but most cases of bursitis or tendonitis are considered chronic, and ice is not helpful. When ice is needed, an ice pack can be applied to the affected area for 15 to 20 minutes every four to six hours for three to five days. Longer use of ice and a stretching program may be recommended by a health care provider.

Activity involving the affected joint is also restricted to encourage healing and prevent further injury.

In some cases (for example, in tennis elbow), elbow bands may be used to compress the forearm muscle to provide some pain relief, limiting the pull of the tendon on the bone. Other protective devices, such as foot orthoses for the ankle and foot or splints for the knee or hand, may temporarily reduce stress to the affected tendon or bursa and facilitate quicker healing times, while allowing general activity levels to continue as usual.

The doctor or therapist may use ultrasound (gentle sound-wave vibrations) to warm deep tissues and improve blood flow. Iontophoresis may also be used. This involves using an electrical current to push a corticosteroid medication through the skin directly over the inflamed bursa or tendon. Gentle stretching and strengthening exercises are added gradually. Massage of the soft tissue may be helpful. These may be preceded or followed by use of an ice pack. The type of exercises recommended may vary depending on the location of the affected bursa or tendon.

If there is no improvement, the doctor may inject a corticosteroid medicine into the area surrounding the inflamed bursa or tendon. While corticosteroid injections are a common treatment, they must be used with caution because they may lead to weakening or rupture of the tendon (especially weight-bearing tendons such as the Achilles [ankle], posterior tibial [arch of the foot], and patellar [knee] tendons). If there is still no improvement after 6–12 months, the doctor may perform either arthroscopic or open surgery to repair damage and relieve pressure on the tendons and bursae.

If the bursitis is caused by an infection, the doctor will prescribe antibiotics.

If a tendon is completely torn, surgery may be needed to repair the damage. After surgery on a quadriceps or patellar tendon, for example, the patient will wear a cast for three to six weeks and use crutches. For a partial tear, the doctor might apply a cast without performing surgery.

Rehabilitating a partial or complete tear of a tendon requires an exercise program to restore the ability to bend and straighten the knee and to strengthen the leg to prevent repeat injury. A rehabilitation program may last six months, although the patient can return to many activities before then.

Can bursitis and tendonitis be prevented?

The following tips can help prevent inflammation or reduce the severity of its recurrence:

- Warm up or stretch before physical activity.
- Strengthen muscles around the joint.
- Take breaks from repetitive tasks often.

- Cushion the affected joint. Use foam for kneeling or elbow pads. Increase the gripping surface of tools with gloves or padding. Apply grip tape or an oversized grip to golf clubs.

- Use two hands to hold heavy tools; use a two-handed backhand in tennis.

- Don't sit still for long periods.

- Practice good posture and position the body properly when going about daily activities.

- Begin new activities or exercise regimens slowly. Gradually increase physical demands following several well-tolerated exercise sessions.

- If a history of tendonitis is present, consider seeking guidance from your doctor or therapist before engaging in new exercises and activities.

Chapter 40

Eye Injuries

Eye Injuries Can Be Serious If Untreated

While eye injuries in sports are not common, they can be serious when they occur.

While the risk of eye injury is related to sport, most injuries can be prevented with protective eyewear.

Injuries to the eye range from foreign bodies (dirt, sand, etc.) to orbital fractures. These injuries have increased in past years due to the popularity of baseball and softball. Foreign bodies and abrasions (scratches) to the eyes are among the more common injuries during athletics.

Athletes often say they "feel something in their eye." It is important to know that foreign bodies in the eye and abrasion injuries produce the same symptoms. These symptoms include pain, increased tearing and the sensation of something in the eye. Do not rub the eye, as this will make matters worse. Have the athlete close the eye until the initial pain subsides. Most of the time the increased tearing will wash out the foreign object. Rinsing with water may also help remove the foreign object.

If you try to wash out the object and it does not come out, do not try to remove it by using your fingernail, Q-tip, or other small object. Cover the eye and take the athlete to the doctor or emergency room to have the object removed. Sometimes these objects can become imbedded in the eye and attempts to remove them can make matters worse.

If you do remove the object and the athlete still complains of "something in there," there may be an abrasion of the eye. In this case, the athlete needs to see a doctor. This injury can also occur from getting a finger in the eye.

Even though the eye is well protected within the eye socket, it can be bruised during sports. The injury can be as mild as a bruise or as severe as an orbital fracture.

Most of the injuries to the eye are of the mild type, commonly, the "dreaded" black eye. A blow to this area can cause damage to the tissue surrounding the eye causing the black eye. Use ice after a black eye to help control swelling and pain in the area. Don't blow your nose following a black eye as this will cause increased swelling.

Symptoms that indicate a serious eye injury include: blurred vision that does not clear when blinking, loss of part or all vision in the affected eye, a sharp stabbing or throbbing pain in the eye or double vision. *If any these symptoms occur, the athlete should cover the eye and be taken to the emergency room.*

Eye injuries should be taken seriously. Athletes should not return to sports until pain-free full vision is obtained. If a physician saw the athlete, a medical clearance must be obtained to return to activity. Eye injuries are not very commonplace, but can be serious if left untreated.

Table 40.1. Sports Eye Injuries In The U.S.

Sport	Percent
Baseball	27
Racquet Sports	20
Basketball	20
Football & Soccer	7
Ice Hockey	4

"Modern Principles of Athletic Training, 9th Edition," by Daniel Arnheim & William Prentice

First Aid For Eye Emergencies

"First Aid for Eye Emergencies," © 2011 Prevent Blindness America (www.preventblindness.org). Reprinted with permission.

Knowing what to do for an eye emergency can save valuable time and possibly prevent vision loss. Here are some instructions for basic eye injury first aid.

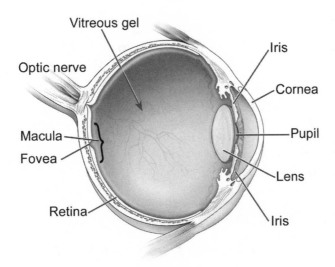

Figure 40.1. Eye Diagram (National Eye Institute).

Be Prepared

- Wear eye protection for all hazardous activities and sports-at school, home, and on the job.

- Stock a first aid kit with a rigid eye shield and commercial eyewash before an eye injury happens.

- DO NOT assume that any eye injury is harmless. When in doubt, see a doctor immediately.

Chemical Burns To The Eye

- In all cases of eye contact with chemicals:

- Immediately flush the eye with water or any other drinkable liquid. Hold the eye under a faucet or shower, or pour water into the eye using a clean container. Keep the eye open and as wide as possible while flushing. Continue flushing for at least 15 minutes.

- DO NOT use an eyecup.

- If a contact lens is in the eye, begin flushing over the lens immediately. This may wash away the lens.

- DO NOT bandage the eye.

- Seek immediate medical treatment after flushing.

Specks In The Eye

- DO NOT rub the eye

- Try to let tears wash the speck out or use an eyewash.

- Try lifting the upper eyelid outward and down over the lower lid.

- If the speck does not wash out, keep the eye closed, bandage it lightly, and see a doctor.

Blows To The Eye

- Apply a cold compress without putting pressure on the eye. Crushed ice in a plastic bag can be taped to the forehead to rest gently on the injured eye.

- In cases of pain, reduced vision, or discoloration (black eye), seek emergency medical care. Any of these symptoms could mean internal eye damage.

Cuts And Punctures Of The Eye Or Eyelid

- DO NOT wash out the eye with water or any other liquid.

- DO NOT try to remove an object that is stuck in the eye.

- Cover the eye with a rigid shield without applying pressure. The bottom half of a paper cup can be used.

- See a doctor at once.

Chapter 41

Facial Injuries

Broken Nose (Nasal Fracture)

Overview

What are the most common causes of a broken nose (nasal fracture)?

A broken nose (nasal fracture) usually occurs from an athlete getting hit in the face by either an opponent or sports equipment such as hockey sticks, baseballs, or softballs. Fractures can occur either from a direct blow to the front of the nose or from a sideways blow.

Who gets a broken nose (nasal fracture)?

A broken nose (nasal fracture) is common in sports where there is direct physical contact between athletes. A broken nose is common in the sports of basketball and soccer from head-to-head contact, head-to- elbow contact, or head-to- shoulder contact.

Any sport in which a small ball is flying at high speeds is a sport in which a broken nose is common. For example, take the sport of softball. Fractures can occur in a number of ways including fouling off an inside fastball or curveball directly to the nose, taking a grounder off of a bad hop directly to the nose, or missing a fly ball with the glove and catching it with the nose.

Symptoms

What are the signs and symptoms of a broken nose?

Most broken noses are going to immediately result in nasal bleeding. The blood can be coming from both the inside of the nose from the fracture and outside of the nose from lacerations and/or abrasions incurred during the impact.

One of the best indicators of a broken nose is the alignment of the nose. Have the athlete look into a mirror as soon after the impact as possible and prior to the swelling setting in. Have the athlete check the bridge of the nose to see if it looks straight.

The nose may also look flattened or asymmetrical. The nasal airway may be obstructed making it difficult for the athlete to breathe through both nostrils.

As time passes, the tissue around the nose and below the eyes will begin to swell. Discoloration will also begin to set in and will increase in color during the 48 hours post-injury.

Treatment

What is the immediate treatment for a broken nose?

Care must first be given to the athlete to ensure that the athlete did not sustain a serious head injury. Any force that can fracture a bone in the face can also cause a concussion or brain injury.

If the athlete is conscious and bleeding, the first step is to stop the bleeding. Gauze can be applied to the nose with mild pressure. The athlete should be placed in a sitting position with his/her head tilted forward. This will cause the blood to drain out of the nose and not down the back of the athlete's throat.

If the athlete is conscious and is lying on the ground and bleeding, gently roll the athlete on to his/her side to allow the blood to drain out and onto the ground. If a neck or serious head injury is suspected, leave the athlete in the position that you find him/her and call emergency medical services.

Once the gauze is in place, determine if the athlete has any signs and symptoms of concussion. Check for the following:

- Dizziness

- Headache

- Confusion

- Nausea

- Ringing in the ears

- Inability to answer simple questions

If any of the above symptoms are present, continue assisting the athlete and call emergency medical services.

Once the bleeding has stopped, a small ice pack can be applied to the nose and face to reduce the swelling. If a fracture is suspected, the athlete should be transported to a local hospital for x-rays and a thorough medical evaluation.

Should I have the broken nose reset?

If a broken nose is present, the athlete may have his/her nose repositioned if needed by an emergency room physician or may be referred to an ear, nose, and throat specialist. To have the fracture repositioned without surgical repair, this should be done either immediately after the injury or three to seven days later when the swelling has reduced.

If significant time has passed and the fracture has begun to heal (seven days post-injury), then surgical repair may be required to reset the fracture.

Is it safe to return to sports after a broken nose?

Athletes can safely return to sport when they have been cleared by a physician to return and only if they wear a protective splint or face guard. These can be purchased by sports medicine companies or can be custom made for the individual. The athlete should wear the face guard for at least six weeks post-injury or until the physician states that it is safe.

If you suspect that you have a broken nose (nasal fracture), it is critical to seek the urgent consultation of a local sports injuries doctor for appropriate care. To locate a top doctor or physical therapist in your area, please visit http://www.sportsmd.com/SportsMD_DoctorSearch/d/doctors.aspx.

Orbital Blowout Fracture

Overview

What is an orbital blowout fracture?

The orbit is the frontal part of the skull that provides structure and a bony pocket for the eyeball to sit in. Fractures can occur anywhere around the orbital walls but are most common to the orbital floor because it has the weakest bone structure.

What injuries can happen to the eye as a result of an orbital blowout fracture?

Several serious injuries can occur to the eye as a result of the blunt force directly to the eyeball. The injuries include:

- Hyphema (hemorrhage into the anterior chamber)
- Retinal detachment

A hyphema can result from the impact of a small ball directly into the eye. Within a few hours of impact, blood settles into the anterior chamber of the eyeball. This is a very serious eye injury requiring hospitalization, bed rest, bilateral patching of the eyes, and sedation. This condition usually resolves itself within a few days.

A retinal detachment is another serious injury that can occur from blunt trauma to the eye, but may occur several months or years post-injury. The retina is the nerve bundle connecting the eyeball to the brain. Without it, the athlete would not be able to see.

A retinal detachment may include the athlete seeing "flashes of light" or the appearance of a "curtain" dropping. The athlete may also complain of "floaters" in his/her vision. Athletes with these symptoms should be immediately treated by covering both eyes with patches and referred to an ophthalmologist for surgical repair.

Symptoms

What are the signs and symptoms of an orbital blowout fracture?

Any time an athlete receives a high force direct blow to the eye, a fracture should be suspected. The signs and symptoms of an orbital blowout fracture include:

- Immediate severe swelling
- Bleeding
- Recessed eyeball
- Inferiorly positioned eyeball
- Limited ocular movements (inability to look up)
- Absent eye movements
- Double vision
- Numbness of the cheek

Causes

Who gets an orbital blowout fracture?

The most common cause of an orbital blowout fracture is blunt force contact with an object larger than the orbit. Sports with these types of objects include tennis, racquetball, baseball, cricket, squash, and softball. The orbit can "blow-out" and fracture when one of these balls directly hits the eye at high speed effectively blowing the contents of the eye inward resulting in a fracture of the orbital floor.

An orbital blowout fracture can also occur to athletes in contact team sports when an athlete runs full force into a fist or elbow as in the sport of basketball. A direct blow to the face in fighting sports can also cause a "blow-out."

Treatment

What is the immediate treatment of an athlete with a suspected orbital blowout fracture?

Because the amount of force required to fracture the orbit is significant, emergency medical services should be immediately called and care should be taken to also evaluate the athlete for possible concussion and/or brain injury.

To determine if the athlete has any signs and symptoms of concussion check for the following:

- Dizziness
- Headache
- Confusion
- Nausea
- Ringing in the ears
- Inability to answer simple questions

If any of the above symptoms are present, assume that the athlete might also have a concussion.

Gauze should be gently applied to the injured area to help stop any bleeding that may be present. Crushed ice can also be applied to reduce the amount of swelling but care must be taken not to increase the pressure to the eye.

If there is excessive bleeding, place a soft object under the athlete's head and roll the athlete onto his/her side so that the blood can flow easily onto the ground and not back into the throat of the athlete.

Another aspect of immediate treatment for a seriously injured athlete is treating for shock. Athletes with serious injuries may go into shock because of the blood loss and/or the psychological impact of the injury.

Keeping the athlete calm by talking softly and slowly with an even pace is one effective way to comfort an athlete. The conversation should focus on anything but the injury. The goal of care during this time is to keep the athlete's breathing pattern regular. A calm athlete should have respirations between 12 and 15 per minute.

Another way to ensure that the athlete stays calm is to remove all people from the scene who are not directly involved in caring for the athlete. Poorly timed comments or outbursts from teammates can alone send an athlete into psychological shock.

Will I need surgery for the orbital blowout fracture to heal?

Surgery will most likely be required to repair the fracture to the orbital floor and release any muscles and/or nerves that may have been compromised as a result of the fracture.

When is it safe to return to sports after an orbital blowout fracture?

The athlete's safe return to sports will be dependent on the severity of the fracture and/or eye damage. The athlete should follow the specific instructions provided by his/her physician for the type and intensity of activity allowed until a full recovery has been made.

If you suspect that you have an orbital blowout fracture, it is critical to seek the urgent consultation of a local sports injuries doctor for appropriate care. To locate a top doctor or physical therapist in your area, please visit http://www.sportsmd.com/SportsMD_DoctorSearch/d/doctors.aspx.

Broken Jaw (Mandibular Fracture)

Overview

What is a broken jaw (mandibular fracture)?

A broken jaw (mandibular fracture) is the second most common facial fracture in sports because of the anterior location on the skull. The mandible is the jawbone. Because the mandible is exposed and not covered by most protective devices, it is susceptible to injury.

Symptoms

What are the signs and symptoms of a broken jaw?

The mandible usually fractures in more than one place and occurs on opposite sides of the midline of the jaw. These fractures can either be displaced (more severe with bone ends separated and moved apart) or nondisplaced (bone ends aligned).

The signs and symptoms of a displaced broken jaw include:

- Gross deformity
- Malocclusion (teeth do not align when jaw is closed)
- Oral bleeding
- Paresthesia or anesthesia of lower lip and chin
- Changes in speech
- Swelling
- Bruising to the floor of the mouth
- Mucous membrane tears

The signs and symptoms of a nondisplaced broken jaw include:

- Oral bleeding oozing between the teeth
- Point tenderness over the fracture site
- Pain on opening and closing the jaw
- Swelling
- Discoloration

Causes

Who gets a broken jaw?

A broken jaw is most often caused by a blow to the lower jaw from sports equipment (hockey stick, bat). Because of the length of a hockey stick and/or bat, it does not take as much force from the opponent swinging the equipment to create enough force to fracture the jawbone.

Mountain biking is another sport with a high incidence of facial fractures. This type of injury occurs when the athlete goes over the handlebars and falls directly onto the lower jaw or chin hitting a hard surface.

Fighting sports in which direct blows are delivered as part of the sport (boxing, mixed martial arts) also have a high incidence of jawbone fractures.

Treatment

What is the immediate treatment for a broken jaw?

If a broken jaw is suspected, emergency services should immediately be called. Initial treatment should be focused on maintaining an open airway with the athlete in a sitting position with the athlete's hands supporting the lower jaw. This position will allow the blood to flow forward and out of the mouth rather than back into the throat.

Because the amount of force required to fracture the mandible is significant, care must be taken to evaluate the athlete for possible concussion and/or brain injury also.

To determine if the athlete has any signs and symptoms of concussion, check for the following:

- Dizziness

- Headache

- Confusion

- Nausea

- Ringing in the ears

- Inability to answer simple questions

If any of the above symptoms are present, assume that the athlete may also have a concussion. An unconscious athlete or an athlete with a suspected concussion should be placed on their side with head tilt and jaw support after the mouth has been cleared of any broken or dislodged teeth.

The jaw can be immobilized using an ace bandage or roller gauze but care must be taken to ensure that the jaw is not displaced posteriorly which may compromise the airway. The bandages can be wrapped under the chin and over the top of the head.

A crushed ice pack can be applied to the area to reduce the amount of swelling. However, care must be taken that the weight of the ice pack does not displace the fracture.

Is surgery needed to repair a broken jaw?

If the athlete has sustained a nondisplaced jawbone fracture, the healing can be managed conservatively with analgesia and rest. To allow the fracture to heal properly, the athlete should only eat soft foods for up to four weeks or as long as recommended by the treating physician.

Most displaced jawbone fractures will require closed reduction and internal fixation for four to six weeks. While the athlete's jaw is wired shut, the athlete should be consuming high-protein, high-carbohydrate liquid diets. It is normal for an athlete to lose between 5% and 10% of his/her body weight during this time. If there is concern about the amount of weight lost, the athlete should consult with a nutritionist.

When is it safe to return to sports after a broken jaw?

Light activities such as stationary cycling, walking, and light resistance exercises can be performed during the time of fixation to maintain muscle tone. Care should be taken not to increase the heart rate to a level where increased oxygen is needed for the muscles because the athlete is only able to breathe through his/her nose and not able to breathe through his/her mouth to increase the oxygen uptake. It is recommended that the athlete should not return to contact or collision sports until one to two months after the jaw is unwired.

If you suspect that you have a broken jaw (mandibular fracture), it is critical to seek the urgent consultation of a local sports injuries doctor for appropriate care. To locate a top doctor or physical therapist in your area, please visit http://www.sportsmd.com/SportsMD_DoctorSearch/d/doctors.aspx.

Chapter 42

Dental Injuries

What Is Endodontic Treatment?

Endo is the Greek word for "inside" and *odont* is Greek for "tooth." Endodontic treatment involves the inside of the tooth.

To understand endodontic treatment, it helps to know something about the anatomy of the tooth. Inside the tooth, under the white enamel and a hard layer called the dentin, is a soft tissue called the pulp. The pulp contains blood vessels, nerves and connective tissue, and creates the surrounding hard tissues of the tooth during development.

The pulp extends from the crown of the tooth to the tip of the roots where it connects to the tissues surrounding the root. The pulp is important during a tooth's growth and development. However, once a tooth is fully mature it can survive without the pulp, because the tooth continues to be nourished by the tissues surrounding it.

Who Performs Endodontic Treatment?

All dentists, including your general dentist, received training in endodontic treatment in dental school. General dentists can perform endodontic procedures along with other dental procedures, but often they refer patients needing endodontic treatment to endodontists.

Endodontists are dentists with special training in endodontic procedures. They provide only endodontic services in their practices because they are specialists. To become specialists, they complete dental school and an additional two or more years of advanced training

About This Chapter: "Traumatic Dental Injuries," © 2011 American Association of Endodontists (www.aae.org). All rights reserved. Reprinted with permission.

233

in endodontics. They perform routine as well as difficult and very complex endodontic procedures, including endodontic surgery. Endodontists are also experienced at finding the cause of oral and facial pain that has been difficult to diagnose.

How Will My Injury Be Treated?

Chipped teeth account for the majority of all dental injuries. Dislodged or knocked-out teeth are examples of less frequent, but more severe injuries. Treatment depends on the type, location and severity of each injury. Any dental injury, even if apparently mild, requires examination by a dentist or an endodontist immediately. Sometimes, neighboring teeth suffer an additional, unnoticed injury that will only be detected by a thorough dental exam.

Chipped Or Fractured Teeth

Most chipped or fractured tooth crowns can be repaired either by reattaching the broken piece or by placing a tooth-colored filling. If a significant portion of the tooth crown is broken off, an artificial crown or cap may be needed to restore the tooth.

If the pulp is exposed or damaged after a crown fracture, root canal treatment may be needed. These injuries require special attention. If breathing through your mouth or drinking cold fluids is painful, bite on clean, moist gauze or cloth to help relieve symptoms until reaching your dentist's office. Never use topical oral pain medications (such as Anbesol®) or ointments, or place aspirin on the affected areas to eliminate pain symptoms.

Injuries in the back teeth often include fractured cusps, cracked teeth, and the more serious split tooth. If cracks extend into the root, root canal treatment and a full coverage crown may be needed to restore function to the tooth. Split teeth may require extraction.

Dislodged (Luxated) Teeth

During an injury, a tooth may be pushed sideways, out of or into its socket. Your endodontist or general dentist will reposition and stabilize your tooth. Root canal treatment is usually needed for permanent teeth that have been dislodged and should be started a few days following the injury. Medication such as calcium hydroxide may be put inside the tooth as part of the root canal treatment. A permanent root canal filling will be placed at a later date.

Children between seven and 12-years-old may not need root canal treatment since their teeth are still developing. For those patients, an endodontist or dentist will monitor the healing carefully and intervene immediately if any unfavorable changes appear. Therefore, multiple follow-up appointments are likely to be needed. New research indicates that stem cells present in the pulps of young people can be stimulated to complete root growth and heal the pulp following injuries or infection.

Knocked-Out (Avulsed) Teeth

If a tooth is completely knocked out of your mouth, time is of the essence. The tooth should be handled very gently, avoiding touching the root surface itself. If it is dirty, quickly and gently rinse it in water. Do not use soap or any other cleaning agent, and never scrape or brush the tooth. If possible, the tooth should be placed back into its socket as soon as possible. The less time the tooth is out of its socket, the better the chance for saving it. Call a dentist immediately.

If you cannot put the tooth back in its socket, it needs to be kept moist in special solutions that are available at many local drugstores (such as Save-A-Tooth). If those solutions are unavailable, you should put the tooth in milk. Doing this will keep the root cells in your tooth moist and alive for a few hours. Another option is to simply put the tooth in your mouth between your gum and cheek. Do not place the tooth in regular tap water because the root surface cells do not tolerate it.

Once the tooth has been put back in its socket, your dentist will evaluate it and will check for any other dental and facial injuries. If the tooth has not been placed back into its socket, your dentist will clean it carefully and replace it. A stabilizing splint will be placed for a few weeks. Depending on the stage of root development, your dentist or endodontist may start root canal treatment a week or two later. A medication may be placed inside the tooth followed by a permanent root canal filling at a later date.

The length of time the tooth was out of the mouth and the way the tooth was stored before reaching the dentist influence the chances of saving the tooth. Again, immediate treatment is essential. Taking all these factors into account, your dentist or endodontist may discuss other treatment options with you.

Root Fractures

A traumatic injury to the tooth may also result in a horizontal root fracture. The location of the fracture determines the long-term health of the tooth. If the fracture is close to the root tip, the chances for success are much better. However, the closer the fracture is to the gum line, the poorer the long-term success rate. Sometimes, stabilization with a splint is required for a period of time.

Do Traumatic Dental Injuries Differ In Children?

Chipped primary (or "baby") teeth can be esthetically restored. Dislodged primary teeth can, in rare cases, be repositioned. However, primary teeth that have been knocked out typically should not be replanted. This is because the replantation of a knocked-out primary tooth may cause further and permanent damage to the underlying permanent tooth that is growing inside the bone.

Children's permanent teeth that are not fully developed at the time of the injury need special attention and careful follow up, but not all of them will need root canal treatment. In an immature permanent tooth, the blood supply to the tooth and the presence of stem cells in the region may enable your dentist or endodontist to stimulate continued root growth.

Endodontists have the knowledge and skill to treat incompletely formed roots in children so that, in some instances, the roots can continue to develop. Endodontists will do all that is possible to save the natural tooth. These specialists are the logical source of information and expertise for children who are victims of dental trauma.

Will The Tooth Need Any Special Care Or Additional Treatment?

The nature of the injury, the length of time from injury to treatment, how your tooth was cared for after the injury and your body's response all affect the long-term health of the tooth. Timely treatment is particularly important with dislodged or knocked-out teeth in order to prevent root resorption.

Resorption occurs when your body, through its own defense mechanisms, begins to reject your own tooth in response to the traumatic injury. Following the injury, you should return to your dentist or endodontist to have the tooth examined and/or treated at regular intervals for up to five years to ensure that root resorption is not occurring and that surrounding tissues continue to heal. It has to be noted that some types of resorption are untreatable.

Chapter 43

Neck Injuries

Understanding Neck Injury

Damage to one anatomical part in your neck often means damage to others. For example, whiplash may result in one or several diagnoses including muscle strain, ligament sprain, and/or disc injury. This is because the parts of your neck are connected. Bones, joints, soft tissue, and nerves work together to hold up and move your head. As you review the most common neck injuries listed below, remember that you could be suffering from more than one of these conditions simultaneously.

Neck Injuries Affecting Soft Tissue

Most of the time, damage from a neck injury is limited to soft tissue. But nearly every type of neck injury, severe or mild, affects muscles. Below are the most common neck injuries affecting muscles, tendons, and/or ligaments. Remember, some of these, will occur in conjunction with more serious injury.

Crick In The Neck

A "crick" or "kink" is a term often used to describe the pain you wake up with after sleeping with your neck in an awkward position. It may also be due to working at the computer for long hours or sudden movements of the neck. "Crick in the neck" is not a medical diagnosis. Usually a muscle spasm, trigger points, arthritis, or a disc problem is the real culprit. At-home therapies can take care of a crick in the neck most of the time, but if the pain lasts longer than a week or disrupts your usual activities, get it checked by a doctor.

About This Chapter: "Types of Neck Injuries," by Anne Asher. © 2011. Used with permission of About, Inc. which can be found online at www.About.com. All rights reserved.

Muscle Strain

Strain is an injury to muscles that move the spine. Although they sometimes affect the neck, most strains occur in the low back. Bending over at the waist to lift a heavy object is a common cause of muscle strain. Symptoms include muscle spasm, reduced flexibility, and pain. To treat a neck or back strain, most medical experts recommend modifying your activity to accommodate your pain and taking an over-the-counter pain medication. If the pain lasts longer than a week, or if it disrupts your usual activities, see a doctor.

Neck Sprain

Sprains are injuries to ligaments. (Ligaments are strong bands of connective tissue that hold bones together.) Neck sprains are often caused by falls or sudden twists that overload or overstretch the joint. Another cause is repeated stress to the joint. Symptoms include swelling, reduced flexibility, and pain. Sprains can be mild, moderate, or severe. If you suspect someone in your environment has a severe neck injury (of any kind), you should immobilize their spine and call 911 immediately. For minor and moderate sprains, rest. and ice the area, take an anti-inflammatory, and get it checked by a doctor.

Neck Injuries That May Affect Nerves And/Or The Spinal Cord

Certain neck injuries may also do damage to the nervous system by irritating nerve roots or affecting the spinal cord. Others may pinch or stretch a nerve. Generally, neck injuries that affect the nervous system are more complicated to diagnose, treat, and cope with than soft tissue trauma or mild to moderate joint injury. For one thing, diagnosing nerve pain is not always straightforward. And injury to the spinal cord often results in life long disability, paralysis, or even death. Below are common neck injuries that may include damage to one or more parts of the nervous system.

Whiplash, Whiplash Associated Disorders (WAD)

Whiplash is a set of symptoms following an injury in which the head is thrown first into hyperextension and then quickly forward. It's most often due to car accidents, but may be caused by sports injuries, falls or trauma. Like a crick, WAD is not a medical diagnosis. It's an event that may result in neck strain or sprain. Whiplash may also damage joints or discs, which in turn may irritate nerve roots or possibly the spinal cord. Depending on the injury, symptoms can include pain, weakness/numbness/tingling down the arm, stiffness, dizziness, or disturbed sleep. Symptoms may delayed a day or two following the injury. Research has not yet identified the most appropriate treatments for WAD, but medication and wearing a collar are common.

Herniated Disc

Herniated disc occurs when the soft substance on the inside of the disc (nucleus pulposus) is pushed out. Should this substance land on a nerve root, which it often does, you'll likely feel pain and have symptoms such as weakness, numbness, and/or pins and needles down your arm. Tears in the tough outer fibers of the disc may lead to a herniation. These tears may be brought on by either repeated or a sudden, forceful stress to the joint. For example, lifting a heavy load with a twisted spine may cause a disc to herniate. Treatment generally starts with medication and physical therapy, but may proceed to surgery as needed.

Stingers And Burners

Stingers and burners (named for the way they feel) are temporary injuries to the nerve root or brachial plexus. They occur most often in football players (especially tacklers) and other contact sport athletes. They may be caused by either by an abrupt tilt of the head or when the head and shoulder are forced in opposite directions at the same time. Symptoms include burning, stinging, numbness/weakness, or an electrical sensation down one arm. You may feel a warm sensation along with the other symptoms. If a stinger or burner is severe or lasts longer than a few minutes, see a doctor. If you are an athlete with stenosis, your risk is higher and your doctor may suggest that you retire from your sport to avoid a catastrophic neck injury.

Neck Fracture

A neck fracture is a break in a cervical bone. It may be caused by trauma, a fall or degenerative changes in the spine. The angle of force hitting the neck and the head's position at impact often determine the type and severity of the break. Football players who block with their head are at high risk. Elderly people with osteoporosis are particularly at risk for neck fractures because their bones are very fragile. The most serious neck fractures are generally accompanied by a dislocation (see Cervical Dislocation). Treatment depends on a lot of things including your age, other medical conditions, and extent of damage to your spine. If a fracture destabilizes your neck, you may need to wear a halo brace. Prevention is the best treatment strategy.

Cervical Dislocation

Dislocation occurs when a neck bone moves out its normal position, creating spinal instability. Either an injury or degenerative changes disrupt the ligaments that hold the vertebra in place, causing it to separate from the bone below. When brought on by trauma, a dislocation may be accompanied by fracture. In the most severe dislocation, the bone is fully displaced forward (called jumping), and it locks in this position. The ligaments rupture completely. Dislocations may damage the spinal cord and/or require surgery. Less severe forms occur when the bone does not move all the way out or when only one side fully displaces. Mild dislocations may go back in place on their own, and the soft tissue treated by wearing a collar.

Spinal Cord Injury

A spinal cord injury (SCI) occurs when a fracture, dislocation, or other neck injury damages the spinal cord. If the spinal cord is damaged at the third cervical vertebra or above, the person may die or need a respirator to live. People living with SCI often endure a lifelong disability with complete or incomplete paralysis below the level of injury. The timeliness of emergency care and the type of medical treatment given immediately after the injury are especially critical to survival and subsequent quality of life. If someone in your environment has a traumatic incident, you should assume they have a serious or even life-threatening neck injury and follow Red Cross guidelines.

Chapter 44

Spine Injuries

What Is A Spinal Cord Injury?

Although the hard bones of the spinal column protect the soft tissues of the spinal cord, vertebrae can still be broken or dislocated in a variety of ways and cause traumatic injury to the spinal cord. Injuries can occur at any level of the spinal cord. The segment of the cord that is injured, and the severity of the injury, will determine which body functions are compromised or lost. Because the spinal cord acts as the main information pathway between the brain and the rest of the body, a spinal cord injury can have significant physiological consequences.

Catastrophic falls, being thrown from a horse or through a windshield, or any kind of physical trauma that crushes and compresses the vertebrae in the neck can cause irreversible damage at the cervical level of the spinal cord and below. Paralysis of most of the body including the arms and legs, called quadriplegia, is the likely result. Automobile accidents are often responsible for spinal cord damage in the middle back (the thoracic or lumbar area), which can cause paralysis of the lower trunk and lower extremities, called paraplegia.

Other kinds of injuries that directly penetrate the spinal cord, such as gunshot or knife wounds, can either completely or partially sever the spinal cord and create life-long disabilities.

Most injuries to the spinal cord don't completely sever it. Instead, an injury is more likely to cause fractures and compression of the vertebrae, which then crush and destroy the axons, extensions of nerve cells that carry signals up and down the spinal cord between the brain and the rest of the body. An injury to the spinal cord can damage a few, many, or almost all of these axons. Some injuries will allow almost complete recovery. Others will result in complete paralysis.

About This Chapter: Excerpted from "Spinal Cord Injury: Hope Through Research," National Institute of Neurological Disorders and Stroke, January 2012.

Until World War II, a serious spinal cord injury usually meant certain death, or at best a lifetime confined to a wheelchair and an ongoing struggle to survive secondary complications such as breathing problems or blood clots. But today, improved emergency care for people with spinal cord injuries and aggressive treatment and rehabilitation can minimize damage to the nervous system and even restore limited abilities.

Advances in research are giving doctors and patients hope that all spinal cord injuries will eventually be repairable. With new surgical techniques and exciting developments in spinal nerve regeneration, the future for spinal cord injury survivors looks brighter every day.

How The Spinal Cord Works

To understand what can happen as the result of a spinal cord injury, it helps to know the anatomy of the spinal cord and its normal functions.

Facts And Figures About Spinal Cord Injury

- There are an estimated 10,000 to 12,000 spinal cord injuries every year in the United States.
- A quarter of a million Americans are currently living with spinal cord injuries.
- The cost of managing the care of spinal cord injury patients approaches $4 billion each year.
- 38.5% of all spinal cord injuries happen during car accidents. Almost a quarter, 24.5%, are the result of injuries relating to violent encounters, often involving guns and knives. The rest are due to sporting accidents, falls, and work-related accidents.
- 55% of spinal cord injury victims are between 16 and 30 years old.
- More than 80% of spinal cord injury patients are men.

Spine Anatomy

The soft, jelly-like spinal cord is protected by the spinal column. The spinal column is made up of 33 bones called vertebrae, each with a circular opening similar to the hole in a donut. The bones are stacked one on top of the other and the spinal cord runs through the hollow channel created by the holes in the stacked bones (see Figure 44.1).

The vertebrae can be organized into sections, and are named and numbered from top to bottom according to their location along the backbone:

- Cervical vertebrae (1–7) located in the neck

- Thoracic vertebrae (1–12) in the upper back (attached to the ribcage)
- Lumbar vertebrae (1–5) in the lower back
- Sacral vertebrae (1–5) in the hip area
- Coccygeal vertebrae (1–4 fused) in the tailbone

Although the hard vertebrae protect the soft spinal cord from injury most of the time, the spinal column is not all hard bone. Between the vertebrae are discs of semi-rigid cartilage, and in the narrow spaces between them are passages through which the spinal nerves exit to the rest of the body. These are places where the spinal cord is vulnerable to direct injury.

The spinal cord is also organized into segments and named and numbered from top to bottom. Each segment marks where spinal nerves emerge from the cord to connect to specific regions of the body. Locations of spinal cord segments do not correspond exactly to vertebral locations, but they are roughly equivalent.

- Cervical spinal nerves (C1 to C8) control signals to the back of the head, the neck and shoulders, the arms and hands, and the diaphragm.
- Thoracic spinal nerves (T1 to T12) control signals to the chest muscles, some muscles of the back, and parts of the abdomen.
- Lumbar spinal nerves (L1 to L5) control signals to the lower parts of the abdomen and the back, the buttocks, some parts of the external genital organs, and parts of the leg.
- Sacral spinal nerves (S1 to S5) control signals to the thighs and lower parts of the legs, the feet, most of the external genital organs, and the area around the anus.

The single coccygeal nerve carries sensory information from the skin of the lower back.

Spinal Cord Anatomy

The spinal cord has a core of tissue containing nerve cells, surrounded by long tracts of nerve fibers consisting of axons. The tracts extend up and down the spinal cord, carrying signals to and from the brain. The average size of the spinal cord varies in circumference along its length from the width of a thumb to the width of one of the smaller fingers. The spinal cord extends down through the upper two thirds of the vertebral canal, from the base of the brain to the lower back, and is generally 15 to 17 inches long depending on an individual's height.

The interior of the spinal cord is made up of neurons, their support cells called glia, and blood vessels. The neurons and their dendrites (branching projections that help neurons communicate with each other) reside in an H-shaped region called grey matter.

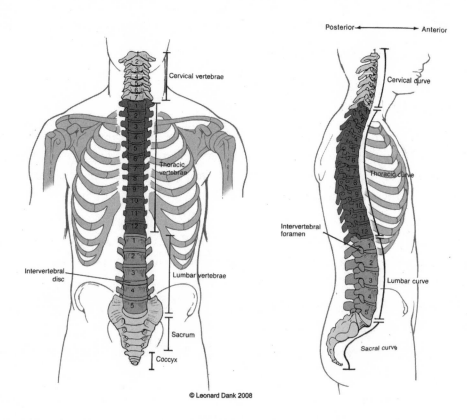

Figure 44.1. Spinal Column. (© 2008 Leonard Dank; reprinted with permission)

The H-shaped grey matter of the spinal cord contains motor neurons that control movement, smaller interneurons that handle communication within and between the segments of the spinal cord, and cells that receive sensory signals and then send information up to centers in the brain.

Surrounding the grey matter of neurons is white matter. Most axons are covered with an insulating substance called myelin, which allows electrical signals to flow freely and quickly. Myelin has a whitish appearance, which is why this outer section of the spinal cord is called white matter.

Axons carry signals downward from the brain (along descending pathways) and upward toward the brain (along ascending pathways) within specific tracts. Axons branch at their ends and can make connections with many other nerve cells simultaneously. Some axons extend along the entire length of the spinal cord.

The descending motor tracts control the smooth muscles of internal organs and the striated (capable of voluntary contractions) muscles of the arms and legs. They also help adjust the autonomic nervous system's regulation of blood pressure, body temperature, and the response to stress. These pathways begin with neurons in the brain that send electrical signals downward to specific levels of the spinal cord. Neurons in these segments then send the impulses out to the rest of the body or coordinate neural activity within the cord itself.

The ascending sensory tracts transmit sensory signals from the skin, extremities, and internal organs that enter at specific segments of the spinal cord. Most of these signals are then relayed to the brain. The spinal cord also contains neuronal circuits that control reflexes and repetitive movements, such as walking, which can be activated by incoming sensory signals without input from the brain.

The circumference of the spinal cord varies depending on its location. It is larger in the cervical and lumbar areas because these areas supply the nerves to the arms and upper body and the legs and lower body, which require the most intense muscular control and receive the most sensory signals.

The functions of these nerves are determined by their location in the spinal cord. They control everything from body functions such as breathing, sweating, digestion, and elimination, to gross and fine motor skills, as well as sensations in the arms and legs.

The Nervous System

Together, the spinal cord and the brain make up the central nervous system.

The central nervous system controls most functions of the body, but it is not the only nervous system in the body. The peripheral nervous system includes the nerves that project to the limbs, heart, skin, and other organs outside the brain. The peripheral nervous system controls the somatic nervous system, which regulates muscle movements and the response to sensations of touch and pain, and the autonomic nervous system, which provides nerve input to the internal organs and generates automatic reflex responses. The autonomic nervous system is divided into the sympathetic nervous system, which mobilizes organs and their functions during times of stress and arousal, and the parasympathetic nervous system, which conserves energy and resources during times of rest and relaxation.

The spinal cord acts as the primary information pathway between the brain and all the other nervous systems of the body. It receives sensory information from the skin, joints, and muscles of the trunk, arms, and legs, which it then relays upward to the brain. It carries messages downward from the brain to the peripheral nervous system, and contains motor neurons, which direct voluntary movements and adjust reflex movements. Because of the central role it plays in coordinating muscle movements and interpreting sensory input, any kind of injury to the spinal cord can cause significant problems throughout the body.

When The Spinal Cord Is Injured

A spinal cord injury usually begins with a sudden, traumatic blow to the spine that fractures or dislocates vertebrae. The damage begins at the moment of injury when displaced bone fragments, disc material, or ligaments bruise or tear into spinal cord tissue. Axons are cut off or damaged beyond repair, and neural cell membranes are broken. Blood vessels may rupture and cause heavy bleeding in the central grey matter, which can spread to other areas of the spinal cord over the next few hours.

Within minutes, the spinal cord swells to fill the entire cavity of the spinal canal at the injury level. This swelling cuts off blood flow, which also cuts off oxygen to spinal cord tissue. Blood pressure drops, sometimes dramatically, as the body loses its ability to self-regulate. As blood pressure lowers even further, it interferes with the electrical activity of neurons and axons. All these changes can cause a condition known as spinal shock that can last from several hours to several days.

Although there is some controversy among neurologists about the extent and impact of spinal shock, and even its definition in terms of physiological characteristics, it appears to occur in approximately half the cases of spinal cord injury, and it is usually directly related to the size and severity of the injury. During spinal shock, even undamaged portions of the spinal cord become temporarily disabled and can't communicate normally with the brain. Complete paralysis may develop, with loss of reflexes and sensation in the limbs.

The crushing and tearing of axons is just the beginning of the devastation that occurs in the injured spinal cord and continues for days. The initial physical trauma sets off a cascade of biochemical and cellular events that kills neurons, strips axons of their myelin insulation, and triggers an inflammatory immune system response. Days or sometimes even weeks later, after this second wave of damage has passed, the area of destruction has increased—sometimes to several segments above and below the original injury—and so has the extent of disability.

Changes In Blood Flow Cause Ongoing Damage

Changes in blood flow in and around the spinal cord begin at the injured area, spread out to adjacent, uninjured areas, and then set off problems throughout the body.

246

Immediately after the injury, there is a major reduction in blood flow to the site, which can last for as long as 24 hours and becomes progressively worse if untreated. Because of differences in tissue composition, the impact is greater on the interior grey matter of the spinal cord than on the outlying white matter.

Blood vessels in the grey matter also begin to leak, sometimes as early as five minutes after injury. Cells that line the still-intact blood vessels in the spinal cord begin to swell, for reasons that aren't yet clearly understood, and this continues to reduce blood flow to the injured area. The combination of leaking, swelling, and sluggish blood flow prevents the normal delivery of oxygen and nutrients to neurons, causing many of them to die.

The body continues to regulate blood pressure and heart rate during the first hour to hour-and-a-half after the injury, but as the reduction in the rate of blood flow becomes more widespread, self-regulation begins to turn off. Blood pressure and heart rate drop.

Excessive Release Of Neurotransmitters Kills Nerve Cells

After the injury, an excessive release of neurotransmitters (chemicals that allow neurons to signal each other) can cause additional damage by overexciting nerve cells.

Glutamate is an excitatory neurotransmitter, commonly used by nerve cells in the spinal cord to stimulate activity in neurons. But when spinal cells are injured, neurons flood the area with glutamate for reasons that are not yet well understood. Excessive glutamate triggers a destructive process called excitotoxicity, which disrupts normal processes and kills neurons and other cells called oligodendrocytes that surround and protect axons.

An Invasion Of Immune System Cells Creates Inflammation

Under normal conditions, the blood-brain barrier (which tightly controls the passage of cells and large molecules between the circulatory and central nervous systems) keeps immune system cells from entering the brain or spinal cord. But when the blood-brain barrier is broken by blood vessels bursting and leaking into spinal cord tissue, immune system cells that normally circulate in the blood, primarily white blood cells, can invade the surrounding tissue and trigger an inflammatory response. This inflammation is characterized by fluid accumulation and the influx of immune cells—neutrophils, T-cells, macrophages, and monocytes.

Neutrophils are the first to enter, within about 12 hours of injury, and they remain for about a day. Three days after the injury, T-cells arrive. Their function in the injured spinal cord is not clearly understood, but in the healthy spinal cord they kill infected cells and regulate the immune response. Macrophages and monocytes enter after the T-cells and scavenge cellular debris.

The up side of this immune system response is that it helps fight infection and cleans up debris. But the down side is that it sets off the release of cytokines—a group of immune system messenger molecules that exert a malign influence on the activities of nerve cells.

For example, microglial cells, which normally function as a kind of on-site immune cell in the spinal cord, begin to respond to signals from these cytokines. They transform into macrophage-like cells, engulf cell debris, and start to produce their own pro-inflammatory cytokines, which then stimulate and recruit other microglia to respond.

Injury also stimulates resting astrocytes to express cytokines. These reactive astrocytes may ultimately participate in the formation of scar tissue within the spinal cord.

Whether or not the immune response is protective or destructive is controversial among researchers. Some speculate that certain types of injury might evoke a protective immune response that actually reduces the loss of neurons.

Free Radicals Attack Nerve Cells

Another consequence of the immune system's entry into the central nervous system is that inflammation accelerates the production of highly reactive forms of oxygen molecules called free radicals.

Free radicals are produced as a by-product of normal cell metabolism. In the healthy spinal cord their numbers are small enough that they cause no harm. But injury to the spinal cord, and the subsequent wave of inflammation that sweeps through spinal cord tissue, signals particular cells to overproduce free radicals.

Free radicals then attack and disable molecules that are crucial for cell function—for example, those found in cell membranes—by modifying their chemical structure. Free radicals can also change how cells respond to natural growth and survival factors, and turn these protective factors into agents of destruction.

Nerve Cells Self-Destruct

Researchers used to think that the only way in which cells died during spinal cord injury was as a direct result of trauma. But recent findings have revealed that cells in the injured spinal cord also die from a kind of programmed cell death called apoptosis, often described as cellular suicide, that happens days or weeks after the injury.

Apoptosis is a normal cellular event that occurs in a variety of tissues and cellular systems. It helps the body get rid of old and unhealthy cells by causing them to shrink and implode.

Nearby scavenger cells then gobble up the debris. Apoptosis seems to be regulated by specific molecules that have the ability to either start or stop the process.

For reasons that are still unclear, spinal cord injury sets off apoptosis, which kills oligodendrocytes in damaged areas of the spinal cord days to weeks after the injury. The death of oligodendrocytes is another blow to the damaged spinal cord, since these are the cells that form the myelin that wraps around axons and speeds the conduction of nerve impulses. Apoptosis strips myelin from intact axons in adjacent ascending and descending pathways, which further impairs the spinal cord's ability to communicate with the brain.

Secondary Damage Takes A Cumulative Toll

All of these mechanisms of secondary damage-restricted blood flow, excitotoxicity, inflammation, free radical release, and apoptosis-increase the area of damage in the injured spinal cord. Damaged axons become dysfunctional, either because they are stripped of their myelin or because they are disconnected from the brain. Glial cells cluster to form a scar, which creates a barrier to any axons that could potentially regenerate and reconnect. A few whole axons may remain, but not enough to convey any meaningful information to the brain.

Researchers are especially interested in studying the mechanisms of this wave of secondary damage because finding ways to stop it could save axons and reduce disabilities. This could make a big difference in the potential for recovery.

Immediate Treatments For Spinal Cord Injury

The outcome of any injury to the spinal cord depends upon the number of axons that survive: the higher the number of normally functioning axons, the less the amount of disability. Consequently, the most important consideration when moving people to a hospital or trauma center is preventing further injury to the spine and spinal cord.

Spinal cord injury isn't always obvious. Any injury that involves the head (especially with trauma to the front of the face), pelvic fractures, penetrating injuries in the area of the spine, or injuries that result from falling from heights should be suspect for spinal cord damage.

Until imaging of the spine is done at an emergency or trauma center, people who might have spinal cord injury should be cared for as if any significant movement of the spine could cause further damage. They are usually transported in a recumbent (lying down) position, with a rigid collar and backboard immobilizing the spine.

Respiratory complications are often an indication of the severity of spinal cord injury. About one third of those with injury to the neck area will need help with breathing and require respiratory support via intubation, which involves inserting a tube connected to an oxygen tank through the nose or throat and into the airway.

Methylprednisolone, a steroid drug, became standard treatment for acute spinal cord injury in 1990 when a large-scale clinical trial supported by the National Institute of Neurological Disorders and Stroke showed significantly better recovery in patients who were given the drug within the first eight hours after their injury. Methylprednisolone appears to reduce the damage to nerve cells and decreases inflammation near the injury site by suppressing activities of immune cells.

Realignment of the spine using a rigid brace or axial traction is usually done as soon as possible to stabilize the spine and prevent additional damage.

Spinal cord injuries are classified as either complete or incomplete, depending on how much cord width is injured. An incomplete injury means that the ability of the spinal cord to convey messages to or from the brain is not completely lost. People with incomplete injuries retain some motor or sensory function below the injury.

A complete injury is indicated by a total lack of sensory and motor function below the level of injury.

Spinal Cord Injury Affects The Rest Of The Body

People who survive a spinal cord injury will most likely have medical complications such as chronic pain and bladder and bowel dysfunction, along with an increased susceptibility to respiratory and heart problems. Successful recovery depends upon how well these chronic conditions are handled day to day.

Breathing

Any injury to the spinal cord at or above the C3, C4, and C5 segments, which supply the phrenic nerves leading to the diaphragm, can stop breathing. People with these injuries need immediate ventilatory support. When injuries are at the C5 level and below, diaphragm function is preserved, but breathing tends to be rapid and shallow and people have trouble coughing and clearing secretions from their lungs because of weak thoracic muscles. Once pulmonary function improves, a large percentage of those with C4 injuries can be weaned from mechanical ventilation in the weeks following the injury.

Pneumonia

Respiratory complications, primarily as a result of pneumonia, are a leading cause of death in people with spinal cord injury. In fact, intubation increases the risk of developing ventilator-associated pneumonia by one to three percent per day of intubation. More than a quarter of the deaths caused by spinal cord injury are the result of ventilator-associated pneumonia. Spinal cord injury patients who are intubated have to be carefully monitored for ventilator-associated pneumonia and treated with antibiotics if symptoms appear.

Irregular Heart Beat And Low Blood Pressure

Spinal cord injuries in the cervical region are often accompanied by blood pressure instability and heart arrhythmias. Because of interruptions to the cardiac accelerator nerves, the heart can beat at a dangerously slow pace, or it can pound rapidly and irregularly. Arrhythmias usually appear in the first two weeks after injury and are more common and severe in the most serious injuries.

Low blood pressure also often occurs due to loss of tone in blood vessels, which widen and cause blood to pool in the small arteries far away from the heart. This is usually treated with an intravenous infusion to build up blood volume.

Blood Clots

People with spinal cord injuries are at triple the usual risk for blood clots. The risk for clots is low in the first 72 hours, but afterwards anticoagulation drug therapy can be used as a preventive measure.

Spasm

Many of our reflex movements are controlled by the spinal cord but regulated by the brain. When the spinal cord is damaged, information from the brain can no longer regulate reflex activity. Reflexes may become exaggerated over time, causing spasticity. If spasms become severe enough, they may require medical treatment. For some, spasms can be as much of a help as they are a hindrance, since spasms can tone muscles that would otherwise waste away. Some people can even learn to use the increased tone in their legs to help them turn over in bed, propel them into and out of a wheelchair, or stand.

Autonomic Dysreflexia

Autonomic dysreflexia is a life-threatening reflex action that primarily affects those with injuries to the neck or upper back. It happens when there is an irritation, pain, or stimulus to the nervous system below the level of injury. The irritated area tries to send a signal to the brain, but since the signal isn't able to get through, a reflex action occurs without the brain's regulation. Unlike spasms that affect muscles, autonomic dysreflexia affects vascular and organ systems controlled by the sympathetic nervous system.

Anything that causes pain or irritation can set off autonomic dysreflexia: the urge to urinate or defecate, pressure sores, cuts, burns, bruises, sunburn, pressure of any kind on the body, ingrown toenails, or tight clothing. For example, the impulse to urinate can set off high blood pressure or rapid heartbeat that, if uncontrolled, can cause stroke, seizures, or death. Symptoms such as flushing or sweating, a pounding headache, anxiety, sudden high blood pressure, vision changes, or goosebumps on the arms and legs can signal the onset of autonomic dysreflexia. Treatment should be swift. Changing position, emptying the bladder or bowels, and removing or loosening tight clothing are just a few of the possibilities that should be tried to relieve whatever is causing the irritation.

Pressure Sores (Or Pressure Ulcers)

Pressure sores are areas of skin tissue that have broken down because of continuous pressure on the skin. People with paraplegia and quadriplegia are susceptible to pressure sores because they can't move easily on their own.

Places that support weight when someone is seated or recumbent are vulnerable areas. When these areas press against a surface for a long period of time, the skin compresses and reduces the flow of blood to the area. When the blood supply is blocked for too long, the skin will begin to break down.

Since spinal cord injury reduces or eliminates sensation below the level of injury, people may not be aware of the normal signals to change position, and must be shifted periodically by a caregiver. Good nutrition and hygiene can also help prevent pressure sores by encouraging healthy skin.

Pain

People who are paralyzed often have what is called neurogenic pain resulting from damage to nerves in the spinal cord. For some survivors of spinal cord injury, pain or an intense burning or stinging sensation is unremitting due to hypersensitivity in some parts of the body. Others are prone to normal musculoskeletal pain as well, such as shoulder pain due to overuse of the shoulder joint from pushing a wheelchair and using the arms for transfers. Treatments for chronic pain include medications, acupuncture, spinal or brain electrical stimulation, and surgery.

Bladder And Bowel Problems

Most spinal cord injuries affect bladder and bowel functions because the nerves that control the involved organs originate in the segments near the lower termination of the spinal cord and are cut off from brain input. Without coordination from the brain, the muscles of the bladder and urethra can't work together effectively, and urination becomes abnormal. The bladder can empty suddenly without warning, or become over-full without releasing. In some cases the bladder releases, but urine backs up into the kidneys because it isn't able to get past the urethral sphincter. Most people with spinal cord injuries use either intermittent catheterization or an indwelling catheter to empty their bladders.

Bowel function is similarly affected. The anal sphincter muscle can remain tight, so that bowel movements happen on a reflex basis whenever the bowel is full. Or the muscle can be permanently relaxed, which is called a "flaccid bowel," and result in an inability to have a bowel movement. This requires more frequent attempts to empty the bowel and manual removal of stool to prevent fecal impaction. People with spinal cord injuries are usually put on a regularly scheduled bowel program to prevent accidents.

Rehabilitation Helps People Recover From Spinal Cord Injuries

No two people will experience the same emotions after surviving a spinal cord injury, but almost everyone will feel frightened, anxious, or confused about what has happened. It's common for people to have very mixed feelings: relief that they are still alive, but disbelief at the nature of their disabilities.

Rehabilitation programs combine physical therapies with skill-building activities and counseling to provide social and emotional support. The education and active involvement of the newly injured person and his or her family and friends is crucial.

A rehabilitation team is usually led by a doctor specializing in physical medicine and rehabilitation (called a physiatrist), and often includes social workers, physical and occupational therapists, recreational therapists, rehabilitation nurses, rehabilitation psychologists, vocational counselors, nutritionists, and other specialists. A caseworker or program manager coordinates care.

In the initial phase of rehabilitation, therapists emphasize regaining leg and arm strength since mobility and communication are the two most important areas of function. For some, mobility will only be possible with the assistance of devices such as a walker, leg braces, or a wheelchair. Communication skills, such as writing, typing, and using the telephone, may also require adaptive devices.

Physical therapy includes exercise programs geared toward muscle strengthening. Occupational therapy helps redevelop fine motor skills. Bladder and bowel management programs teach basic toileting routines, and patients also learn techniques for self-grooming. People acquire coping strategies for recurring episodes of spasticity, autonomic dysreflexia, and neurogenic pain.

Vocational rehabilitation begins with an assessment of basic work skills, current dexterity, and physical and cognitive capabilities to determine the likelihood for employment. A vocational rehabilitation specialist then identifies potential work places, determines the type of assistive equipment that will be needed, and helps arrange for a user-friendly workplace. For those whose disabilities prevent them from returning to the workplace, therapists focus on encouraging productivity through participation in activities that provide a sense of satisfaction and self-esteem. This could include educational classes, hobbies, memberships in special interest groups, and participation in family and community events.

Recreation therapy encourages patients to build on their abilities so that they can participate in recreational or athletic activities at their level of mobility. Engaging in recreational outlets and athletics helps those with spinal cord injuries achieve a more balanced and normal lifestyle and also provides opportunities for socialization and self-expression.

Chapter 45

Burners And Stingers

The spinal cord extends from the base of the brain down the neck; large nerves branch off the spinal cord along its course. When one or more of these nerves are stretched or pinched, this mild injury to the nerves causes tingling and numbness in the arm and fingers; some athletes notice weakness in their arm as well. The terms "stinger" and "burner" are two terms sometimes used to describe this stretched or pinched condition.

How It Occurs

A stinger can occur by one of two mechanisms. Either the athlete's head is pulled away from his shoulder, which stretches the nerves, or his head is forced towards the shoulder which pinches the nerves. A common scenario is that an athlete's head is forced to the opposite side while going in to make a tackle or block during football. These injuries are fairly common especially in football players, wrestlers, and divers. Up to 70% of college football players have experienced a stinger by the end of their college careers.

Signs And Symptoms

Athletes with a stinger often describe a sensation of "electricity," warmth, discomfort, and/or numbness. They may often report arm weakness. Symptoms tend to be brief, lasting seconds to minutes. With more significant injury, symptoms can last hours or even days and weeks.

About This Chapter: "Stinger or Burner (brachial plexus injury from sports)," reprinted with permission from Ann & Robert H. Lurie Children's Hospital of Chicago (www.luriechildrens.org). © 2012. All rights reserved.

Diagnosis

Your doctor will usually be able to make the diagnosis based on a description of the way the injury occurred and your symptoms. A physical exam helps evaluate the extent of injury. Stingers do not cause significant neck pain or involvement of both arms so if you are experiencing these symptoms, your doctor will likely recommend additional testing to determine the cause. Doctors often recommend tests such as x-rays, nerve studies and/or MRI scans for patients who have multiple stingers.

Treatment

Most patients who experience a stinger will feel fine by the time after a few minutes. In patients with symptoms lasting more than a few hours, rest and anti-inflammatory medications, such as ibuprofen or naproxen, are the main interventions until the symptoms resolve on their own. Patients with prolonged symptoms need to be re-evaluated by a physician. Patients with frequent stingers may need further evaluation to rule out the possibility of underlying spinal column narrowing which could make return to contact sports unsafe.

Returning To Activity And Sports

No athlete should return to activity until the initial symptoms have resolved and arm strength has returned. If symptoms are very brief and arm strength is normal, athletes can often return to competition very quickly. However, if symptoms persist, as they do in 5–10% of cases, the athlete will need further evaluation prior to returning to their sports. Football players with recurrent stingers may benefit from the use of high shoulder pads or a "cowboy collar," which prevents the nerves from being stretched.

Preventing Stingers Or Burners

Proper equipment, use of good technique and neck strengthening exercises can make an athlete less likely to get stingers. For football players, "spearing"(attempting to make a tackle while leading with the crown of the head) and poor form tackling should be avoided. Shoulder pads must be fitted properly. As noted above, additional equipment such as a soft neck roll or 'cowboy collar' may help prevent stingers. Finally, players with recurrent stingers may benefit from physical therapy focusing on neck, shoulder, and back stretching and strengthening.

Chapter 46

Shoulder Injuries

Common Shoulder Problems

The most movable joint in the body, the shoulder is also one of the most potentially unstable joints. As a result, it is the site of many common problems. They include sprains, strains, dislocations, separations, tendinitis, bursitis, torn rotator cuffs, frozen shoulder, fractures, and arthritis.

According to the Centers for Disease Control and Prevention, nearly 1.5 million people in the United States visited an emergency room in 2006 for shoulder problems.

Structures Of The Shoulder

To better understand shoulder problems and how they occur, it helps to begin with an explanation of the shoulder's structure and how it functions (see Figure 39.2 on p. 214).

The shoulder joint is composed of three bones—the clavicle (collarbone), the scapula (shoulder blade), and the humerus (upper arm bone) (see diagram). Two joints facilitate shoulder movement. The acromioclavicular joint is located between the acromion (part of the scapula that forms the highest point of the shoulder) and the clavicle. The glenohumeral joint, commonly called the shoulder joint, is a ball-and-socket-type joint that helps move the shoulder forward and backward and allows the arm to rotate in a circular fashion or hinge out and up away from the body. (The "ball," or humerus, is the top, rounded portion of the upper arm bone; the "socket," or glenoid, is a dish-shaped part of the outer edge of the scapula into which

About This Chapter: From "Questions and Answers about Shoulder Problems," National Institute of Arthritis and Musculoskeletal and skin Diseases (www.niams.nih.gov), May 2010.

What's It Mean?

Acromioclavicular (AC) Joint: The joint of the shoulder located between the acromion (part of the scapula that forms the highest point of the shoulder) and the clavicle (collarbone).

Acromion: The part of the scapula (shoulder blade) that forms the highest point of the shoulder.

Arthrogram: A diagnostic test in which a contrast fluid is injected into the shoulder joint and an x-ray is taken to view the fluid's distribution in the joint. Leaking of fluid into an area where it does not belong may indicate a tear or opening.

Bursae: Filmy sac-like structures that permit smooth gliding between bone, muscle, and tendon. Two bursae cushion and protect the rotator cuff from the bony arch of the acromion.

Capsule: A soft tissue envelope that encircles the glenohumeral joint and is lined by a thin, smooth, synovial membrane.

Clavicle: The collarbone.

Corticosteroids: Powerful anti-inflammatory hormones made naturally in the body or manmade for use as medicine. Injections of corticosteroid drugs are sometimes used to treat inflammation in the shoulder.

Glenohumeral Joint: The joint where the rounded upper portion of the humerus (upper arm bone) joins the glenoid (socket in the shoulder blade). This is commonly referred to as the shoulder joint.

Glenoid: The dish-shaped part of the outer edge of the scapula into which the top end of the humerus fits to form the glenohumeral shoulder joint.

Humerus: The upper arm bone.

Impingement Syndrome: Squeezing of the rotator cuff, usually under the acromion.

Osteoarthritis: The most common form of arthritis. It is characterized by the breakdown of joint cartilage, leading to pain, stiffness, and disability.

Rotator Cuff: Composed of tendons that work with associated muscles, this structure holds the ball at the top of the humerus in the glenoid socket and provides mobility and strength to the shoulder joint.

Scapula: The shoulder blade.

Synovial Fluid: Lubricating fluid secreted by the synovial membrane that lines a joint.

Synovium: The membrane that lines the joint and secretes a lubricating liquid called synovial fluid.

Transcutaneous Electrical Nerve Stimulation (TENS): A technique that uses a small battery-operated unit to send electrical impulses to the nerves to block pain signals to the brain.

the ball fits.) The capsule is a soft tissue envelope that encircles the glenohumeral joint. It is lined by a thin, smooth synovial membrane.

In contrast to the hip joint, which more closely approximates a true ball-and-socket joint, the shoulder joint can be compared to a golf ball and tee, in which the ball can easily slip off the flat tee. Because the bones provide little inherent stability to the shoulder joint, it is highly dependent on surrounding soft tissues such as capsule ligaments and the muscles surrounding the rotator cuff to hold the ball in place. Whereas the hip joint is inherently quite stable because of the encircling bony anatomy, it also is relatively immobile. The shoulder, on the other hand, is relatively unstable but highly mobile, allowing an individual to place the hand in numerous positions. It is, in fact, one of the most mobile joints in the human body.

The bones of the shoulder are held in place by muscles, tendons, and ligaments. Tendons are tough cords of tissue that attach the shoulder muscles to bone and assist the muscles in moving the shoulder. Ligaments attach shoulder bones to each other, providing stability. For example, the front of the joint capsule is anchored by three glenohumeral ligaments. The rotator cuff is a structure composed of tendons that work along with associated muscles to hold the ball at the top of the humerus in the glenoid socket and provide mobility and strength to the shoulder joint. Two filmy sac-like structures called bursae permit smooth gliding between bones, muscles, and tendons. They cushion and protect the rotator cuff from the bony arch of the acromion.

Origins And Causes Of Shoulder Problems

The shoulder is easily injured because the ball of the upper arm is larger than the shoulder socket that holds it. To remain stable, the shoulder must be anchored by its muscles, tendons, and ligaments.

Although the shoulder is easily injured during sporting activities and manual labor, the primary source of shoulder problems appears to be the natural age-related degeneration of the surrounding soft tissues such as those found in the rotator cuff. The incidence of rotator cuff problems rises dramatically as a function of age and is generally seen among individuals who are more than 60 years old. Often, the dominant and nondominant arm will be affected to a similar degree. Overuse of the shoulder can lead to more rapid age-related deterioration.

Shoulder pain may be localized or may be felt in areas around the shoulder or down the arm. Disease within the body (such as gallbladder, liver, or heart disease, or disease of the cervical spine of the neck) also may generate pain that travels along nerves to the shoulder. However, these other causes of shoulder pain are beyond the scope of this chapter, which will focus on problems within the shoulder itself.

Diagnosing Shoulder Problems

As with any medical issue, a shoulder problem is generally diagnosed using a three-part process:

- **Medical history:** The patient tells the doctor about any injury or other condition that might be causing the pain.

- **Physical examination:** The doctor examines the patient to feel for injury and to discover the limits of movement, location of pain, and extent of joint instability.

- **Tests:** The doctor may order one or more of the tests listed below to make a specific diagnosis.

These tests may include the following:

- **Standard x-ray:** A familiar procedure in which low-level radiation is passed through the body to produce a picture called a radiograph. An x-ray is useful for diagnosing fractures or other problems of the bones. Soft tissues, such as muscles and tendons, do not show up on x-rays.

- **Arthrogram:** A diagnostic record that can be seen on an x-ray after injection of a contrast fluid into the shoulder joint to outline structures such as the rotator cuff. In disease or injury, this contrast fluid may either leak into an area where it does not belong, indicating a tear or opening, or be blocked from entering an area where there normally is an opening.

- **Ultrasound:** A noninvasive, patient-friendly procedure in which a small, hand-held scanner is placed on the skin of the shoulder. Just as ultrasound waves can be used to

---

Treat Shoulder Injuries With RICE (Rest, Ice, Compression, And Elevation)

If you injure a shoulder, try the following:

- **Rest:** Reduce or stop using the injured area for 48 hours.
- **Ice:** Put an ice pack on the injured area for 20 minutes at a time, four to eight times per day. Use a cold pack, ice bag, or a plastic bag filled with crushed ice that has been wrapped in a towel.
- **Compression:** Compress the area with bandages, such as an elastic wrap, to help stabilize the shoulder. This may help reduce the swelling.
- **Elevation:** Keep the injured area elevated above the level of the heart. Use a pillow to help elevate the injury.

If pain and stiffness persist, see a doctor.

visualize the fetus during pregnancy, they can also be reflected off the rotator cuff and other structures to form a high-quality image of them. The accuracy of ultrasound for the rotator cuff is particularly high.

- **MRI (magnetic resonance imaging):** A noninvasive procedure in which a machine with a strong magnet passes a force through the body to produce a series of cross-sectional images of the shoulder.

Other diagnostic tests, such as one that involves injecting an anesthetic into and around the shoulder joint, are discussed in detail in other parts of this chapter.

Specific Shoulder Problems, Symptoms, And Treatment

The symptoms of shoulder problems, as well as their diagnosis and treatment, vary widely, depending on the specific problem. The following is important information to know about some of the most common shoulder problems.

Dislocation

The shoulder joint is the most frequently dislocated major joint of the body. In a typical case of a dislocated shoulder, either a strong force pulls the shoulder outward (abduction) or extreme rotation of the joint pops the ball of the humerus out of the shoulder socket. Dislocation commonly occurs when there is a backward pull on the arm that either catches the muscles unprepared to resist or overwhelms the muscles. When a shoulder dislocates frequently, the condition is referred to as shoulder instability. A partial dislocation in which the upper arm bone is partially in and partially out of the socket is called a subluxation.

- **Signs And Symptoms:** The shoulder can dislocate either forward, backward, or downward. When the shoulder dislocates, the arm appears out of position. Other symptoms include pain, which may be worsened by muscle spasms, swelling, numbness, weakness, and bruising. Problems seen with a dislocated shoulder are tearing of the ligaments or tendons reinforcing the joint capsule and, less commonly, bone and/or nerve damage.

- **Diagnosis:** Doctors usually diagnose a dislocation by a physical examination; x-rays may be taken to confirm the diagnosis and to rule out a related fracture.

- **Treatment:** Doctors treat a dislocation by putting the ball of the humerus back into the joint socket, a procedure called a closed reduction. The arm is then stabilized for several weeks in a sling or a device called a shoulder immobilizer. Usually the doctor recommends resting the shoulder and applying ice three or four times a day. After pain and swelling have been controlled, the patient enters a rehabilitation program that includes exercises. The goal is to restore the range of motion of the shoulder, strengthen the muscles, and prevent future dislocations. These exercises may progress from simple motion to the use of weights.

After treatment and recovery, a previously dislocated shoulder may remain more susceptible to reinjury, especially in young, active individuals. Ligaments may have been stretched or torn, and the shoulder may tend to dislocate again. A shoulder that dislocates severely or often, injuring surrounding tissues or nerves, usually requires surgical repair to tighten stretched ligaments or reattach torn ones.

Sometimes the doctor performs surgery through a tiny incision into which a small scope (arthroscope) is inserted to observe the inside of the joint. After this procedure, called arthroscopic surgery, the shoulder is generally stabilized for about six weeks. Full recovery takes several months. In other cases, the doctor may repair the dislocation using a traditional open surgery approach.

Separation

A shoulder separation occurs where the collarbone (clavicle) meets the shoulder blade (scapula). When ligaments that hold the joint together are partially or completely torn, the outer end of the clavicle may slip out of place, preventing it from properly meeting the scapula. Most often, the injury is caused by a blow to the shoulder or by falling on an outstretched hand.

- **Signs And Symptoms:** Shoulder pain or tenderness and, occasionally, a bump in the middle of the top of the shoulder (over the acromioclavicular (AC) joint) are signs that a separation may have occurred.

- **Diagnosis:** Doctors may diagnose a separation by performing a physical examination. They may confirm the diagnosis and determine the severity of the separation by taking an x-ray. While the x-ray is being taken, the patient makes the separation more pronounced by holding a light weight that pulls on the muscles.

- **Treatment:** A shoulder separation is usually treated conservatively by rest and wearing a sling. Soon after injury, an ice bag may be applied to relieve pain and swelling. After a period of rest, a therapist helps the patient perform exercises that put the shoulder through its range of motion. Most shoulder separations heal within two or three months without further intervention. However, if ligaments are severely torn, surgical repair may be required to hold the clavicle in place. A doctor may wait to see if conservative treatment works before deciding whether surgery is required.

Torn Rotator Cuff

Rotator cuff tendons often become inflamed from overuse, aging, or a fall on an outstretched hand or another traumatic cause. Sports or occupations requiring repetitive overhead motion or heavy lifting can also place a significant strain on rotator cuff muscles and tendons. Over time, as a function of aging, tendons become weaker and degenerate. Eventually, this degeneration can lead to complete tears of both muscles and tendons. These tears are surprisingly common. In fact, a tear of the rotator cuff is not necessarily an abnormal situation in older individuals if there is no significant pain or disability. Fortunately, these tears do not lead to any pain or disability in most people. However, some individuals can develop very significant pain as a result of these tears and they may require treatment.

- **Signs And Symptoms:** Typically, a person with a rotator cuff injury feels pain over the deltoid muscle at the top and outer side of the shoulder, especially when the arm is raised or extended out from the side of the body. Motions like those involved in getting dressed can be painful. The shoulder may feel weak, especially when trying to lift the arm into a horizontal position. A person may also feel or hear a click or pop when the shoulder is moved. Pain or weakness on outward or inward rotation of the arm may indicate a tear in a rotator cuff tendon. The patient also feels pain when lowering the arm to the side after the shoulder is moved backward and the arm is raised.

- **Diagnosis:** A doctor may detect weakness but may not be able to determine from a physical examination where the tear is located. X-rays, if taken, may appear normal. An MRI or ultrasound can help detect a full tendon tear or a partial tendon tear.

- **Treatment:** Doctors usually recommend that patients with a rotator cuff injury rest the shoulder, apply heat or cold to the sore area, and take medicine to relieve pain and inflammation. Other treatments might be added, such as electrical stimulation of muscles and nerves, ultrasound, or a cortisone injection near the inflamed area of the rotator cuff. If surgery is not an immediate consideration, exercises are added to the treatment program to build flexibility and strength and restore the shoulder's function. If there is no improvement with these conservative treatments and functional impairment persists, the doctor may perform arthroscopic or open surgical repair of the torn rotator cuff.

Treatment for a torn rotator cuff usually depends on the severity of the injury, the age and health status of the patient, and the length of time a given patient may have had the condition. Patients with rotator cuff tendinitis or bursitis that does not include a complete tear of the tendon can usually be treated without surgery. Nonsurgical treatments include the use of anti-inflammatory medication and occasional steroid injections into the area of the inflamed rotator cuff, followed by rehabilitative rotator cuff strengthening exercises. These treatments are best undertaken with the guidance of a health care professional such as a physical therapist, who works in conjunction with the treating physician.

Surgical repair of rotator cuff tears is best for the following patients:

- Younger patients, especially those with small tears. Surgery leads to a high degree of successful healing and reduces concerns about the tear getting worse over time.

- Individuals whose rotator cuff tears are caused by an acute, severe injury. These people should seek immediate treatment that includes surgical repair of the tendon.

Generally speaking, individuals who are older and have had shoulder pain for a longer period of time can be treated with nonoperative measures even in the presence of a complete rotator cuff tear. These people are often treated similarly to those who have pain, but do not have a rotator cuff tear. Again, anti-inflammatory medication, use of steroid injections, and rehabilitative exercises can be very effective. When treated surgically, rotator cuff tears can be repaired by either arthroscopic or traditional open surgical techniques.

Frozen Shoulder (Adhesive Capsulitis)

As the name implies, movement of the shoulder is severely restricted in people with a "frozen shoulder." This condition, which doctors call adhesive capsulitis, is frequently caused by injury that leads to lack of use due to pain. Rheumatic disease progression and recent shoulder surgery can also cause frozen shoulder. Intermittent periods of use may cause inflammation. Adhesions (abnormal bands of tissue) grow between the joint surfaces, restricting motion. There is also a lack of synovial fluid, which normally lubricates the gap between the arm bone and socket to help the shoulder joint move. It is this restricted space between the capsule and ball of the humerus that distinguishes adhesive capsulitis from a less complicated painful, stiff shoulder. People with diabetes, stroke, lung disease, rheumatoid arthritis, and heart disease, or those who have been in an accident, are at a higher risk for frozen shoulder. People between the ages of 40 and 70 are most likely to experience it.

- **Signs And Symptoms:** With a frozen shoulder, the joint becomes so tight and stiff that it is nearly impossible to carry out simple movements, such as raising the arm. Stiffness and discomfort may worsen at night.

- **Diagnosis:** A doctor may suspect a frozen shoulder if a physical examination reveals limited shoulder movement. X-rays usually appear normal.

- **Treatment:** Treatment focuses on restoring joint movement and reducing shoulder pain. Usually, treatment begins with nonsteroidal anti-inflammatory drugs and the application of heat, followed by gentle stretching exercises, which may be performed in the home with the help of a physical therapist. These are the treatment of choice. In some cases, transcutaneous electrical nerve stimulation (TENS) with a small battery-operated unit may be used to reduce pain by blocking nerve impulses. If these measures are unsuccessful, an intra-articular injection of steroids into the glenoid humeral joint can result in marked improvement. In those rare people who do not improve from nonoperative measures, manipulation of the shoulder under general anesthesia and an arthroscopic procedure to cut the remaining adhesions can be highly effective in most cases.

Fracture

A fracture involves a partial or total crack through a bone. The break in a bone usually occurs as a result of an impact injury, such as a fall or blow to the shoulder. A fracture usually involves the clavicle or the neck (area below the ball) of the humerus.

- **Signs And Symptoms:** A shoulder fracture is usually accompanied by severe pain. There may be redness and bruising around the area. Sometimes the bones appear out of position.

- **Diagnosis:** X-rays can confirm the diagnosis and the degree of its severity.

- **Treatment:** When a fracture occurs, the doctor tries to bring the bones into a position that will promote healing and restore arm movement. If someone's clavicle is fractured, he or she must initially wear a strap and sling around the chest to keep the clavicle in place. After removing the strap and sling, the doctor will prescribe exercises to strengthen the shoulder and restore movement. Surgery is occasionally needed for certain clavicle fractures.

Fracture of the neck of the humerus is usually treated with a sling or shoulder stabilizer. If the bones are out of position, surgery may be necessary to reset them. Exercises are also part of restoring shoulder strength and motion.

Arthritis Of The Shoulder

Arthritis is a degenerative disease caused by either wear and tear of the cartilage (osteoarthritis) or an inflammation (rheumatoid arthritis) of one or more joints. Arthritis not only affects joints, but may also affect supporting structures such as muscles, tendons, and ligaments.

265

- **Signs And Symptoms:** The usual signs of arthritis of the shoulder are pain, particularly over the acromioclavicular joint, and a decrease in shoulder motion.

- **Diagnosis:** A doctor may suspect the patient has arthritis when there is both pain and swelling in the joint. The diagnosis may be confirmed by a physical examination and x-rays. Blood tests may be helpful for diagnosing rheumatoid arthritis, but other tests may be needed as well. Analysis of synovial fluid from the shoulder joint may be helpful in diagnosing some kinds of arthritis. Although arthroscopy permits direct visualization of damage to cartilage, tendons, and ligaments, and may confirm a diagnosis, it is usually done only if a repair procedure is to be performed.

- **Treatment:** Treatment of shoulder arthritis depends in part on the type of arthritis. Osteoarthritis of the shoulder is usually treated with nonsteroidal anti-inflammatory drugs, such as aspirin and ibuprofen. Rheumatoid arthritis may require physical therapy and additional medications such as corticosteroids.

When nonoperative treatment of arthritis of the shoulder fails to relieve pain or improve function, or when there is severe wear and tear of the joint causing parts to loosen and move out of place, shoulder joint replacement (arthroplasty) may provide better results. In this operation, a surgeon replaces the shoulder joint with an artificial ball for the top of the humerus and a cap (glenoid) for the scapula. Passive shoulder exercises (where someone else moves the arm to rotate the shoulder joint) are started soon after surgery. Patients begin exercising on their own about three to six weeks after surgery. Eventually, stretching and strengthening exercises become a major part of the rehabilitation program. The success of the operation often depends on the condition of rotator cuff muscles prior to surgery and the degree to which the patient follows the exercise program.

Chapter 47

Elbow Injuries

Little League, Golfer's Or Javelin Thrower's Elbow (Medial Epicondylitis)

This is an irritation and inflammation of the medial epicondyle (the inside part of the elbow/forearm on the pinkie side). This injury is usually caused by sports activities that require repeated forceful flexion of the wrist. The most common offending activities are golfing or throwing. Medial epicondylitis/Little League elbow is common among young pitchers. While many people attribute Little League elbow to throwing specialty pitches such as curveballs, the most common cause is overuse from throwing too much.

Too often, young players throw quite a few pitches in practices or games. They will then play other positions that require throwing. This is further aggravated by playing catch on off days. The result is cumulative overuse. This is irritated further by poor or faulty mechanics and pitchers who are skeletally and muscularly immature, have poor shoulder or elbow flexibility, and those who tend to use excessive wrist flexion in order to try to spin the baseball to make it curve.

Tennis Elbow (Lateral Epicondylitis)

Tennis elbow is an irritation and inflammation of the lateral epicondyle (the outside part of the elbow/forearm on the thumb side). This injury is usually caused by sports activities that involve repeated forceful extension or twisting of the wrist. This is often seen when tennis players have bad mechanics with their backhand strokes or use rackets with grips that are too large or that are strung too tightly.

Signs and symptoms of epicondylitis usually involve pain/point tenderness around the epicondyles or may radiate down the arm with some mild swelling. These are initially present only after activity. As the condition worsens, the pain occurs during activity. If left unattended, constant pain ensues.

More Severe Elbow Injuries

Commonly caused by more severe hyperextension or valgus stresses, more severe elbow injuries can occur acutely if the mild symptoms of tendonitis or epicondylitis are ignored.

Sprains of the elbow usually involve damage to the ulnar collateral ligament (UCL) at the inner aspect of the elbow. There can also be a disruption to the growth plate of the elbow in young athletes. A severe overuse injury can result in bony destruction at the outer part of the elbow. All of these can be very debilitating.

A tear or rupture of the UCL ligament normally requires surgery, which is most commonly known to baseball players as "Tommy John surgery." Growth plate injury can require prolonged immobilization. Bony destruction can require surgery and could be a career-ending injury. For these reasons, it is important to take elbow pain seriously.

Keep these things in mind:

- Follow the pain closely
- Rest and begin conservative measures at the onset of symptoms (see below)
- Seek medical care if pain persists or worsens
- Never "play through the pain"
- Evaluate equipment, technique, strength and flexibility as possible underlying causes of pain
- Avoid having pitchers play positions requiring long, hard and/or repetitive throwing (outfield, left side of infield) on off days
- Keep a careful pitch count on pitchers

Conservative Treatments

- Rest
- Moist heat followed by stretching then ice massage
- Ice massage after activity

- Ibuprofen, Advil, or other non-steroidal anti-inflammatory drugs (NSAIDs), as prescribed by a physician (do not use before exercise—this covers up the pain and gives a false sense of wellness)

- Bracing, applied just below the point of maximum pain

- Gentle massage

- Decrease or elimination of the activity that caused the injury until symptoms improve

Athletes can continue to condition and perform non-painful activities during recovery. Once pain-free, athletes can gradually return to their sport, as pain allows. Seek care from your athletic trainer or physician if pain is severe or does not respond to conservative measures.

Chapter 48

Hand And Wrist Injuries

With so many bones, ligaments, tendons, and joints keeping hands and wrists working, there is ample opportunity for injury. In fact, injuries to the hand and wrists are some of the most common ailments facing athletes. If managed properly, however, most athletes can expect their injury to heal without any significant long-term disability.

What are the most common sports-related hand and wrist injuries?

There are a number of injuries that may occur in an athlete's hands or wrists. They can be classified into two main categories: traumatic (acute) and overuse (chronic).

Traumatic injuries are more likely to occur in athletes who participate in sports that require higher levels of contact (that is, football, hockey, or wrestling), whereas overuse injuries result in athletes who participate in sports that require them to "overdo" a particular movement (that is, baseball, tennis, or golf).

Some common traumatic injuries in athletes include joint dislocations, sprains, muscle strains, broken bones, tendon inflammation, and ligament tears. The most common fracture injury in the athletic population occurs in the fingers.

Overuse injuries are stress-induced and include tendon inflammation and dislocation, nerve injury, and over use stress fractures. Long-term disability is less likely to occur from overuse injuries than from traumatic injuries. However, if left untreated, an athlete's sports performance may be significantly diminished. Surgical treatment may be required if an injury persists.

What should I do if I injure my hand or wrist?

Should you sustain a hand or wrist injury while participating in a game where an attending team physician is not present, seek immediate medical care if any of the following symptoms are present:

- Severe pain

- Severe swelling

- Numbness

- Coldness or grayness in the finger, hand, or wrist

- Abnormal twisting or bending of the finger or hand

- A clicking, grating, or shifting noise while moving your finger, hand, or wrist

- Bleeding that does not slow and persists for more than 15 minutes

Contact your physician during regular practice hours if mild wrist pain, bruising, or swelling after an injury persists and does not improve after two weeks.

For minor hand injuries, home treatment, including rest, ice, compression, and elevation to the effected limb can help relieve pain, swelling, and stiffness. An anti-inflammatory medication such as ibuprofen or naproxen may also be taken to help with the pain and inflammation.

What treatment options are available for hand and wrist injuries?

Treatment depends on the location, type, duration, and severity of the injury. While surgery is needed for some injuries, such as ligament tears, medication, "buddy-taping" (taping the injured finger to a neighboring one for support), splints, braces, casts, or physical therapy may be used as a treatment option. Your doctor will determine the best option, taking into consideration short and long-term damage; deformities, and stiffness.

How can I prevent a hand or wrist injury?

Wearing wrist guards, gloves, and stretching are just a few ways to help prevent a traumatic hand or wrist injury. You can prevent overuse injuries by taking breaks to rest the hands or wrists, using proper posture and technique, and utilizing protective equipment.

Common Hand And Wrist Injuries

Jammed Finger

- **Causes/Description:** Striking the end of the finger while fully extended
- **Symptoms:** Pain, swelling at the joint, difficult to bend, tenderness over the joint
- **Treatment:** Ice, rest, buddy tape to adjacent finger
- **Return To Play:** As tolerated with buddy tape

Finger Fracture

- **Causes/Description:** Force of contact overwhelms strength of bone (ball, ground, helmet)
- **Symptoms:** Pain, tenderness over the bone, deformity may be present
- **Treatment:** Ice, splint, doctor evaluation, x-rays
- **Return To Play:** Only after proper evaluation, realignment from a physician, and wearing appropriate protection until healed

Mallet Finger

- **Causes/Description:** Impact on tip of finger leads to rupture of tendon that holds fingertip straight
- **Symptoms:** Unable to hold small joint at fingertip out straight, tender just behind nail
- **Treatment:** Doctor evaluation, splinting finger in full extension eight weeks
- **Return To Play:** May return as tolerated in splint which must be worn at all times for eight weeks

Nail Bed Injury

- **Causes/Description:** Impact or crushing injury on top of nail
- **Symptoms:** Blood under nail, tender, may represent tear in nailbed under nail
- **Treatment:** If blood covers more than 50% of nail, need doctor evaluation may need repair of nail bed
- **Return To Play:** As tolerated

Finger Dislocation

- **Causes/Description:** Force on finger overwhelms ligaments and joint displaces
- **Symptoms:** Most common at middle joint of finger, with visible displacement
- **Treatment:** Relocation of joint best performed by doctor, may require local anesthesia and x-ray evaluation. May require surgery.
- **Return To Play:** After proper evaluation, use buddy tape or splint as determined by physician

Tendon Tear "Jersey Finger"

- **Causes/Description:** Force of grasp with object (jersey) pulling away, ruptures tendon
- **Symptoms:** Most commonly seen in ring finger, unable to flex the joint at finger tip
- **Treatment:** Needs medical evaluation within 24–48 hours, requires surgery, possibly within 10 days
- **Return To Play:** Only after surgical repair is fully healed. Early return to play places the athlete at risk of long-term problems with finger function and motion

Wrist Bone Fracture "Scaphoid"

- **Causes/Description:** Fall on outstretched hand
- **Symptoms:** Pain with wrist motion, tenderness in wrist at the base of thumb
- **Treatment:** Needs doctor evaluation may require special x-ray (CT scan). May require surgery.
- **Return To Play:** Not allowed until thorough evaluation by physician. If fracture present may be able to return with proper protection (cast) which is worn until healed.

Wrist Ligament Tear

- **Causes/Description:** Impaction or twisting injury of wrist
- **Symptoms:** Pain in wrist with gripping rotation of wrist
- **Treatment:** Needs physician evaluation, x-rays, possible MRI
- **Return To Play:** Not allowed until thorough evaluation by physician. Evaluation and early treatment can prevent long-term problems.

Ulnar Collateral Ligament Tear "Skiers Thumb"

- **Causes/Description:** Tear of ligament that stabilizes the thumb with grasping
- **Symptoms:** Pain and instability of thumb with grasping objects
- **Treatment:** Needs physician evaluation, x-rays, may need surgery or casting
- **Return To Play:** May return to play in cast protection.

Tendonitis

- **Causes/Description:** Repetitive activity of one specific movement
- **Symptoms:** Tenderness over the tendon may feel "grading" over tendon with finger or wrist motion
- **Treatment:** Rest, ice, limitation of repetitive motion, nonsteroidal anti-inflammatory drugs (NSAIDs)
- **Return To Play:** As tolerated

Stress Fractures

- **Causes/Description:** Repetitive activity overcomes strength of bones and leads to small fractures
- **Symptoms:** Pain with activity, most commonly in lower extremities (running, jumping)
- **Treatment:** Physician evaluation, x-rays, bone scans, may need casting, surgery, must have rest, nutritional evaluation
- **Return To Play:** Must rest and cease offending activity until fully healed. May need bone growth stimulator, casting, surgery

Growth Plate Stress

- **Causes/Description:** Over stressing bone of still growing children, most commonly seen in gymnastics (wrist bone), baseball pitchers (shoulder, elbow)
- **Symptoms:** Persistent pain, tenderness swelling over growing bone, bone pain/tenderness
- **Treatment:** Physician evaluation rest, ice, must cease offending activity
- **Return To Play:** Athlete cannot return to play until fully healed as growing problems can have long-term problems

Chapter 49

Groin Injuries

It was late in the third period of Wayne's fourth hockey game in five days, and he was exhausted, but he wasn't going to let it show. He was still going all out and sprinting after every loose puck. But on one play, he was skating fast and tried to make a sudden change in direction when he felt a sharp pain in his right groin and could barely make it off the ice.

The next day Wayne's groin felt tight and painful, and there appeared to be some swelling in the area, so he went to see a doctor. The doctor asked some questions, examined him, and told Wayne he had a grade 2 groin strain.

What is a groin strain?

A groin strain—also known as a groin pull—is a partial or complete tear of one or more of the muscles that help you squeeze your legs together.

There are five of these muscles, called the adductor muscles: The pectineus, adductor brevis and adductor longus (the short adductors) run from your pelvis to your thighbone. The gracilis and adductor magnus (long adductors) run from your pelvis to your knee.

Groin strains are a common injury in hockey and skiing, as well as sports like football and track and field that require running or jumping. They can range from grade 1, which is a mild injury with few symptoms and a short recovery time, to grade 3, which is a complete or nearly complete tear of a groin muscle.

About This Chapter: "Groin Strain," April 2011, reprinted with permission from www.kidshealth.org. Copyright © 2011 The Nemours Foundation. This information was provided by KidsHealth, one of the largest resources online for medically reviewed health information written for parents, kids, and teens. For more articles like this one, visit www.KidsHealth.org or www.TeensHealth.org.

What are the symptoms of a groin strain?

The symptoms of a groin strain vary somewhat depending on the grade of the strain. All groin strains will cause pain and tenderness in the affected area, and many will hurt when you bring your legs together or raise your knee. If a strain is severe, you may feel a popping or snapping sensation during the injury and severe pain afterward.

Here's what you'll likely notice for different grades of groin sprain:

- **Grade 1:** Mild pain that may not be noticeable until after you finish exercising, followed by tightness and tenderness. With this type of strain, a person probably won't have trouble walking, and activity will usually not be limited.

- **Grade 2:** Moderate pain and tightness in the groin, along with some minor swelling and bruising. With a grade 2 strain, the leg may feel weak, and you'll probably feel increased pain when you stretch the muscle. Walking may be affected and running can be difficult.

- **Grade 3:** Severe pain, considerable swelling and bruising, and an inability to squeeze the legs together. Someone who's had a complete tear might be able to feel a gap in the muscle. Walking will be very difficult.

How is a groin strain diagnosed?

If you see a doctor for a strained groin, he or she will ask about your symptoms and what you were doing when the injury happened. The doctor will examine the affected area to check for swelling, bruising, and tenderness—and to rule out another condition with similar symptoms, such as a sports hernia. In rare instances, the doctor may send you for an MRI scan to determine the extent of the tear.

The doctor will grade your strain. Grade 1 means that less than 10% of the muscle fibers are torn. Grade 2 strains are those where 10% to 90% of the fibers are torn. (Because of the big range in grade 2 strains, a doctor might grade strains on a scale from 2- to 2+.) Grade 3 means that the muscle is either completely or almost completely torn or ruptured.

What causes a groin strain?

Groin strains usually happen when the adductor muscles get stretched too far and begin to tear. Strains also can occur when the adductor muscles suddenly have stress put on them when they aren't ready for it (as when someone doesn't go through a proper warm-up before playing) or when there's a direct blow to one of the muscles.

Some of the risk factors that can make a groin pull more likely include:

- **Sports That Require Sprinting, Bursts Of Speed, Or Sudden Changes In Direction:** Examples include track and field, particularly the hurdle and long jump events, basketball, soccer, football, rugby, hockey, and skiing.

- **Tight Muscles:** Muscles that haven't been warmed up and stretched properly are more likely to tear. This is especially true in cold weather.

- **Poor Conditioning Or Fatigue:** Weak muscles are less able to handle the stress of exercise, and muscles that are tired lose some of their ability to absorb energy, making them more likely to get injured.

- **Returning To Activities Too Quickly After An Injury:** Groin strains need time and rest to heal completely. Trying to come back from a strain too soon will make you more likely to injure your groin again.

How can you prevent a groin strain?

The main thing you can do to help prevent a strained groin is to warm up and stretch before any exercise or intense physical activity. Jog in place for a minute or two, or do some jumping jacks to get your muscles warmed up. Then do some dynamic stretching (ask a coach, athletic trainer, or sports medicine specialist to show you how to do this type of stretching).

Some other things you can do to try and prevent groin strains include:

- **Keep Your Muscles Strong And Flexible Year Round:** Get regular exercise (even in the off-season) and follow a good stretching program.

- **Increase The Duration And Intensity Of Your Exercise Slowly:** A good rule of thumb is to make sure you add no more than 10% each week to the miles you run or the time you spend playing a sport.

- **If You Feel Pain In Your Groin, Stop Your Exercise Or Activity Immediately:** If you're worried that you might have strained your groin, give it time to rest, and don't resume your activity until you are pain-free and your injured adductor muscles feel as strong as the uninjured ones.

- **Learn And Use Proper Technique When Exercising Or Playing Sports:** Your coach or trainer can give you pointers and tips for your sport.

- **Wear Shoes Or Skates That Fit Correctly And Offer Your Feet Good Support:** Replace shoes with a new pair when they show signs of wear or the soles start to lose their shape. The same goes for skates—you want to be sure they maintain good ankle and foot support.

How should you treat a groin strain?

Most groin strains will heal on their own in time. The key is patience because it can take a while to fully recover. Even if you feel better, a groin strain may not be fully healed, and you risk starting over with the injury if you get back in the game too soon.

Mild to moderate strains will need around four to eight weeks of proper rehabilitation. More severe strains will take longer to heal. Only the most severe muscle tears require surgery. To treat a groin strain, take these steps and be sure to follow your doctor's advice:

- **Take Anti-Inflammatory Medications:** Painkillers such as ibuprofen and acetaminophen can help relieve pain and reduce swelling in the affected area.

- **Follow A Rehabilitation Exercise Program:** Once the pain and swelling go away, talk with your doctor about a rehabilitation and exercise program to improve strength and flexibility in your groin. This type of program is an absolute must when it comes to groin strains. Without this step, an injury can last and really interfere with an athlete's performance.

In the event of a complete muscle tear, or if the treatments above don't help after a few months, a doctor may call for surgery as a last resort. In this case, a surgeon will either attempt to reattach a torn tendon to a bone or stitch torn muscle tissue back together. Some people are able to return to previous levels of activity after surgery. A doctor will only choose this option as a last resort—and fortunately it's rarely needed.

Use The RICE Formula

Rest: Limit the amount of walking and physical activity you do. If you have a lot of pain, you may need to use crutches.

Ice: Use a bag of ice or cold compress to help reduce swelling. This should be done as soon as possible after the injury and then three or four times a day for 20 to 30 minutes at a time until the swelling and pain are gone.

Compress: Use bandages or wraps to help support your groin and keep the swelling down.

Elevate: This may be difficult with a groin strain, but if you are lying down, try putting pillows under your pelvis to elevate your hips and thighs.

Most groin strains heal on their own as long as the athlete follows a doctor's or physical therapist's instructions about rest and rehabilitation. The key is patience.

It can be frustrating to wait the full time needed to get back in the game, but this is one kind of injury you don't want to mess with. Get your doctor's signoff for any kind of exercise.

The good news is that once you're fully healed, you should be able to play as you used to.

Chapter 50

Testicular Injuries

It hurts to even think about it. A baseball takes an unexpected bounce when you're crouched and waiting to field a grounder, an opponent misses a kick on the soccer field and his foot has only one place to go, or you're speeding along on your bike and you hit a big bump. All result in one really painful thing—a shot to the testicles, one of the most tender areas on a guy's body.

Testicular injuries are relatively uncommon, but guys should be aware that they can happen. So how can you avoid injury?

Why Do Testicular Injuries Happen And What Can You Do?

If you're a guy who plays sports, likes to lift weights and exercise a lot, or leads an all-around active life, you've probably come to find out that the testicles are kind of vulnerable and can be injured in a variety of ways.

Because they hang in a sac outside the body (the scrotum), the testicles are not protected by bones and muscles like other parts of your reproductive system and most of your other organs. Also, the location of the testicles makes them prime targets to be accidentally struck on the playing field or injured during strenuous exercise and activity.

The good news is that because the testicles are loosely attached to the body and are made of a spongy material, they're able to absorb most collisions without permanent damage. Testicles, although sensitive, can bounce back pretty quickly and minor injuries rarely have long-term effects. Also, sexual function or sperm production will most likely not be affected if you have a testicular injury.

You'll definitely feel pain if your testicles are struck or kicked, and you might also feel nauseated for a short time. If it's a minor testicular injury, the pain should gradually subside in less than an hour and any other symptoms should go away.

In the meantime, you can do a few things to help yourself feel better such as take pain relievers, lie down, gently support the testicles with supportive underwear, and apply ice packs to the area. At any rate, it's a good idea to avoid strenuous activity for a while and take it easy for a few days.

However, if the pain doesn't subside or you experience extreme pain that lasts longer than an hour; if you have swelling or bruising of the scrotum or a puncture of the scrotum or testicle; if you continue to have nausea and vomiting; or if you develop a fever, get to a doctor immediately. These are symptoms of a much more serious injury that needs to be addressed as soon as possible.

Serious Testicular Injuries

Examples of serious testicular injury are testicular torsion and testicular rupture. In the case of testicular torsion, the testicle twists around, cutting off its blood supply. This can happen due to a serious trauma to the testicles, strenuous activity, or even for no apparent reason.

Testicular torsion isn't common, but when it does happen, it most often occurs in guys ages 12 to 18. If it occurs, it is crucial to see a doctor as soon as possible—within six hours of the time the pain starts. Unfortunately, after six hours, there is a much greater possibility that complications could result, including reduced sperm production or the loss of the testicle. The problem may be fixed by a doctor manually untwisting the testicle. If that doesn't work, surgery will be necessary.

Testicular rupture can also happen, but it is a rare type of testicular trauma. This can happen when the testicle receives a forceful direct blow or when the testicle is crushed against the pubic bone (the bone that forms the front of the pelvis), causing blood to leak into the scrotum. Testicular rupture, like testicular torsion and other serious injuries to the testicles, causes extreme pain, swelling in the scrotum, nausea, and vomiting. To fix the problem, surgery is necessary to repair the ruptured testicle.

Seeing A Doctor

If you have to see a doctor, he or she will first need to know how long you have been experiencing pain and how severe your discomfort is. To rule out a hernia or other problem as the cause of the pain, the doctor will examine your abdomen and groin.

In addition, the doctor will look at your scrotum for swelling, color, and damage to the skin and examine the testicle itself. Because infections of the reproductive system or urinary tract can sometimes cause similar pain, your doctor may do a urine test to rule out a urinary tract infection or infection of the reproductive organs.

Preventing Testicular Injuries

It's wise to take precautions to avoid testicular injuries, especially if you play sports, exercise a lot, or just live an all-around active life. Here are some tips to keep your testicles safe and sound:

- **Protect Your Testicles:** Always wear an athletic cup or athletic supporter when playing sports or participating in strenuous activity. Athletic cups are usually made of hard plastic, are worn over the groin area, and provide a good degree of shielding and safety for the testicles. Cups are best used when participating in sports where your testicles might get hit or kicked, like football, hockey, soccer, or karate. An athletic supporter, or jock strap, is basically a cloth pouch that you wear to keep your testicles close to your body. Athletic supporters are best used when participating in strenuous exercise, cycling, or doing any heavy lifting.

- **Check Your Fit:** Make sure the athletic cup and/or athletic supporter is the right size. Safety equipment that's too small or too big won't protect you as effectively.

- **Keep Your Doctor Informed:** If you play sports, you probably have regular physical exams by a doctor. If you experience testicular pain even occasionally, talk to your doctor about it.

- **Be Aware Of The Risks Of Your Sport Or Activity:** If you play a sport or participate in an activity with a high risk of injury, talk to your coach or doctor about any additional protective gear you should use.

Participating in sports and living an active life are great ways to stay fit and relieve stress. But it's important to make sure your testicles are protected. When you're exercising or playing sports, make sure that using protective gear is part of your routine and you'll be able to play hard without fear of testicular injury.

Chapter 51

Hip Injuries

Apophysitis Of The Pelvis/Hip

An apophysis is a growth plate that provides a point for a muscle to attach. Growth plates are made up of cartilage cells, which are softer and more vulnerable to injury than mature bone. When the muscle attached to the apophysis is excessively tight or overworked, it can put increased tension and stress on the apophysis, which results in irritation and inflammation, a condition called apophysitis. There are several apophyses at the hip and pelvis that can be affected. Pelvic/hip apophysitis most commonly affects adolescents between 14 and 18 years of age.

How It Occurs

Apophysitis is an overuse injury that typically occurs after repetitive activities of the muscles attached to the apophysis. Adolescents with excessively tight hip and thigh muscles are more prone to pelvis/hip apophysitis. The apophyses most commonly affected are the anterior superior iliac spine (ASIS), the anterior inferior iliac spine (AIIS) and the iliac crest. The muscles that attach to these apophyses flex the hip and rotate and twist the pelvis and trunk. Apophysitis of the pelvis/hip usually affects runners, sprinters, dancers, soccer players, and ice hockey players.

Signs And Symptoms

There may be dull pain in the groin or the front or side of the hip that worsens with activity. There will be tenderness over the injury site and sometimes some swelling. Apophysitis may be mistaken for a muscle strain.

About This Chapter: "Apophysitis of the Pelvis/Hip" and "Internal Snapping Hip Syndrome," reprinted with permission from Ann & Robert H. Lurie Children's Hospital of Chicago (www.luriechildrens.org). © 2012. All rights reserved.

Diagnosis

Your doctor will review your symptoms and examine the injured area. Your doctor may order an x-ray to determine whether there has been a fracture to the apophysis.

Treatment

The doctor will recommend rest from irritating activities until the pain and tenderness go away. Ice should be applied to the painful area for 15–20 minutes as often as every two to three hours until the pain goes away. After daily activities can be tolerated without pain, gentle stretching and strengthening the muscles that attach to the affected apophysis (the hip flexors and abdominal muscles) can begin. Once flexibility and strength have improved, sport-specific activities such as jogging can begin with gradual progress to full activity.

Return To Activity And Sports

The goal is to return to sport or activity as quickly and safely as possible. Returning to activities too soon or playing with pain may cause the injury to worsen. This could lead to chronic pain and difficulty with sports. Everyone recovers from injury at a different rate. Returning to sport or activity will be determined by how soon an individual's injured area recovers, not by how many days or weeks it has been since the injury occurred. In general, the longer an individual has symptoms before starting treatment the longer it will take to get better. Safe return to sport and activity may happen when each of the following is true (begin at the top of the list and progress to the bottom):

- Full range of motion in the injured leg compared to the uninjured leg

- Regained normal strength in the injured leg compared to the uninjured leg

- Ability to jog straight ahead without pain or limping

- Ability to sprint straight ahead without pain or limping

- Ability to perform 45-degree cuts, first at half-speed, then at full-speed

- Ability to perform 20-yard figure-of-eight runs

- Ability to perform 90-degree cut

- Ability to perform 10-yard figure-of-eight runs

- Ability to jump on both legs without pain and can hop on the injured leg without pain

Preventing Apophysitis Of The Pelvis/Hip

- Perform a proper warm-up before starting any activity. Ten minutes of light jogging, cycling, or calisthenics before practice will increase circulation to cold muscles, making them more pliable so that they put less stress and tension on their attachment sites (apophyses). Studies have shown that an active warm-up is associated with better athletic performance than a warm-up that consists only of static stretching.

- Stretch tight muscle groups. The ideal time to stretch is after your workout. Be sure to include all major muscle groups. Hold each stretch for 30 seconds. Don't bounce.

- Do not play through pain. Pain is a sign of injury, stress, or overuse. Rest is required to allow time for the injured area to heal. If pain does not resolve after a couple days of rest, consult your physician. The sooner an injury is identified, the sooner proper treatment can begin. The result is shorter healing time and faster return to sport.

Internal Snapping Hip Syndrome

When there is a snapping sound that occurs with flexion or extension of the hip, it is called internal snapping hip syndrome, or coxa saltans internal type. The snapping sound comes from the tendon of the iliopsoas (hip flexor) muscle as it moves through its normal motion across the bony structures of the hip joint (iliopectineal eminence, femoral head, or lesser trochanter). Internal snapping hip syndrome is usually painless, but for some people it can become painful. This condition typically affects athletes in their mid-adolescence or adulthood. Females seem to be affected more frequently. It is most commonly seen activities that involve repetitive hip flexion, such as dance, soccer, gymnastics, and running.

How It Occurs

Internal snapping hip syndrome is an overuse injury that is caused by repetitive flexion and external rotation of the hip. Athletes with tight hip flexors and unbalanced strength in their pelvic, hip, and abdominal muscles are more prone to this condition.

Signs And Symptoms

A snapping or clicking sound is heard with flexion or extension of the hip. Athletes are usually able to voluntarily reproduce the snapping sound by extending and rotating their hip. The snapping is usually painless, but can sometimes generate pain in the groin area. Symptoms tend to worsen with activity.

Diagnosis

Your doctor will ask about your symptoms and examine your hip and pelvis. Findings that suggest internal snapping hip syndrome include tenderness over the iliopsoas tendon, tightness in the iliopsoas muscle, and a snapping sound with hip extension and rotation. An x-ray may be performed to rule out more serious causes of hip pain. An ultrasound can sometimes demonstrate the movement of the iliopsoas tendon over the iliopectineal eminence but it is not required for making the diagnosis.

Treatment

Internal snapping hip syndrome that is painless does not require any treatment. Painful cases are treated with temporary rest from irritating activities until the pain resolves. A short course of anti-inflammatory medicines might also be prescribed. Physical therapy that includes stretching and soft tissue massage for the iliopsoas muscle and strengthening of all the hip muscles can help to reduce pain and speed return to activity. Once pain has resolved and flexibility and strength have improved, gradual return to sports and activities is allowed.

Returning To Activity And Sports

The goal is to return you to your sport or activity as quickly and safely as possible. If you return to activities too soon or play with pain, the injury may worsen. This could lead to chronic pain and difficulty with sports. Everyone recovers from injury at a different rate. Return to your sport or activity will be determined by how soon your injured area recovers, not by how many days or weeks it has been since the injury occurred. In general, the longer you have symptoms before starting treatment the longer it will take to get better. You may return safely to your sport or activity when each of the following is true (begin at the top of the list and progress to the bottom):

- You have full range of motion in the injured leg compared to the uninjured leg.
- You have regained normal strength in the injured leg compared to the uninjured leg.
- You are able to jog straight ahead without pain or limping.
- You are able to sprint straight ahead without pain or limping.
- You are able to do 45-degree cuts, first at half-speed, then at full-speed.
- You can do 20-yard figure-of-eight runs.
- You can do 90-degree cuts.

- You can do 10-yard figure-of-eight runs.

- You are able to jump on both legs without pain and can hop on the injured leg without pain.

Preventing Internal Snapping Hip Syndrome

- Perform a proper warm-up before starting any activity. Ten minutes of light jogging, cycling, or calisthenics before exercise will increase circulation to cold muscles, making them more pliable and less prone to injury.

- Stretch your iliopsoas muscle regularly (1–2 times per day). The ideal time to stretch is after your muscles are warmed-up. Hold each stretch for 30 seconds. Don't bounce.

- Maintain balanced strength in the hip muscles.

- Do not play through pain. Pain is a sign of injury, stress, or overuse. Rest is required to allow time for the injured area to heal. If pain does not resolve after a couple days of rest, consult your physician. The sooner an injury is identified, the sooner proper treatment can begin. The result is shorter healing time and faster return to sport.

Chapter 52

Knee Injuries

Anterior Cruciate Ligament (ACL) Injury

Ligaments are ropes that hold bones together. The knee has four major ligaments. Two collateral ligaments run along the sides of the knee. There are also two cruciate ligaments which cross in the middle of the knee (the term *cruciate* comes from the Latin word for cross). The anterior cruciate ligament (ACL) is an important stabilizing ligament of the knee. It courses from back of the femur (thigh bone) to the front of the tibia (shin bone). The primary function is to keep the tibia from sliding forward, especially with twisting or pivoting motions.

How It Occurs

ACL injuries can occur by a variety of mechanisms. ACL injuries can be due to physical contact, occurring with a blow to the outer aspect of the knee (for example, getting tackled from the side in football). Non-contact injuries can also cause an ACL tear. This type of injury occurs when an athlete is running or jumping and then suddenly slows and changes direction or twists.

Bones And Cartilage

Signs And Symptoms

You may feel or hear a "pop" in your knee at the time of injury. Most people with an ACL tear feel an initial sharp pain and have significant swelling which develops in the first few

About This Chapter: This chapter begins with "Anterior Cruciate Ligament (ACL) Injury," "Patellar Dislocation (Kneecap Dislocation)," and "Patellofemoral Pain Syndrome (Runner's Knee)," reprinted with permission from Ann & Robert H. Lurie Children's Hospital of Chicago (www.luriechildrens.org). © 2012. All rights reserved. The concluding questions and answers are excerpted from "Questions and Answers about Knee Problems," National Institute of Arthritis and Musculoskeletal and Skin Diseases, May 2011.

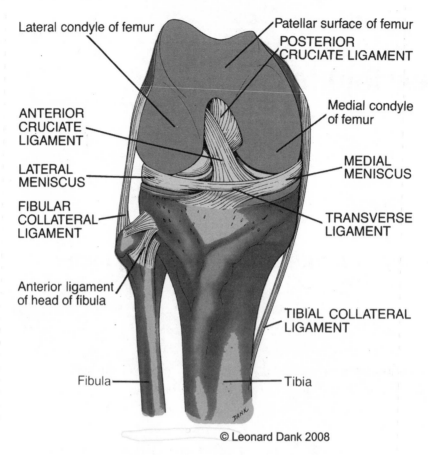

Lateral condyle of femur

Patellar surface of femur

POSTERIOR
CRUCIATE LIGAMENT

ANTERIOR
CRUCIATE
LIGAMENT

Medial condyle
of femur

LATERAL
MENISCUS

MEDIAL
MENISCUS

FIBULAR
COLLATERAL
LIGAMENT

TRANSVERSE
LIGAMENT

Anterior ligament
of head of fibula

TIBIAL COLLATERAL
LIGAMENT

Fibula

Tibia

© Leonard Dank 2008

Figure 52.1. Knee: Cruciate Ligaments. (© Leonard Dank 2008; reprinted with permission).

hours after injury. Swelling can make the knee feel "full" and stiff. Over days or weeks, the swelling resolves; pain generally improves as well. After the initial phase of healing, athletes are often left with a feeling that their knee is unstable and have a sense that it will "give out" with certain motions. Movements such as squatting, pivoting, walking down stairs, and moving to the side are most often affected.

Risk Factors

Women engaging in pivoting sports, such as soccer and basketball, sustain non-contact ACL injuries at higher rates than men performing the same activities. There are many possible explanations for this finding. Girls use and control their muscles in a different way than boys

294

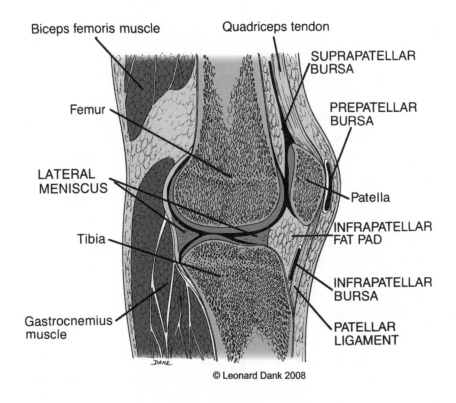

Biceps femoris muscle   Quadriceps tendon

SUPRAPATELLAR BURSA

PREPATELLAR BURSA

Femur

LATERAL MENISCUS

Patella

INFRAPATELLAR FAT PAD

Tibia

INFRAPATELLAR BURSA

Gastrocnemius muscle

PATELLAR LIGAMENT

© Leonard Dank 2008

Figure 52.2. Knee Joint. (© Leonard Dank 2008; reprinted with permission).

do which seems to contribute to the risk of ACL injuries. Other risk factors for ACL injuries include increased knee joint laxity (looseness), weakness in the hamstring muscles, increased body mass index (BMI), genetic factors, and playing on surfaces with increased traction (for example, synthetic gym floors).

Diagnosis

Your doctor will perform a detailed physical examination of the knee including maneuvers that test the ACL. The unaffected knee will also be tested for comparison. Your doctor may perform x-rays to see if there are any injuries to the bone; x-rays are excellent for assessing bony injuries but they do not show the cartilage or ligaments. If your doctor is suspicious of an ACL injury based on the physical exam, he or she may order an MRI. The MRI helps confirm the diagnosis and determine if there is any associated injury to the cartilage.

Treatment

In the initial period after the injury, ice and compression can help decrease swelling and assist with pain. Ice can be applied to the area for 15–20 minutes as often as every two to three hours until the pain goes away. A brace may also be provided to add support to your knee. Your doctor may provide you with crutches initially until you have the strength and confidence to put weight on your knee. Your doctor may also prescribe physical therapy to help you regain full motion of your knee and to help you gain strength in your thigh muscles.

If your ACL is torn, then your doctor will discuss possible treatment options. Unfortunately, if the ACL is truly torn, the body cannot repair it. Therefore, in most cases, your doctor will recommend surgery to replace/reconstruct the ACL. The ACL cannot be sewn back together; surgery involves using another tendon from your body or a graft from a cadaver. The exact method of surgery can vary depending on many factors including your age. Your surgeon will discuss various options with you.

Returning To Activity And Sports

The goal is to return your sport as quickly and safely as possible. If you have a complete ACL tear and you elect to delay surgery, you may not be able to safely return to pivoting/twisting sports until your ligament is reconstructed. Generally patients who have surgery return to full activities about six months later.

Preventing ACL Injuries

ACL injuries can be prevented through a strengthening, agility and flexibility program which emphasizes proper biomechanics. Your doctor may recommend that you participate in a specific exercise program if you play a high-risk sport. The programs will help strengthen the lower body and core muscles and teach specific landing, cutting, and stopping maneuvers. Well-designed knee injury prevention programs have been shown in research studies to decrease the risk of ACL injuries.

Patellar Dislocation (Kneecap Dislocation)

With a patellar dislocation, the patella (kneecap) pops out of its usual place in the groove at the end of the femur (thigh bone). Normally, the kneecap moves up and down within this groove when the knee is bent or straightened. During dislocation, the kneecap slips out of this groove, most often moving to the outer aspect of the knee. There is often sudden onset of pain and swelling associated with patellar dislocation. In some cases, there may be injury to the soft cartilage (soft bone) surface overlying the patella or femur.

How It Occurs

Many patellar dislocations occur in a non-contact manner when a person's foot is planted on the ground and they twist or quickly change direction. In this type of injury there may be an underlying looseness (laxity) of the knee joint. Often individuals who sustain this type of injury have a particular structure of the bones such as a shallow or uneven groove for the patella or a patella that sits a little high on the femur (patella alta), which make dislocation more likely. These factors determine how the kneecap moves in its groove and may make it easier for the kneecap to slip out of place.

Additionally, a kneecap may dislocate after a direct blow to the knee. This type of injury requires a strong force to the knee and therefore often causes more damage to the surrounding structures.

Up to 25% of people with this injury have a family history of patellar dislocations. This condition is seen most often in adolescent and young adults.

Signs And Symptoms

Patellar dislocations often cause severe pain and swelling. People may have stiffness and difficulty straightening the knee. They may notice the kneecap has slipped off to the side. There may be a popping or creaking sound when they move their knee or a sensation that the kneecap is unstable. There may be tenderness along the inside border of the kneecap. Often, the kneecap will spontaneously pop back into place when the knee is straightened.

Diagnosis

People who have suspected patellar dislocations should be evaluated by a sports medicine specialist or orthopedic surgeon. The physician will take a complete medical history and ask about how the injury occurred. He or she will carefully examine the knee and observe how the kneecap moves in the patellar groove and evaluate the ligaments, tendons and muscles of the knee. The physician will generally obtain x-rays to look at the shape of the kneecap and patellar groove, to evaluate for small chips of bone which may have dislodged with injury and to rule out fractures of the kneecap or thigh bone. Further imaging with an MRI may be recommended if there is concern for other injuries to the ligaments, tendons, or cartilage of the knee.

Treatment

After a patellar dislocation, the kneecap will often return to its normal position spontaneously. When a kneecap remains dislocated, a trained specialist may be able to gently push the

Other Common Knee Injuries And Problems

Chondromalacia

Chondromalacia, also called chondromalacia patellae, refers to softening of the articular cartilage of the kneecap. This disorder occurs most often in young adults and can be caused by injury, overuse, misalignment of the patella, or muscle weakness. Instead of gliding smoothly across the lower end of the thigh bone, the kneecap rubs against it, thereby roughening the cartilage underneath the kneecap. The damage may range from a slightly abnormal surface of the cartilage to a surface that has been worn away to the bone. Chondromalacia related to injury occurs when a blow to the kneecap tears off either a small piece of cartilage or a large fragment containing a piece of bone (osteochondral fracture).

Meniscal Injuries (Injuries To The Menisci)

The menisci can be easily injured by the force of rotating the knee while bearing weight. A partial or total tear may occur when a person quickly twists or rotates the upper leg while the foot stays still (for example, when dribbling a basketball around an opponent or turning to hit a tennis ball). If the tear is tiny, the meniscus stays connected to the front and back of the knee; if the tear is large, the meniscus may be left hanging by a thread of cartilage. The seriousness of a tear depends on its location and extent.

Cruciate Ligament Injuries

Cruciate ligament injuries are sometimes referred to as sprains. They don't necessarily cause pain, but they are disabling. The anterior cruciate ligament is most often stretched or torn (or both) by a sudden twisting motion (for example, when the feet are planted one way and the knees are turned another). The posterior cruciate ligament is most often injured by a direct impact, such as in an automobile accident or football tackle.

Medial And Lateral Collateral Ligament Injuries

The medial collateral ligament is more easily injured than the lateral collateral ligament. The cause of collateral ligament injuries is most often a blow to the outer side of the knee that stretches and tears the ligament on the inner side of the knee. Such blows frequently occur in contact sports such as football or hockey.

Tendon Injuries

Knee tendon injuries range from tendinitis (inflammation of a tendon) to a ruptured (torn) tendon. If a person overuses a tendon during certain activities such as dancing, cycling, or running, the tendon stretches and becomes inflamed. Tendinitis of the patellar tendon is sometimes called "jumper's knee" because in sports that require jumping, such as basketball, the muscle contraction and force of hitting the ground after a jump strain the tendon. After repeated stress, the tendon may become inflamed or tear.

Osgood-Schlatter Disease

Osgood-Schlatter disease is a condition caused by repetitive stress or tension on part of the growth area of the upper tibia (the apophysis). It is characterized by inflammation of the patellar tendon and surrounding soft tissues at the point where the tendon attaches to the tibia. The disease may also be associated with an injury in which the tendon is stretched so much that it tears away from the tibia and takes a fragment of bone with it. The disease most commonly affects active young people, particularly boys between the ages of 10 and 15, who play games or sports that include frequent running and jumping.

Iliotibial Band Syndrome

Iliotibial band syndrome is an inflammatory condition caused when a band of tissue rubs over the outer bone (lateral condyle) of the knee. Although iliotibial band syndrome may be caused by direct injury to the knee, it is most often caused by the stress of long-term overuse, such as sometimes occurs in sports training and, particularly, in running.

Osteochondritis Dissecans

Osteochondritis dissecans results from a loss of the blood supply to an area of bone underneath a joint surface. It usually involves the knee. The affected bone and its covering of cartilage gradually loosen and cause pain. This problem usually arises spontaneously in an active adolescent or young adult. It may be caused by a slight blockage of a small artery or to an unrecognized injury or tiny fracture that damages the overlying cartilage. A person with this condition may eventually develop osteoarthritis.

Lack of a blood supply can cause bone to break down (osteonecrosis). The involvement of several joints or the appearance of osteochondritis dissecans in several family members may indicate that the disorder is inherited.

Plica Syndrome

Plica syndrome occurs when plicae (bands of synovial tissue) are irritated by overuse or injury. Synovial plicae are the remains of tissue pouches found in the early stages of fetal development. As the fetus develops, these pouches normally combine to form one large synovial cavity. If this process is incomplete, plicae remain as four folds or bands of synovial tissue within the knee. Injury, chronic overuse, or inflammatory conditions are associated with this syndrome.

Source: Excerpted from "Questions and Answers about Knee Problems," National Institute of Arthritis and Musculoskeletal and Skin Diseases, May 2011.

kneecap back into its groove; in some cases, this procedure requires sedating medications and monitoring. Treatment for an initial patellar dislocation involves a stepwise process of rehabilitation. Initially, use of a brace will keep the patella in its groove; crutches may be needed for walking more comfortably. Rest, ice and elevating the affected leg will help reduce pain and swelling in the knee. Rehabilitation exercises focusing on improving range of motion and strengthening the hip and thigh muscles to keep the kneecap aligned are added gradually.

The final phase of the rehabilitation process includes skill-specific training to prepare for return to sports. Recurrence of patellar dislocation is relatively common, particularly in younger patients. Some patients with loose bone or cartilage fragments or recurrent dislocations require surgical treatment. The type of surgery varies depending on the underlying cause of the dislocations.

Returning To Activity And Sports

Most people with patellar dislocations are able to return to sports after a supervised, stepwise rehabilitation program. A physician should assess strength and balance to determine when it is safe to return to sports. Use of a brace with sports is generally recommended for individuals following a patellar dislocation.

Preventing Patellar Dislocations

Young athletes who have experienced a patellar dislocation in the past should maintain their core, hip, and leg strength and consider use a brace to lessen the chances another dislocation.

Patellofemoral Pain Syndrome (Runner's Knee)

Patellofemoral pain is a common knee problem. People with this condition feel pain under and around your kneecap. The patellofemoral joint is made of the patella (kneecap), femur (thigh bone), and soft tissue supporting structures (patellar ligaments, bursae, and tendons). The pain usually comes from these supporting structures. The two most common causes of knee pain in runners is patellofemoral pain syndrome and iliotibial (IT) band friction syndrome.

How It Occurs

For most people with patellofemoral pain syndrome there are a collection of factors that cause the pain. Anything that increases the strain on the soft tissue supporting structures around the kneecap can lead to a problem with how the patella moves through its groove in the thigh bone as you bend and straighten the knee. Even though it is sometimes called runner's knee, patellofemoral pain syndrome can also affect people who do not play sports.

Patellofemoral pain syndrome can result from direct trauma such as falling onto the kneecap or hitting the knee on the dashboard in a car accident. It most commonly occurs from overuse of the knee in sports or activities that involve intense and repetitive running and jumping. Activities of daily living such as prolonged sitting or standing and going up and down steps create extra pressure between the patella and the femur causing more stress and irritation.

Some variants of normal hip, knee, and foot alignment can put additional strain on the patellofemoral joint and supporting structures. People who are "flat-footed," "knock-kneed," or "pigeon-toed" tend to have higher rates of patellofemoral pain syndrome. Weak hip and thigh muscles are an important cause of patellofemoral pain. These muscles support the patella. When they are weak, the patella will not glide smoothly through its groove. This increases the strain on the patella's supporting structures which causes pain. A tight IT band (a tendon that runs along the outside of your thigh from your hip to your shin bone) is another risk factor for patellofemoral pain, since it also helps to control the movement of the patella in its groove. Finally, tight hamstrings are a frequent cause of patellofemoral pain, especially in growing bodies. Since muscles grow faster than bones, it is common for larger muscles to become relatively tight during growth spurts. Tight hamstrings increase the pressure behind the kneecap, which can lead to pain.

Signs And Symptoms

The most common symptoms are pain during and/or after activity and pain or stiffness after prolonged sitting or standing. There may also be a grinding or popping feeling under the kneecap, and some people may experience mild swelling. The pain is usually dull and achy, and may shift from one side of the kneecap to the other. People may have pain in both knees or only in one knee. The pain is usually worse when kneeling, walking downhill, or going up and down stairs.

Diagnosis

Your doctor will review your symptoms and examine your knee. X-rays, MRIs, and other imaging studies are not valuable in diagnosing patellofemoral syndrome, but may be helpful to rule out other sources of knee pain.

Treatment

Treatment includes temporarily reducing irritating activities until the pain is better controlled. For example, you might want to bike or swim instead of run. The mainstay of treatment is a customized physical therapy program to strengthen and stretch the hip and thigh muscles so that they can help the patella move smoothly through its groove. Ice often helps to reduce the pain. Ice should be applied for no more than 15 minutes at a time, and can be used as often as every hour. Anti-inflammatory medications, such as ibuprofen are typically not very helpful except when there is swelling. Your doctor may recommend shoe inserts if you have flat feet that are contributing to the knee pain. A patellofemoral brace can provide support to the patella, and may reduce pain during activity.

Returning To Activity And Sports

The goal of treatment is to return to your sport or activity as soon as it is safely possibly. Everyone recovers from injury at a different rate. Return to your sport or activity will be determined by how soon your knee recovers, not by how many days or weeks it has been since the pain started. In general, the longer you have symptoms before you start treatment, the longer it will take to get better.

You may begin to return safely to your activity when each of the following is true:

- You can fully straighten and bend your knee without pain

- Swelling is resolved

- Your knee and leg have normal strength and flexibility

- You are able to walk and perform daily activities without pain.

- You are able to jog straight without limping and without pain.

- You are able to jump on both legs without pain and jump on the injured leg without pain.

Preventing Patellofemoral Pain Syndrome

- Maintain strong and flexible thigh and hip muscles.

- Make sure you wear shoes that fit well, have good support, and are appropriate for the activity.

- Begin any new activity slowly and increase the intensity, duration, and frequency gradually. (Runners should increase their mileage by no more than 10% per week).

- Do not play through significant knee pain. If pain persists despite rest for a few days, see your physician.

Knees And Arthritis

There are some 100 different forms of arthritis, rheumatic diseases, and related conditions. Virtually all of them have the potential to affect the knees in some way. However, the following are the most common:

- *Osteoarthritis:* Some people with knee problems have a form of arthritis called osteoarthritis. In this disease, the cartilage gradually wears away and changes occur in the adjacent bone. Osteoarthritis may be caused by joint injury or being overweight. It is associated with aging and most typically begins in people age 50 or older. A young person who develops osteoarthritis typically has had an injury to the knee or may have an inherited form of the disease.

- *Rheumatoid Arthritis:* Rheumatoid arthritis, which generally affects people at a younger age than does osteoarthritis, is an autoimmune disease. This means it occurs as a result of the immune system attacking components of the body. In rheumatoid arthritis, the primary site of the immune system's attack is the synovium, the membrane that lines the joint. This attack causes inflammation of the joint. It can lead to destruction of the cartilage and bone and, in some cases, muscles, tendons, and ligaments as well.

Other Rheumatic Diseases

These include the following:

- *Gout:* An acute and intensely painful form of arthritis that occurs when crystals of the bodily waste product uric acid are deposited in the joints

- *Systemic Lupus Erythematosus (Lupus):* An autoimmune disease characterized by destructive inflammation of the skin, internal organs, and other body systems, as well as the joints

- *Ankylosing Spondylitis:* An inflammatory form of arthritis that primarily affects the spine, leading to stiffening and in some cases fusing into a stooped position

- *Psoriatic Arthritis:* A condition in which inflamed joints produce symptoms of arthritis for patients who have or will develop psoriasis

- *Infectious Arthritis:* A term describing forms of arthritis that are caused by infectious agents, such as bacteria or viruses. Prompt medical attention is essential to treat the infection and minimize damage to joints, particularly if fever is present.

Source: Excerpted from "Questions and Answers about Knee Problems," National Institute of Arthritis and Musculoskeletal and Skin Diseases, May 2011.

Questions And Answers About Knee Problems

What do the knees do? How do they work?

The knee is the joint where the bones of the upper leg meet the bones of the lower leg, allowing hinge-like movement while providing stability and strength to support the weight of the body. Flexibility, strength, and stability are needed for standing and for motions like walking, running, crouching, jumping, and turning.

Several kinds of supporting and moving parts, including bones, cartilage, muscles, ligaments, and tendons, help the knees do their job. Each of these structures is subject to disease and injury. When a knee problem affects your ability to do things, it can have a big impact on your life. Knee problems can interfere with many things, from participation in sports to simply getting up from a chair and walking.

Joint Basics

The point at which two or more bones are connected is called a joint. In all joints, the bones are kept from grinding against each other by a lining called cartilage. Bones are joined to bones by strong, elastic bands of tissue called ligaments. Muscles are connected to bones by tough cords of tissue called tendons. Muscles pull on tendons to move joints. Although muscles are not technically part of a joint, they're important because strong muscles help support and protect joints.

Source: Excerpted from "Questions and Answers about Knee Problems," National Institute of Arthritis and Musculo-skeletal and Skin Diseases, May 2011.

What are the parts of the knee?

Like any joint, the knee is composed of bones and cartilage, ligaments, tendons, and muscles.

The knee joint is the junction of three bones: the femur (thigh bone or upper leg bone), the tibia (shin bone or larger bone of the lower leg), and the patella (kneecap). The patella is two to three inches wide and three to four inches long. It sits over the other bones at the front of the knee joint and slides when the knee moves. It protects the knee and gives leverage to muscles.

The ends of the three bones in the knee joint are covered with articular cartilage, a tough, elastic material that helps absorb shock and allows the knee joint to move smoothly. Separating the bones of the knee are pads of connective tissue called menisci. The menisci are two crescent-shaped discs, each called a meniscus, positioned between the tibia and femur on the outer and inner sides of each knee. The two menisci in each knee act as shock absorbers, cushioning the lower part of the leg from the weight of the rest of the body as well as enhancing stability.

Muscles

There are two groups of muscles at the knee. The four quadriceps muscles on the front of the thigh work to straighten the knee from a bent position. The hamstring muscles, which run along the back of the thigh from the hip to just below the knee, help to bend the knee.

Tendons And Ligaments

The quadriceps tendon connects the quadriceps muscle to the patella and provides the power to straighten the knee. The following four ligaments connect the femur and tibia and give the joint strength and stability:

- The medial collateral ligament, which runs along the inside of the knee joint, provides stability to the inner (medial) part of the knee.

- The lateral collateral ligament, which runs along the outside of the knee joint, provides stability to the outer (lateral) part of the knee.

- The anterior cruciate ligament, in the center of the knee, limits rotation and the forward movement of the tibia.

- The posterior cruciate ligament, also in the center of the knee, limits backward movement of the tibia.

- The knee capsule is a protective, fiber-like structure that wraps around the knee joint. Inside the capsule, the joint is lined with a thin, soft tissue called synovium.

How are knee problems diagnosed?

Doctors diagnose knee problems based on the findings of a medical history, physical exam, and diagnostic tests.

Medical History

During the medical history, the doctor asks how long symptoms have been present and what problems you are having using your knee. In addition, the doctor will ask about any injury, condition, or health problem that might be causing the problem.

Physical Examination

The doctor bends, straightens, rotates (turns), or presses on the knee to feel for injury and to determine how well the knee moves and where the pain is located. The doctor may ask you to stand, walk, or squat to help assess the knee's function.

Diagnostic Tests

Depending on the findings of the medical history and physical exam, the doctor may use one or more tests to determine the nature of a knee problem. Some of the more commonly used tests include the following:

- *X-ray (Radiography):* A procedure in which an x-ray beam is passed through the knee to produce a two-dimensional picture of the bones.

- *Computerized Axial Tomography (CT) Scan:* A painless procedure in which x-rays are passed through the knee at different angles, detected by a scanner, and analyzed by a computer. CT scan images show soft tissues such as ligaments or muscles more clearly than do conventional x-rays. The computer can combine individual images to give a three-dimensional view of the knee.

- *Bone Scan (Radionuclide Scanning):* A technique for creating images of bones on a computer screen or on film. Before the procedure, a harmless radioactive material is injected into your bloodstream. The material collects in the bones, particularly in abnormal areas of the bones, and is detected by a scanner.

- *Magnetic Resonance Imaging (MRI):* A procedure that uses a powerful magnet linked to a computer to create pictures of areas inside the knee. During the procedure, your leg is placed in a cylindrical chamber where energy from a powerful magnet (rather than x-rays) is passed through the knee. An MRI is particularly useful for detecting soft tissue damage.

- *Arthroscopy:* A surgical technique in which the doctor manipulates a small, lighted optic tube (arthroscope) that has been inserted into the joint through a small incision in the knee. Images of the inside of the knee joint are projected onto a television screen.

- *Joint Aspiration:* A procedure that uses a syringe to remove fluid buildup in a joint to reduce swelling and relieve pressure. A laboratory analysis of the fluid can determine the presence of a fracture, an infection, or an inflammatory response.

- *Biopsy:* A procedure in which tissue is removed from the body and studied under a microscope.

What kinds of doctors evaluate and treat knee problems?

After an examination by your primary care doctor, he or she may refer you to a rheumatologist, an orthopaedic surgeon, or both. A rheumatologist specializes in nonsurgical treatment of arthritis and other rheumatic diseases. An orthopaedic surgeon, or orthopaedist, specializes in nonsurgical and surgical treatment of bones, joints, and soft tissues such as ligaments, tendons, and muscles.

You may also be referred to a physiatrist. Specializing in physical medicine and rehabilitation, physiatrists seek to restore optimal function to people with injuries to the muscles, bones, tissues, and nervous system.

Minor injuries or arthritis may be treated by an internist (a doctor trained to diagnose and treat nonsurgical diseases) or your primary care doctor.

How can people prevent knee problems?

Some knee problems, such as those resulting from an accident, cannot be foreseen or prevented. However, people can prevent many knee problems by following these suggestions:

- Before exercising or participating in sports, warm up by walking or riding a stationary bicycle, then do stretches. Stretching the muscles in the front of the thigh (quadriceps) and back of the thigh (hamstrings) reduces tension on the tendons and relieves pressure on the knee during activity.

- Strengthen the leg muscles by doing specific exercises (for example, by walking up stairs or hills or by riding a stationary bicycle). A supervised workout with weights is another way to strengthen the leg muscles that support the knee.

- Avoid sudden changes in the intensity of exercise. Increase the force or duration of activity gradually.

- Wear shoes that fit properly and are in good condition. This will help maintain balance and leg alignment when walking or running. Flat feet or overpronated feet (feet that roll inward) can cause knee problems. People can often reduce some of these problems by wearing special shoe inserts (orthotics).

- Maintain a healthy weight to reduce stress on the knee. Obesity increases the risk of osteoarthritis of the knee.

What types of exercise are best for people with knee problems?

Ideally, everyone should get three types of exercise regularly:

- Range-of-motion exercises to help maintain normal joint movement and relieve stiffness.

- Strengthening exercises to help keep or increase muscle strength. Keeping muscles strong with exercises, such as walking up stairs, doing leg lifts or dips, or riding a stationary bicycle, helps support and protect the knee.

- Aerobic or endurance exercises to improve function of the heart and circulation and to help control weight. Weight control can be important to people who have arthritis because extra weight puts pressure on many joints. Some studies show that aerobic exercise can reduce inflammation in some joints.

If you already have knee problems, your doctor or physical therapist can help with a plan of exercise that will help the knee(s) without increasing the risk of injury or further damage. As a general rule, you should choose gentle exercises such as swimming, aquatic exercise, or walking rather than jarring exercises such as jogging or high-impact aerobics.

Chapter 53

Shin Splints

Description

The term *shin splints* refers to pain and tenderness along or just behind the inner edge of the tibia, the large bone in the lower leg. Shin splints—or medial tibial stress syndrome as it is called by orthopaedists—usually develops after physical activity, such as vigorous exercise or sports. Repetitive activity leads to inflammation of the muscles, tendons, and periosteum (thin layer of tissue covering a bone) of the tibia, causing pain. The bone tissue itself is also involved.

Risk Factors

- Flatfeet or abnormally rigid arches

- Running/jogging

- Dancing

- Sudden increase in training or new vigorous impact training

- Military training

Certain factors seem to contribute to shin splints. The condition commonly affects runners, aerobic dancers, and people in the military. Shin splints often develop after sudden changes in physical activity, such as running longer distances or on hills, or increasing the number of days you exercise each week. Flat feet are another factor that can contribute to increased stress on the lower leg muscles during exercising.

About This Chapter: "Shin Splints," reproduced with permission from *Your Orthopaedic Connection* © American Academy of Orthopaedic Surgeons (www.aaos.org), Rosemont, IL, 2007. Reviewed by David A. Cooke, MD, FACP, April 2012.

Treatment
Nonsurgical Treatment

Nonsurgical treatment for shin splints includes several weeks of rest from the activity that caused it. Other forms of conditioning can be substituted. The doctor may recommend that you take anti-inflammatory medications, or use cold packs and mild compression to feel better. Stretching exercises can also help.

In most people, the pain is not so bad with ordinary walking. After several weeks of rest, low-level training may begin. Be sure to warm up and stretch thoroughly before you exercise. Increase training slowly. If you start to feel the same pain, stop exercising immediately. Use a cold pack and rest for a day or two. Return to training again at a lower level of intensity. Increase training even more slowly than before.

Surgical Treatment

Very few people need surgery for shin splints. Surgery has been done in very severe cases of shin splints that do not respond to nonsurgical treatment. It is not clear how effective surgery is, however.

An accurate diagnosis is very important. Sometimes, other problems may exist, which will have an impact on healing.

Other Causes of Shin Pain
Stress Fracture

When shin splints are not responsive to treatment, your doctor may want to make sure you do not have a stress fracture. A bone scan and magnetic resonance imaging (MRI) can often show if a fracture is present. The diagnostic tests, causes of shin splints, and treatment regimens all bear a similarity and relationship to stress fractures. It is possible that there is a relationship between shin splints and stress fracture, but this has not been clearly identified.

Tendonitis

Tendonitis can be present, especially if there is a partial tear of the involved tendon. MRI can also help the doctor diagnose the presence of tendonitis.

Chronic Exertional Compartment Syndrome

An uncommon condition called chronic exertional compartment syndrome involves swelling of muscle with exertion. This happens within the muscle's usually tight compartment in the leg. These compartments are nonyielding. Swelling can raise pressure within the compartment to levels so high that blood will not flow into the muscle. This causes severe pain and is best treated surgically. The tests that are used to diagnose chronic exertional compartment syndrome are highly specialized and not easily available. They involve measuring the pressure within the leg compartments immediately after exercise.

Chapter 54

Foot And Ankle Injuries

General Foot Health

A Biological Masterpiece, But Subject To Many Ills

The human foot is a biological masterpiece. Its strong, flexible, and functional design enables it to do its job well and without complaint—if you take care of it and don't take it for granted.

The foot can be compared to a finely tuned racecar, or a space shuttle, vehicles whose function dictates their design and structure. And like them, the human foot is complex, containing within its relatively small size 26 bones (the two feet contain a quarter of all the bones in the body), 33 joints, and a network of more than 100 tendons, muscles, and ligaments, to say nothing of blood vessels and nerves.

Tons Of Pressure

The components of your feet work together, sharing the tremendous pressures of daily living. An average day of walking, for example, brings a force equal to several hundred tons to bear on the feet. This helps explain why your feet are more subject to injury than any other part of your body.

Foot ailments are among the most common of our health problems. Although some can be traced to heredity, many stem from the cumulative impact of a lifetime of abuse and neglect. Studies show that most Americans experience foot problems of a greater or lesser degree of seriousness at some time in their lives; nowhere near that many seek medical treatment, apparently because they mistakenly believe that discomfort and pain are normal and expectable.

There are a number of systemic diseases that are sometimes first detected in the feet, such as diabetes, circulatory disorders, anemia, and kidney problems. Arthritis, including gout, often attacks foot joints first.

Specialized Care

Your feet, like other specialized structures, require specialized care. A doctor of podiatric medicine can make an important contribution to your total health, whether it is regular preventive care or surgery to correct a deformity.

In order to keep your feet healthy, you should be familiar with the most common ills that affect them. Remember, though, that self-treatment can often turn a minor problem into a major one and is generally not advisable. You should see a podiatric physician when any of the following conditions occur or persist.

- **Athlete's foot** is a skin disease, usually starting between the toes or on the bottom of the feet, which can spread to other parts of the body. It is caused by a fungus that commonly attacks the feet, because the wearing of shoes and hosiery fosters fungus growth. The signs of athlete's foot are dry scaly skin, itching, inflammation, and blisters. You can help prevent infection by washing your feet daily with soap and warm water; drying carefully, especially between the toes; and changing shoes and hose regularly to decrease moisture. Athlete's foot is not the only infection, fungal or otherwise, which afflicts the foot, and other dry skin/dermatitis conditions can be good reasons to see a doctor of podiatric medicine if a suspicious condition persists.

- **Blisters** are caused by skin friction. Don't pop them. Apply moleskin or an adhesive bandage over a blister, and leave it on until it falls off naturally in the bath or shower. Keep your feet dry and always wear socks as a cushion between your feet and shoes. If a blister breaks on its own, wash the area, apply an antiseptic, and cover with a sterile bandage.

- **Bunions** are misaligned big toe joints, which can become swollen and tender. The deformity causes the first joint of the big toe to slant outward, and the big toe to angle toward the other toes. Bunions tend to run in families, but the tendency can be aggravated by shoes that are too narrow in the forefoot and toe. There are conservative and preventive steps that can minimize the discomfort of a bunion, but surgery is frequently recommended to correct the problem.

- **Corns and calluses** are protective layers of compacted, dead skin cells. They are caused by repeated friction and pressure from skin rubbing against bony areas or against an irregularity in a shoe. Corns ordinarily form on the toes and calluses on the soles of the feet. The friction and pressure can burn or otherwise be painful and may be relieved by moleskin or padding on the affected areas. Never cut corns or calluses with any instrument, and never apply home remedies, except under a podiatrist's instructions.

- **Foot odor** results from excessive perspiration from the more than 250,000 sweat glands in the foot. Daily hygiene is essential. Change your shoes daily to let each pair air out, and change your socks, perhaps even more frequently than daily. Foot powders and antiperspirants, and soaking your feet in vinegar and water, can help lessen odor.

- **Hammertoe** is a condition in which any of the toes are bent in a claw-like position. It occurs most frequently with the second toe, often when a bunion slants the big toe toward and under it, but any of the other three smaller toes can be affected. Although the condition usually stems from muscle imbalance, it is often aggravated by ill-fitting shoes or socks that cramp the toes. Avoid pressure on the toes as much as possible. Surgery may be necessary to realign the toes to their proper position.

- **Heel pain** can generally be traced to faulty biomechanics which place too much stress on the heel bone, ligaments, or nerves in the area. Stress could result while walking or jumping on hard surfaces, or from poorly made footwear. Overweight is also a major contributing factor. Some general health conditions—arthritis, gout, and circulatory problems, for example—also cause heel pain.

- **Heel spurs** are growths of bone on the underside of the heel bone. They can occur without pain; pain may result when inflammation develops at the point where the spur forms. Both heel pain and heel spurs are often associated with plantar fasciitis, an inflammation of the long band of connective tissue running from the heel to the ball of the foot. Treatments may range from exercise and custom-made orthotics to anti-inflammatory medication or cortisone injections.

- **Ingrown nails** are nails whose corners or sides dig painfully into the skin, often causing infection. They are frequently caused by improper nail trimming but also by shoe pressure, injury, fungus infection, heredity, and poor foot structure. Toenails should be trimmed straight across, slightly longer than the end of the toe, with toenail clippers. If the ingrown portion of the nail is painful or infected, your podiatric physician may remove the affected portion; if the condition reoccurs frequently, your podiatrist may permanently remove the nail.

- **Neuromas** are enlarged, benign growths of nerves, most commonly between the third and fourth toes. They are caused by bones and other tissue rubbing against and irritating the nerves. Abnormal bone structure or pressure from ill-fitting shoes also can create the condition, which can result in pain, burning, tingling, or numbness between the toes and in the ball of the foot. Conservative treatment can include padding, taping, orthotic devices, and cortisone injections, but surgical removal of the growth is sometimes necessary.

- **Warts** are caused by a virus, which enters the skin through small cuts and infects the skin. Children, especially teenagers, tend to be more susceptible to warts than adults. Most warts are harmless and benign, even though painful and unsightly. Warts often come from walking barefooted on dirty surfaces or littered ground. There are several simple procedures, which your podiatric physician might use to remove warts.

Your podiatric physician/surgeon has been trained specifically and extensively in the diagnosis and treatment of all manner of foot conditions. This training encompasses all of the intricately related systems and structures of the foot and lower leg including neurological, circulatory, skin, and the musculoskeletal system, which includes bones, joints, ligaments, tendons, muscles, and nerves.

Foot And Ankle Injuries

"Foot and Ankle Injuries," © 2011 American Podiatric Medical Association. All rights reserved. Reprinted with permission. For additional information, visit http://www.apma.org.

Immediate Treatment

Foot and ankle emergencies happen every day. Broken bones, dislocations, sprains, contusions, infections, and other serious injuries can occur at any time. Early attention is vitally important. Whenever you sustain a foot or ankle injury, you should seek immediate treatment from a podiatric physician.

This advice is universal, even though there are lots of myths about foot and ankle injuries. Some of them follow.

Myths

- "It can't be broken, because I can move it." False; this widespread idea has kept many fractures from receiving proper treatment. The truth is that often you can walk with certain kinds of fractures. Some common examples: Breaks in the smaller, outer bone of the

Top Ten Foot Health Tips

Diseases, disorders, and disabilities of the foot or ankle affect the quality of life and mobility of millions of Americans. However, the general public and even many physicians are unaware of the important relationship between foot health and overall health and well-being. With this in mind, the American Podiatric Medical Association (APMA) would like to share a few tips to help keep feet healthy.

1. Don't ignore foot pain—it's not normal. If the pain persists, see a podiatric physician.

2. Inspect your feet regularly. Pay attention to changes in color and temperature of your feet. Look for thick or discolored nails (a sign of developing fungus), and check for cracks or cuts in the skin. Peeling or scaling on the soles of feet could indicate athlete's foot. Any growth on the foot is not considered normal.

3. Wash your feet regularly, especially between the toes, and be sure to dry them completely.

4. Trim toenails straight across, but not too short. Be careful not to cut nails in corners or on the sides; it can lead to ingrown toenails. Persons with diabetes, poor circulation, or heart problems should not treat their own feet because they are more prone to infection.

5. Make sure that your shoes fit properly. Purchase new shoes later in the day when feet tend to be at their largest and replace worn out shoes as soon as possible.

6. Select and wear the right shoe for the activity that you are engaged in (that is, running shoes for running).

7. Alternate shoes—don't wear the same pair of shoes every day.

8. Avoid walking barefooted—your feet will be more prone to injury and infection. At the beach or when wearing sandals, always use sunblock on your feet just as on the rest of your body.

9. Be cautious when using home remedies for foot ailments; self-treatment can often turn a minor problem into a major one.

10. If you are a person with diabetes, it is vital that you see a podiatric physician at least once a year for a check-up.

lower leg, small chip fractures of either the foot or ankle bones, and the often neglected fracture of the toe.

- "If you break a toe, immediate care isn't necessary." False; a toe fracture needs prompt attention. If x-rays reveal it to be a simple, displaced fracture, care by your podiatric physician usually can produce rapid relief. However, x-rays might identify a displaced or angulated break. In such cases, prompt realignment of the fracture by your podiatric physician will help prevent improper or incomplete healing. Often, fractures do not show up in the initial x-ray. It may be necessary to x-ray the foot a second time, seven to ten days later. Many patients develop post-fracture deformity of a toe, which in turn results in a deformed toe with a painful corn. A good general rule is: Seek prompt treatment for injury to foot bones.

- "If you have a foot or ankle injury, soak it in hot water immediately." False; don't use heat or hot water on an area suspect for fracture, sprain, or dislocation. Heat promotes blood flow, causing greater swelling. More swelling means greater pressure on the nerves, which causes more pain. An ice bag wrapped in a towel has a contracting effect on blood vessels, produces a numbing sensation, and prevents swelling and pain. Your podiatric physician may make additional recommendations upon examination.

- "Applying an elastic bandage to a severely sprained ankle is adequate treatment." False; ankle sprains often mean torn or severely overstretched ligaments, and they should receive immediate care. X-ray examination, immobilization by casting or splinting, and physiotherapy to ensure a normal recovery all may be indicated. Surgery may even be necessary.

- "The terms *fracture*, *break*, and *crack* are all different." False; all of those words are proper in describing a broken bone.

Before Seeing The Podiatrist

If an injury or accident does occur, the steps you can take to help yourself until you can reach your podiatric physician are easy to remember if you can recall the word "rice."

- **Rest:** Restrict your activity and get off your foot/ankle.

- **Ice:** Gently place a plastic bag of ice wrapped in a towel on the injured area in a 20-minute-on, 40-minute-off cycle.

- **Compression:** Lightly wrap an Ace bandage around the area, taking care not to pull it too tight.

- **Elevation:** To reduce swelling and pain, sit in a position that allows you to elevate the foot/ankle higher than your waist.

For bleeding cuts, cleanse well, apply pressure with gauze or a towel, and cover with a clean dressing. See your podiatrist as soon as possible. It's best not to use any medication on the cut before you see the doctor.

Leave blisters unopened if they are not painful or in a weight-bearing area of the foot. A compression bandage placed over a blister can provide relief.

Foreign materials in the skin—such as slivers, splinters, and sand—can be removed carefully, but a deep foreign object, such as broken glass or a needle, must be removed professionally.

Treatment for an abrasion is similar to that of a burn, since raw skin is exposed to the air and can easily become infected. It is important to remove all foreign particles with thorough cleaning. Sterile bandages should be applied, along with an antibiotic cream or ointment.

Prevention

- Wear the correct shoes for your particular activity.

- Wear hiking shoes or boots in rough terrain.

- Don't continue to wear any sports shoe if it is worn unevenly.

- The toe box in steel-toe shoes should be deep enough to accommodate your toes comfortably.

- Always wear hard-top shoes when operating a lawn mower or other grass-cutting equipment.

- Don't walk barefoot on paved streets or sidewalks.

- Watch out for slippery floors at home and at work. Clean up obviously dangerous spills immediately.

- If you get up during the night, turn on a light. Many fractured toes and other foot injuries occur while attempting to find one's way in the dark.

Ankle Sprains

"Ankle Sprains," by Mark A. Jenkins, MD, © 2005 SportsMed Web (www.rice.edu/~jenky/). Reprinted with permission. Reviewed by David A. Cooke, MD, FACP, April 2012.

The most common type of ankle injury is a sprain. A sprain is stretching and tearing of ligaments (fibrous bands connecting adjacent bones in a joint.) There are many ligaments around the ankle and these can become damaged when the ankle is forced into a position not normally encountered.

The most frequently seen sprain occurs when weight is applied to a foot, which is on an uneven surface, and the foot "rolls in" (inversion). Because the sole of the foot is pointing inward as force is applied, the ligaments stabilizing the lateral—or outside—part of the ankle are stressed. Many patients report hearing a "snap" or "pop" at the time of the injury. This is usually followed by pain and swelling on the lateral aspect of the ankle.

The most important initial management of a sprain is R: Rest; I: Ice; C: Compression; and E: Elevation.

Many of the problems resulting from sprains are due to blood and edema in and around the ankle. Minimizing swelling helps the ankle heal faster. The RICE regimen facilitates this.

- **Rest:** No weight bearing for the first 24 hours after the injury (Possibly longer, depending upon severity)

- **Ice:** Apply ice packs using a towel over a plastic bag to the area that is painful. Be careful to avoid frostbite. Ice should be intermittently applied for the first 24 hours.

- **Compression:** An ACE bandage or other soft elastic material should be applied to the ankle to help prevent the accumulation of edema.

- **Elevation:** Elevating the ankle helps in removing edema. By having the foot higher than the hip (or heart), gravity is used to pull edema out of the ankle.

In the initial 24 hours, it is very important to avoid things, which might increase swelling. Avoid:

- Hot showers

- Heat rubs (methylsalicylate counterirritants such as Ben Gay, etc.)

- Hot packs

- Drinking alcohol

- Aspirin prolongs the clotting time of blood and may cause more bleeding into the ankle. (Tylenol or Ibuprofen may be taken to help with pain, but will not speed up the healing process.)

When To Seek Medical Attention

If the ankle is obviously fractured or dislocated, then medical attention should be sought immediately. If you are fairly certain that it is sprained then use the RICE regimen and get a professional opinion regarding diagnosis and treatment. Rice University students [Ed. Note: Rice University is the producer of this information; the name is not related to the RICE regimen] are encouraged to make an appointment with one of the physicians at the student health service to assess the severity of the injury, determine if x-rays are necessary, and to receive instruction on proper rehabilitation of the injury.

In some instances a fracture of one of the bones in the leg or ankle may occur along with a sprain. Pain alone is not necessarily a reliable guide of the presence or absence of a fracture. Fractures can usually be diagnosed with an x-ray examination.

A student who sprains his or her ankle on a Friday night can usually follow the RICE regimen, and see a physician on Monday or Tuesday.

Because it is not possible to predict or discuss every possible situation that might arise, it is recommended that the student use common sense in dealing with his or her injury.

Degree Of Severity Of Ankle Sprains

- **Grade I:** Stretch and/or minor tear of the ligament without laxity (loosening)
- **Grade II:** Tear of ligament plus some laxity
- **Grade III:** Complete tear of the affected ligament (very loose)

Treatment

After the initial 24-hours the patient can begin partial weight bearing using crutches, gradually progressing to full weight bearing over several days as tolerated. The patient should try to use a normal heel-toe gait. An ankle brace may be necessary to protect the joint from reinjury. As soon as pain allows, rehabilitation exercises should be done. The rehabilitation exercises are the most important aspect of recovering full function of the ankle.

One simple exercise that can be begun early in the course of treatment is the "alphabet" exercise. This is non-weight bearing and involves trying to draw the letters of the alphabet with your toes.

Most sprains heal completely within a few weeks. The more severe the injury, the longer the time to heal. Often it is necessary to continue rehab exercises for a month or two following the injury. Grade III injuries are usually managed conservatively—rehabilitation exercises, etc.—but a small percentage may require surgery.

Ankle Injuries: To Tape or Not to Tape?

Opinions abound about ankle wrapping, taping or bracing as prevention against ankle injuries that include sprains, strains, and fracture. Ankle injuries are common in soccer and can lead to days or weeks lost from competition or practice. As a result, leagues across the country are taking steps to better protect athletes from injury: improving shoes and playing fields, and educating coaches and certified athletic trainers about conditioning and injury prevention techniques that include ankle strengthening and appropriate use of external ankle supports.

To the last, what does the research reveal about the usefulness of external ankle support in preventing injuries, or in helping to prevent another ankle injury?

Ankle Taping As Injury Prevention

Ankle taping has been used for years as a method to *prevent ankle injuries*, despite a lack of significant evidence supporting its use. Only in recent years has research more closely examined the effectiveness of this technique.

In sum, most research shows little evidence supporting ankle wrapping or taping for injury prevention. Contrary to popular belief, some studies found that wrapping reduced proprioceptive feedback (the sense of where the ankle and foot is in space) associated with ankle stability and maintenance of a normal position when faced with an unstable or abnormal position.

Other studies found that the peroneal muscles located on the outside of the ankle bone that help to control ankle motion did not react as quickly when wrapped or taped. Still other studies reported a decrease in performance when the tape or wrap was applied inappropriately. Last, several studies found that most tape loosens within 10 to 60 minutes of application, providing no measurable support.

Ankle Taping To Prevent Re-injury

Research supports use of ankle taping, wrapping, and bracing (orthosis) by athletes who have experienced one or more ankle injuries. The external support provides backup for ankle muscles, ligaments, and tendons.

First-line treatment for ankle injuries includes a rehabilitation program supervised by a physical therapist and a certified athletic trainer, followed by use of a brace for up to six months after injury. A progressive strengthening, proprioceptive, and flexibility program should follow an ankle injury.

Ankle wrap or tape should be regularly used in practice and competition, and can be applied by coaches and parents who are trained in appropriate techniques.

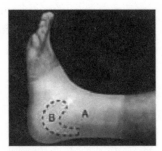

Step 1

Preparation: Shave the ankle region before taping. Or, use a pre-taping underwrap to prevent painful hair removal from the skin. This wrap also eliminates possible skin reactions caused by adhesive.

• Use pre-taping underwrap in a traditional Figure 8 "overwrapping" style if you are unable to shave or are sensitive to the adhesive properties of tape.

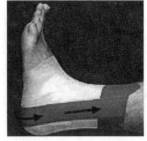

Step 2

Anchors are next applied (top). Their function is to firmly attach the Stirrups (side, first stirrup). Sports tape 38mm is the most popular tape for this technique.

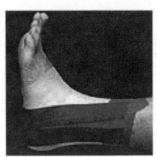

Step 3

Three Stirrups are generally applied (side, Stirrups 2 and 3). These attach to the anchors starting from medial (inside) to lateral (outside) in a U-shape formation. They provide excellent support.

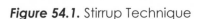

Figure 54.1. Stirrup Technique

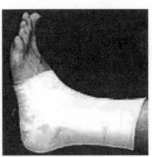

Step 4

The ankle taping technique is completed with Figure 8s and a spiral to completely encase the rigid tape.

What About Bracing?

Bracing is a good choice for players who require additional support following an injury and is an option in lieu of taping by a trained professional. Braces are less expensive than taping and tend not to irritate or breakdown the skin. Players can tighten the brace during competition and practice.

Ankle Wrapping Techniques

The Stirrup (see Figure 54.1) and Figure 8 (see illustration online at http://www.mshssca .org/resources/tapingankles.pdf) taping techniques are most useful in preventing ankle re-injury. Athletes who routinely use ankle tape may rely on coaches and parents to help apply tape strips, anchors, or pre-wrap.

Stirrup Technique

As A Precaution: Ask the athlete to walk around to check for any discomfort. Pain, numbness, pins and needles or excessive redness in the foot/ankle region may indicate circulation difficulties. The tape will have to be adjusted if any of these symptoms are present. If the athlete advises of a pinching pain around the base of the fifth metatarsal, scissors will be required to cut through to relieve pain.

Research Gaps

There is still much to learn about preventing ankle injuries. What conditioning and in-season training programs are best to prevent ankle injuries? Will these programs equally protect men and women, or do gender needs differ? What is best intervention for an athlete who has already experienced an ankle injury? These questions and more will be addressed in coming years.

Chapter 55

Plantar Fasciitis And Bone Spurs

Plantar fasciitis (fashee-EYE-tiss) is the most common cause of pain on the bottom of the heel. Approximately two million patients are treated for this condition every year.

Plantar fasciitis occurs when the strong band of tissue that supports the arch of your foot becomes irritated and inflamed.

Anatomy

The plantar fascia is a long, thin ligament that lies directly beneath the skin on the bottom of your foot. It connects the heel to the front of your foot and supports the arch of your foot.

Cause

The plantar fascia is designed to absorb the high stresses and strains we place on our feet. But, sometimes, too much pressure damages or tears the tissues. The body's natural response to injury is inflammation, which results in the heel pain and stiffness of plantar fasciitis.

Risk Factors

In most cases, plantar fasciitis develops without a specific, identifiable reason. There are, however, many factors that can make you more prone to the condition:

- Tighter calf muscles that make it difficult to flex your foot and bring your toes up toward your shin

About This Chapter: "Plantar Fasciitis and Bone Spurs," reproduced with permission from *Your Orthopaedic Connection.* © American Academy of Orthopaedic Surgeons (www.aaos.org), Rosemont, IL, 2010.

325

- Obesity
- Very high arch
- Repetitive impact activity (running/sports)
- New or increased activity

Heel Spurs

Although many people with plantar fasciitis have heel spurs, spurs are not the cause of plantar fasciitis pain. One out of 10 people have heel spurs, but only one out of 20 people (5%) with heel spurs has foot pain. Because the spur is not the cause of plantar fasciitis, the pain can be treated without removing the spur.

Heel spurs do not cause plantar fasciitis pain.

Symptoms

The most common symptoms of plantar fasciitis include:

- Pain on the bottom of the foot near the heel
- Pain with the first few steps after getting out of bed in the morning, or after a long period of rest, such as after a long car ride. The pain subsides after a few minutes of walking
- Greater pain after (not during) exercise or activity

Doctor Examination

After you describe your symptoms and discuss your concerns, your doctor will examine your foot. Your doctor will look for these signs:

- A high arch
- An area of maximum tenderness on the bottom of your foot, just in front of your heel bone
- Pain that gets worse when you flex your foot and the doctor pushes on the plantar fascia. The pain improves when you point your toes down
- Limited "up" motion of your ankle

Tests

Your doctor may order imaging tests to help make sure your heel pain is caused by plantar fasciitis and not another problem.

X-Rays

X-rays provide clear images of bones. They are useful in ruling out other causes of heel pain, such as fractures or arthritis. Heel spurs can be seen on an x-ray.

Other Imaging Tests

Other imaging tests, such as magnetic resonance imaging (MRI) and ultrasound, are not routinely used to diagnose plantar fasciitis. They are rarely ordered. An MRI scan may be used if the heel pain is not relieved by initial treatment methods.

Treatment

Nonsurgical Treatment

More than 90% of patients with plantar fasciitis will improve within 10 months of starting simple treatment methods.

- **Rest:** Decreasing or even stopping the activities that make the pain worse is the first step in reducing the pain. You may need to stop athletic activities where your feet pound on hard surfaces (for example, running or step aerobics).

- **Ice:** Rolling your foot over a cold water bottle or ice for 20 minutes is effective. This can be done three to four times a day.

- **Nonsteroidal Anti-Inflammatory Medication:** Drugs such as ibuprofen or naproxen reduce pain and inflammation. Using the medication for more than one month should be reviewed with your primary care doctor.

- **Exercise:** Plantar fasciitis is aggravated by tight muscles in your feet and calves. Stretching your calves and plantar fascia is the most effective way to relieve the pain that comes with this condition [see box].

- **Cortisone Injections:** Cortisone, a type of steroid, is a powerful anti-inflammatory medication. It can be injected into the plantar fascia to reduce inflammation and pain. Your doctor may limit your injections. Multiple steroid injections can cause the plantar fascia to rupture (tear), which can lead to a flat foot and chronic pain.

- **Supportive Shoes And Orthotics:** Shoes with thick soles and extra cushioning can reduce pain with standing and walking. As you step and your heel strikes the ground, a significant amount of tension is placed on the fascia, which causes microtrauma (tiny tears in the tissue). A cushioned shoe or insert reduces this tension and the microtrauma that occurs with every step. Soft silicone heel pads are inexpensive and work by elevating and cushioning your heel. Pre-made or custom orthotics (shoe inserts) are also helpful.

- **Night Splints:** Most people sleep with their feet pointed down. This relaxes the plantar fascia and is one of the reasons for morning heel pain. A night splint stretches the plantar fascia while you sleep. Although it can be difficult to sleep with, a night splint is very effective and does not have to be used once the pain is gone.

- **Physical Therapy:** Your doctor may suggest that you work with a physical therapist on an exercise program that focuses on stretching your calf muscles and plantar fascia. In addition to exercises like the ones mentioned in the box, a physical therapy program may involve specialized ice treatments, massage, and medication to decrease inflammation around the plantar fascia.

- **Extracorporeal Shockwave Therapy (ESWT):** During this procedure, high-energy shockwave impulses stimulate the healing process in damaged plantar fascia tissue. ESWT has not shown consistent results and, therefore, is not commonly performed. ESWT is noninvasive—it does not require a surgical incision. Because of the minimal risk involved, ESWT is sometimes tried before surgery is considered.

Calf Stretch

Lean forward against a wall with one knee straight and the heel on the ground. Place the other leg in front, with the knee bent. To stretch the calf muscles and the heel cord, push your hips toward the wall in a controlled fashion. Hold the position for 10 seconds and relax. Repeat this exercise 20 times for each foot. A strong pull in the calf should be felt during the stretch.

Plantar Fascia Stretch

This stretch is performed in the seated position. Cross your affected foot over the knee of your other leg. Grasp the toes of your painful foot and slowly pull them toward you in a controlled fashion. If it is difficult to reach your foot, wrap a towel around your big toe to help pull your toes toward you. Place your other hand along the plantar fascia. The fascia should feel like a tight band along the bottom of your foot when stretched. Hold the stretch for 10 seconds. Repeat it 20 times for each foot. This exercise is best done in the morning before standing or walking.

Surgical Treatment

Surgery is considered only after 12 months of aggressive nonsurgical treatment.

Gastrocnemius Recession: This is a surgical lengthening of the calf (gastrocnemius) muscles. Because tight calf muscles place increased stress on the plantar fascia, this procedure is useful for patients who still have difficulty flexing their feet, despite a year of calf stretches.

In gastrocnemius recession, one of the two muscles that make up the calf is lengthened to increase the motion of the ankle. The procedure can be performed with a traditional, open incision or with a smaller incision and an endoscope, an instrument that contains a small camera. Your doctor will discuss the procedure that best meets your needs.

Complication rates for gastrocnemius recession are low, but can include nerve damage.

Plantar Fascia Release: If you have a normal range of ankle motion and continued heel pain, your doctor may recommend a partial release procedure. During surgery, the plantar fascia ligament is partially cut to relieve tension in the tissue. If you have a large bone spur, it will be removed, as well. Although the surgery can be performed endoscopically, it is more difficult than with an open incision. In addition, endoscopy has a higher risk of nerve damage.

Complications: The most common complications of release surgery include incomplete relief of pain and nerve damage.

Recovery: Most patients have good results from surgery. However, because surgery can result in chronic pain and dissatisfaction, it is recommended only after all nonsurgical measures have been exhausted.

Part Four
Caring For Injured Athletes

Chapter 56

What To Do If A Sports Injury Occurs

First Aid

Accidents happen. Someone chokes on an ice cube or gets stung by a bee. It is important to know when to call 9-1-1. It is for life-threatening emergencies. While waiting for help to arrive, you may be able to save someone's life. Cardiopulmonary resuscitation (CPR) is for people whose hearts or breathing has stopped and the Heimlich maneuver is for people who are choking. CPR should only be done if you have had the training.

You can also learn to handle common injuries and wounds. Cuts and scrapes, for example, should be rinsed with cool water. To stop bleeding, apply firm but gentle pressure, using gauze. If blood soaks through, add more gauze, keeping the first layer in place. Continue to apply pressure.

It is important to have a first aid kit available. It should include a first-aid guide. Read the guide to learn how to use the items, so you are ready in case an emergency happens.

Injuries

An injury is damage to your body. It is a general term that refers to harm caused by accidents, falls, blows, burns, weapons and more. In the U.S., millions of people injure themselves

About This Chapter: The text in this chapter begins with excerpts from "First Aid," "Injuries," and "Wounds," National Library of Medicine (www.nlm.nih.gov/medlineplus), 2012. "If A Sports Injury Occurs" is excerpted from "Handout on Health: Sports Injuries," National Institute of Arthritis and Musculoskeletal and Skin Diseases (NIAMS), April 2009. Brand names included in this chapter are provided as examples only, and their inclusion does not mean that these products are endorsed by the National Institutes of Health or any other government agency. Also, if a particular brand name is not mentioned, this does not mean or imply that the product is unsatisfactory.

every year. These injuries range from minor to life-threatening. Injuries can happen at work or play, indoors or outdoors, driving a car, or walking across the street. Common injuries include burns, dislocations, fractures, sprains, and strains.

Wounds

Wounds include cuts, scrapes, scratches, and punctured skin. They often occur as a result of an accident or injury, but surgical incisions, sutures, and stitches also cause wounds. Minor wounds usually aren't serious, but even cuts and scrapes require care. Take these steps to avoid infection and aid healing:

- Apply pressure with a clean cloth to stop bleeding
- Clean the wound with water
- Use an antibiotic ointment to prevent infection
- Bandage the wound if it's in an area that might get dirty
- Watch for swelling and redness
- Get a tetanus booster if you are due for one

Serious and infected wounds require medical attention. You should also seek attention if the wound is deep, if you cannot close it yourself, if you cannot stop the bleeding or get the dirt out, or if it does not heal.

If A Sports Injury Occurs

What should I do if I suffer an injury?

Whether an injury is acute or chronic, there is never a good reason to try to work through the pain of an injury. When you have pain from a particular movement or activity, STOP! Continuing the activity only causes further harm. Some injuries require prompt medical attention, while others can be self-treated. Here's what you need to know about both types:

When To Seek Medical Treatment: You should call a health professional in these situations:

- The injury causes severe pain, swelling, or numbness.
- You can't tolerate any weight on the area.
- The pain or dull ache of an old injury is accompanied by increased swelling or joint abnormality or instability.

When And How To Treat At Home: If you don't have any of the above symptoms, it's probably safe to treat the injury at home—at least at first. If pain or other symptoms worsen, it's best to check with your health care provider. Use the RICE method described below to relieve pain and inflammation and speed healing. Follow these four steps immediately after injury and continue for at least 48 hours.

- **Rest:** Reduce regular exercise or activities of daily living as needed. If you cannot put weight on an ankle or knee, crutches may help. If you use a cane or one crutch for an ankle injury, use it on the uninjured side to help you lean away and relieve weight on the injured ankle.

- **Ice:** Apply an ice pack to the injured area for 20 minutes at a time, four to eight times a day. A cold pack, ice bag, or plastic bag filled with crushed ice and wrapped in a towel can be used. To avoid cold injury and frostbite, do not apply the ice for more than 20 minutes. Do not use heat immediately after an injury. This tends to increase internal bleeding or swelling. Heat can be used later on to relieve muscle tension and promote relaxation.

- **Compression:** Compression of the injured area may help reduce swelling. Compression can be achieved with elastic wraps, special boots, air casts, and splints. Ask your health care provider for advice on which one to use.

- **Elevation:** If possible, keep the injured ankle, knee, elbow, or wrist elevated on a pillow, above the level of the heart, to help decrease swelling.

The Body's Healing Process: From the moment a bone breaks or a ligament tears, your body goes to work to repair the damage. Here's what happens at each stage of the healing process:

- **At The Moment Of Injury:** Chemicals are released from damaged cells, triggering a process called inflammation. Blood vessels at the injury site become dilated; blood flow increases to carry nutrients to the site of tissue damage.

- **Within Hours Of Injury:** White blood cells (leukocytes) travel down the bloodstream to the injury site where they begin to tear down and remove damaged tissue, allowing other specialized cells to start developing scar tissue.

- **Within Days Of Injury:** Scar tissue is formed on the skin or inside the body. The amount of scarring may be proportional to the amount of swelling, inflammation, or bleeding within. In the next few weeks, the damaged area will regain a great deal of strength as scar tissue continues to form.

- **Within A Month Of Injury:** Scar tissue may start to shrink, bringing damaged, torn, or separated tissues back together. However, it may be several months or more before the injury is completely healed.

Who should I see for my Injury?

Although severe injuries will need to be seen immediately in an emergency room, particularly if they occur on the weekend or after office hours, most sports injuries can be evaluated and, in many cases, treated by your primary health care provider.

Depending on your preference and the severity of your injury or the likelihood that your injury may cause ongoing, long-term problems, you may want to see, or have your primary health care professional refer you to, one of the following:

First Aid Kit

Knowing how to treat minor injuries can make a difference in an emergency. You may consider taking a first aid class, but simply having the following things can help you stop bleeding, prevent infection, and assist in decontamination.

- Two pairs of latex or other sterile gloves if you are allergic to latex
- Sterile dressings to stop bleeding
- Cleansing agent/soap and antibiotic towelettes
- Antibiotic ointment
- Burn ointment
- Adhesive bandages in a variety of sizes
- Eye wash solution to flush the eyes or as general decontaminant
- Thermometer
- Prescription medications you take every day such as insulin, heart medicine and asthma inhalers. You should periodically rotate medicines to account for expiration dates.
- Prescribed medical supplies such as glucose and blood pressure monitoring equipment and supplies
- Non-prescription drugs, such as aspirin or non-aspirin pain relievers, anti-diarrhea medications, antacids, and laxatives.
- Other first aid supplies, including scissors, tweezers, and a tube of petroleum jelly or other lubricant

Source: From "First Aid Kit," Ready.gov, July 15, 2011.

- **Orthopaedic Surgeon:** A doctor specializing in the diagnosis and treatment of the musculoskeletal system, which includes bones, joints, ligaments, tendons, muscles, and nerves.

- **Physical Therapist/Physiotherapist:** A health care professional who can develop a rehabilitation program. Your primary care physician may refer you to a physical therapist after you begin to recover from your injury to help strengthen muscles and joints and prevent further injury.

How are sports injuries treated?

Although using the RICE technique described previously can be helpful for any sports injury, RICE is often just a starting point. Here are some other treatments your doctor or other health care provider may administer, recommend, or prescribe to help your injury heal.

Nonsteroidal Anti-Inflammatory Drugs (NSAIDs): The moment you are injured, chemicals are released from damaged tissue cells. This triggers the first stage of healing: inflammation. Inflammation causes tissues to become swollen, tender, and painful. Although inflammation is needed for healing, it can actually slow the healing process if left unchecked.

To reduce inflammation and pain, doctors and other health care providers often recommend taking an over-the-counter (OTC) nonsteroidal anti-inflammatory drug (NSAID) such as aspirin, ibuprofen (Advil, Motrin IB, Nuprin), ketoprofen (Actron, Orudis KT), or naproxen sodium (Aleve). For more severe pain and inflammation, doctors may prescribe one of several dozen NSAIDs available in prescription strength.

Like all medications, NSAIDs can have side effects. The list of possible adverse effects is long, but major problems are few. The intestinal tract heads the list with nausea, abdominal pain, vomiting, and diarrhea. Changes in liver function frequently occur in children (but not in adults) who use aspirin. Changes in liver function are rare in children using the other NSAIDs. Questions about the appropriate use of NSAIDs should be directed toward your health care provider or pharmacist.

Though not an NSAID, another commonly used OTC medication, acetaminophen (Tylenol), may relieve pain. It has no effect on inflammation, however.

Immobilization: Immobilization is a common treatment for sports injuries that may be done immediately by a trainer or paramedic. Immobilization involves reducing movement in the area to prevent further damage. By enabling the blood supply to flow more directly to the injury (or the site of surgery to repair damage from an injury), immobilization reduces pain, swelling, and muscle spasm and helps the healing process begin. Following are some devices used for immobilization:

- Slings, to immobilize the upper body, including the arms and shoulders.

- Splints and casts, to support and protect injured bones and soft tissue. Casts can be made from plaster or fiberglass. Splints can be custom made or ready-made. Standard splints come in a variety of shapes and sizes and have Velcro straps that make them easy to put on and take off or adjust. Splints generally offer less support and protection than a cast, and therefore may not always be a treatment option.

- Leg immobilizers, to keep the knee from bending after injury or surgery. Made from foam rubber covered with fabric, leg immobilizers enclose the entire leg, fastening with Velcro straps.

Surgery: In some cases, surgery is needed to repair torn connective tissues or to realign bones with compound fractures. The vast majority of sports injuries, however, do not require surgery.

Rehabilitation (Exercise): A key part of rehabilitation from sports injuries is a graduated exercise program designed to return the injured body part to a normal level of function.

Getting Emergency Care

In an emergency, you should call **9-1-1** or go to the nearest emergency room (ER).

What Is An Emergency?

It is an emergency if you reasonably believe that if you don't get care right away, it could be dangerous to your life or to a part of your body. Emergencies include active labor, a bad injury, severe pain, and an illness that is suddenly getting much worse.

How To Get Emergency Care

- If you can, go to the emergency room at a hospital in your health plan's network.

- Try to take your membership card with you.

- If you are not sure if it is an emergency and there is time, call your doctor.

- If you are admitted to a hospital outside your plan's network, call the plan within 24 hours, or as soon as you can. Your plan may move you to a hospital in its network, if it is possible without danger to your health.

When Can I Call An Ambulance?

Health plans only pay for an ambulance when:

- You call 9-1-1 because you think you are having an emergency and cannot get to the hospital safely or quickly enough in a car.

With most injuries, early mobilization—getting the part moving as soon as possible—will speed healing. Generally, early mobilization starts with gentle range-of-motion exercises and then moves on to stretching and strengthening exercise when you can without increasing pain. For example, if you have a sprained ankle, you may be able to work on range of motion for the first day or two after the sprain by gently tracing letters with your big toe. Once your range of motion is fairly good, you can start doing gentle stretching and strengthening exercises. When you are ready, weights may be added to your exercise routine to further strengthen the injured area. The key is to avoid movement that causes pain.

As damaged tissue heals, scar tissue forms, which shrinks and brings torn or separated tissues back together. As a result, the injury site becomes tight or stiff, and damaged tissues are at risk of reinjury. That's why stretching and strengthening exercises are so important. You should continue to stretch the muscles daily and as the first part of your warmup before exercising.

- Your doctor says you need an ambulance and the health plan pre-approves it.

How To Get Urgent Care

Urgent care is care you need soon, usually within 24 hours, for a problem that is serious but is not an emergency. Examples include earache, a sprain, or a minor burn.

Some plans have urgent care clinics you can go to directly. Otherwise, call your primary care doctor and ask what to do.

How To Get Care When You Are Away From Home

Before you leave home, ask your plan how to get care when you are traveling.

- Emergency and urgent care are usually covered anywhere in the world.
- If you have an emergency, call 9-1-1 or go to the nearest ER.
- If you need urgent care, call your primary care doctor or the health plan if you can. If you cannot, go to the nearest clinic or urgent care center.
- Take your membership card with you.
- If you need follow-up care, call your primary care doctor.

Source: "Getting Emergency Care," reprinted with permission from the California Office of the Patient Advocate. Copyright © 2012 State of California. All rights reserved. For additional information, visit http://www.opa.ca.gov.

When planning your rehabilitation program with a health care professional, remember that progression is the key principle. Start with just a few exercises, do them often, and then gradually increase how much you do. A complete rehabilitation program should include exercises for flexibility, endurance, and strength; instruction in balance and proper body mechanics related to the sport; and a planned return to full participation.

Throughout the rehabilitation process, avoid painful activities and concentrate on those exercises that will improve function in the injured part. Don't resume your sport until you are sure you can stretch the injured tissues without any pain, swelling, or restricted movement, and monitor any other symptoms. When you do return to your sport, start slowly and gradually build up to full participation.

Rest: Although it is important to get moving as soon as possible, you must also take time to rest following an injury. All injuries need time to heal; proper rest will help the process. Your health care professional can guide you regarding the proper balance between rest and rehabilitation.

Other Therapies: Other therapies commonly used in rehabilitating sports injuries include the following:

- **Electrostimulation:** Mild electrical current provides pain relief by preventing nerve cells from sending pain impulses to the brain. Electrostimulation may also be used to decrease swelling, and to make muscles in immobilized limbs contract, thus preventing muscle atrophy and maintaining or increasing muscle strength.

- **Cold/Cryotherapy:** Ice packs reduce inflammation by constricting blood vessels and limiting blood flow to the injured tissues. Cryotherapy eases pain by numbing the injured area. It is generally used for only the first 48 hours after injury.

- **Heat/Thermotherapy:** Heat, in the form of hot compresses, heat lamps, or heating pads, causes the blood vessels to dilate and increase blood flow to the injury site. Increased blood flow aids the healing process by removing cell debris from damaged tissues and carrying healing nutrients to the injury site. Heat also helps to reduce pain. It should not be applied within the first 48 hours after an injury.

- **Ultrasound:** High-frequency sound waves produce deep heat that is applied directly to an injured area. Ultrasound stimulates blood flow to promote healing.

- **Massage:** Manual pressing, rubbing, and manipulation soothe tense muscles and increase blood flow to the injury site.

Most of these therapies are administered or supervised by a licensed health care professional.

Chapter 57

What Do Athletic Trainers Do?

Nature Of The Work

Athletic trainers help prevent and treat injuries for people of all ages. Their patients and clients include everyone from professional athletes to industrial workers. Recognized by the American Medical Association as allied health professionals, athletic trainers specialize in the prevention, diagnosis, assessment, treatment, and rehabilitation of muscle and bone injuries and illnesses. Athletic trainers, as one of the first healthcare providers on the scene when injuries occur, must be able to recognize, evaluate, and assess injuries and provide immediate care when needed. Athletic trainers should not be confused with fitness trainers or personal trainers, who are not healthcare workers, but rather train people to become physically fit.

Athletic trainers try to prevent injuries by educating people on how to reduce their risk for injuries and by advising them on the proper use of equipment, exercises to improve balance and strength, and home exercises and therapy programs. They also help apply protective or injury-preventive devices such as tape, bandages, and braces.

Athletic trainers may work under the direction of a licensed physician, and in cooperation with other healthcare providers. The extent of the direction ranges from discussing specific injuries and treatment options with a physician to performing evaluations and treatments as directed by a physician. Some athletic trainers meet with the team physician or consulting physician once or twice a week; others interact with a physician every day. Athletic trainers often have administrative responsibilities. These may include regular meetings with an athletic director, physician practice manager, or other administrative officer to deal with budgets, purchasing, policy implementation, and other business-related issues.

About This Chapter: Excerpted from "Athletic Trainers," *Occupational Outlook Handbook*, U.S. Department of Labor, December 2009.

Work Environment

The industry and individual employer are significant in determining the work environment of athletic trainers. Many athletic trainers work indoors most of the time; others, especially those in some sports-related jobs, spend much of their time working outdoors. The job also might require standing for long periods, working with medical equipment or machinery, and being able to walk, run, kneel, stoop, or crawl. Travel may be required.

Schedules vary by work setting. Athletic trainers in non-sports settings generally have an established schedule—usually about 40 to 50 hours per week—with nights and weekends off. Athletic trainers working in hospitals and clinics may spend part of their time working at other locations doing outreach services. The most common outreach programs include conducting athletic training services and speaking at high schools, colleges, and commercial businesses.

Athletic trainers in sports settings have schedules that are longer and more variable. These athletic trainers must be present for team practices and competitions, which often are on evenings and weekends, and their schedules can change on short notice when games and practices have to be rescheduled. In high schools, athletic trainers who also teach may work 60 to 70 hours a week, or more. In National Collegiate Athletic Association Division I colleges and universities, athletic trainers generally work with one team; when that team's sport is in season, working at least 50 to 60 hours a week is common. Athletic trainers in smaller colleges and universities often work with several teams and have teaching responsibilities. During the off-season, a 40-hour to 50-hour workweek may be normal in most settings. Athletic trainers for professional sports teams generally work the most hours per week. During training camps, practices, and competitions, they may be required to work up to 12 hours a day.

There is some stress involved with being an athletic trainer. The work of athletic trainers requires frequent interaction with others. They consult with physicians as well as have frequent contact with athletes and patients to discuss and administer treatments, rehabilitation programs, injury-preventive practices, and other health-related issues. Athletic trainers are responsible for their clients' health, and sometimes have to make quick decisions that could affect the health or career of their clients. Athletics trainers also can be affected by the pressure to win that is typical of competitive sports teams.

Training And Other Qualifications

A bachelor's degree is usually the minimum requirement, but many athletic trainers hold a master's or doctoral degree. In 2009, 47 States required athletic trainers to be licensed or hold some form of registration.

Education And Training

A bachelor's degree from an accredited college or university is required for almost all jobs as an athletic trainer. In 2009, there were about 350 accredited undergraduate programs nationwide. Students in these programs are educated both in the classroom and in clinical settings. Formal education includes many science and health-related courses, such as human anatomy, physiology, nutrition, and biomechanics.

According to the National Athletic Trainers' Association, almost 70% of athletic trainers have a master's degree or higher. Athletic trainers may need a master's or higher degree to be eligible for some positions, especially those in colleges and universities, and to increase their advancement opportunities. Because some positions in high schools involve teaching along with athletic trainer responsibilities, a teaching certificate or license could be required.

Licensure And Certification

In 2009, 47 States required athletic trainers to be licensed or registered; this requires certification from the Board of Certification, Inc. (BOC). For BOC certification, athletic trainers need a bachelor's or master's degree from an accredited athletic training program and must pass a rigorous examination. To retain certification, credential holders must continue taking medical-related courses and adhere to the BOC standards of practice. In Alaska, California, West Virginia, and the District of Columbia where licensure is not required, certification is voluntary but may be helpful for those seeking jobs and advancement.

Other Qualifications

Because all athletic trainers deal directly with a variety of people, they need good social and communication skills. They should be able to manage difficult situations and the stress associated with them, such as when disagreements arise with coaches, patients, clients, or parents regarding suggested treatment. Athletic trainers also should be organized, be able to manage time wisely, be inquisitive, and have a strong desire to help people.

Chapter 58

Choosing A Doctor

Finding the right doctor or health care provider for you is a big part of your medical care. Don't wait until you get sick to find one. When you look for or change doctors, follow these tips:

- Look for one who accepts your health plan. Check with the plan. Ask the person at work who handles employee benefits.

- If you belong to a managed care plan, get a list of providers who work with the plan. Health Maintenance Organizations (HMOs) and Preferred Provider Organizations (PPOs) are two types of managed care plans. The doctor(s) you see now may be on your HMO or PPO list.

- Make a list of things you want in a doctor or provider, such as close location, certain gender, age, etc.

- Ask relatives and friends for doctors they trust and have given them good medical care.

- Find out if a doctor is taking new patients. Check with your health plan. Call the doctor's office.

- Look for a doctor you can relate to. How do you want medical decisions to be made? The doctor alone? You and the doctor together? Find one that meets your needs.

- Ask about office hours and staffing. Ask how many patients are scheduled to be seen in an hour and how long they usually wait to see the doctor.

About This Chapter: Excerpted from *Healthier at Home: The Proven Guide to Self-Care & Being a Wise Consumer*, by Don Powell, PhD. © 2011 American Institute for Preventive Medicine (www.healthylife.com). All rights reserved. Reprinted with permission.

- Ask how payment is handled. Must you pay for your visit at that time? Can you be billed and pay later?

- Find out what other providers serve as backups when the doctor is away. Ask what you should do at non-office hour times.

- Find out which hospital(s) the doctor or provider sends patients to.

- Look for a doctor who is competent and can care for all your general health needs. Ask if and who the doctor will refer you to for any special health needs.

See Your Primary Doctor Before You See A Specialist

Primary care doctors manage your medical care. If you are a member of a Health Maintenance Organization (HMO), your primary care doctor is the doctor you select from the HMO plan to coordinate your medical care. This person could be a family doctor, internist, obstetrician/gynecologist, etc. Whether or not you belong to an HMO, call or see your primary care doctor before you see a specialist. If your primary care doctor cannot take care of your needs, he or she will refer you to a specialist.

Tell And Ask The Doctor/Provider Checklists

Checklist 1: Before You Call Or See Your Doctor/Provider

- Your signs and symptoms (in the order they occurred and what makes them better or worse)

- Results of home testing, such as temperature

- Medicines you take (prescribed, over-the-counter, herbal products, vitamins, etc.)

- Allergies to medicines, food, etc.

- Family and personal medical history

- Your lifestyle: eating, drinking, sleeping, exercising habits, sexual functioning, etc.

- Concerns you have about your health and/or what you think the problem may be due to

- What you would like the doctor to do for you

- Your pharmacist's phone number and fax number

If needed, have your medical records, results of lab tests and x-rays, etc. from other health care providers sent to your doctor before your visit.

Checklist 2: During The Doctor/Provider Visit Or Call

Tell the doctor what you wrote down in Checklist 1. Take the list with you. Ask your doctor these questions:

- What do you think the problem or diagnosis is?
- What, if any, tests are needed to rule out or confirm your diagnosis?
- What do I need to do to treat the problem?
- Do I need to take medicine?
- How can I prevent the problem in the future?
- When do I need to call or see you again?
- How are costs handled for this visit and for tests?

Checklist 3: After The Doctor/Provider Visit Or Call

- Follow your doctor's advice
- Call the doctor if you feel worse, have other problems or side effects from the medicines, etc.
- Keep return visit appointments

Chapter 59

Guidelines For Medical Decision Making

Key Questions Checklist

Diagnosis

- What is my diagnosis?
- Is my condition chronic or acute?
- Is there anything I can do to cure, treat, and/or prevent it from getting worse?
- Is my condition contagious or genetic?
- How certain are you about this diagnosis?

Treatment

- What is the recommended treatment?
- Is there a support group for my condition?

If You Are Discussing Medications

- What will the medicine do for my particular problem?
- When, how often, and for how long should I take the medicine?
- How long before the medicine starts working?
- Will there be side effects?
- Will there be interactions with other medications I am taking?

About This Chapter: Excerpted from *Healthier at Home: The Proven Guide to Self-Care & Being a Wise Consumer*, by Don Powell, PhD. © 2011 American Institute for Preventive Medicine (www.healthylife.com). All rights reserved. Reprinted with permission.

If You Are Discussing A Test

- What is the test called and how will it help identify the problem? Will it give specific or general information?

- Will more tests be necessary?

- How accurate and reliable is the test?

- How should I prepare for the test?

- Where do I go for the test?

- How and when will I get the test's results?

If You Are Discussing Surgery

- How many of these surgeries have you done and what were the results?

- Can I get a step-by-step account of the procedure, including anesthesia and recovery?

Benefits Vs. Risks

- What are the benefits if I go ahead with the treatment?

- What are the possible risks and complications?

- Do the benefits outweigh the risks?

Success

- What is the success rate for the treatment?

- Are there any personal factors that will affect my odds either way?

- How long will the results of treatment last?

Timing

- When is the best time to begin the treatment?

- When can I expect to see results?

Alternatives

- What will happen if I decide to do nothing?

- What are my other options?

Cost

- What is the cost for the treatment?

- What related costs should I consider (for example: time off work, travel, etc.).

Decision

- You can now make an informed decision.

- You have the right to choose or refuse treatment.

Chart 59.1. Medical Decision Comparison Chart

Make copies as needed. Use this chart to help you compare medical options that are available to you.

Diagnosis:	Option One	Option Two	Option Three
Treatment			
Benefits			
Risks			
Success			
Timing			
Alternatives			
Cost			
Decision	Yes No	Yes No	Yes No

Patient Rights

According to the American Hospital Association (AHA), all hospital patients are entitled to certain standards of care. The AHA developed a voluntary code called The Patient's Bill of Rights. This gives guidelines for both staff and patients. It gives you these rights:

- To considerate and respectful care

- To obtain from your doctor complete, current information about your diagnosis, treatment, and prognosis (these should be given in terms you can understand)

- To receive from your doctor information necessary to give informed consent before the start of any procedure and/or treatment

- To expect reasonable continuity of care

- To refuse treatment to the extent the law permits

- To be informed of the medical effects of your action

- To privacy for your medical care (this includes all communications and records about your care)

- To expect that, within its capacity, a hospital must make a reasonable response to your request for services

- To get information about any connection between your hospital and other health care and educational institutions, as it relates to your care

- To be advised if the hospital proposes to take part in or perform human experiments that could affect your care or treatment

- To examine and receive an explanation of your bill no matter how it is paid

- To know what hospital rules and regulations apply to your conduct as a patient

- To obtain a copy of your written medical records

Informed Consent

Informed consent means that you agree to treatment only after it has been explained to you and that you understand it. You should know the nature of the treatment, its benefits and risks, and the likelihood of its success. You should also be told if your treatment is an experimental one.

The doctor should review any alternatives to surgery or other procedures. There are no guaranteed outcomes in medicine, but informed consent enables you to make a rational and educated decision about your treatment.

With Informed Consent

- You cannot demand services that go beyond what are considered acceptable practices of medicine or that violate professional ethics.

- You must recognize that you may be faced with some uncertainties or unpleasantness.

- You should, if competent, be responsible for your choices. Don't have others make decisions for you.

Chapter 60

Caring For Casts And Splints

Casts and splints support and protect injured bones and soft tissue. When you break a bone, your doctor will put the pieces back together in the right position. Casts and splints hold the bones in place while they heal. They also reduce pain, swelling, and muscle spasm.

In some cases, splints and casts are applied following surgery.

Splints or "half-casts" provide less support than casts. However, splints can be adjusted to accommodate swelling from injuries easier than enclosed casts. Your doctor will decide which type of support is best for you.

Types Of Splints And Casts

Casts are custom-made. They must fit the shape of your injured limb correctly to provide the best support. Casts can be made of plaster or fiberglass—a plastic that can be shaped.

Splints or half-casts can also be custom-made, especially if an exact fit is necessary. Other times, a ready-made splint will be used. These off-the-shelf splints are made in a variety of shapes and sizes, and are much easier and faster to use. They have Velcro straps, which make the splints easy to put on, take off, and adjust.

Materials

Fiberglass or plaster materials form the hard supportive layer in splints and casts.

Fiberglass is lighter in weight, longer wearing, and "breathes" better than plaster. In addition, x-rays can see through fiberglass better than through plaster. This is important because

About This Chapter: "Care of Casts and Splints," reproduced with permission from *Your Orthopaedic Connection.* © American Academy of Orthopaedic Surgeons (www.aaos.org), Rosemont, IL, 2011.

your doctor will probably schedule additional x-rays after your splint or cast has been applied. X-rays can show whether the bones are healing well or have moved out of place.

Plaster is less expensive than fiberglass and shapes better than fiberglass for some uses.

Application

Both fiberglass and plaster splints and casts use padding, usually cotton, as a protective layer next to the skin. Both materials come in strips or rolls which are dipped in water and applied over the padding covering the injured area.

The splint or cast must fit the shape of the injured arm or leg correctly to provide the best possible support. Generally, the splint or cast also covers the joint above and below the broken bone.

In many cases, a splint is applied to a fresh injury first. As swelling subsides, a full cast may replace the splint.

Sometimes, it may be necessary to replace a cast as swelling goes down and the cast gets too big. As a fracture heals, the cast may be replaced by a splint to make it easier to perform physical therapy exercises.

Getting Used To A Splint Or Cast

Swelling due to your injury may cause pressure in your splint or cast for the first 48 to 72 hours. This may cause your injured arm or leg to feel snug or tight in the splint or cast. If you have a splint, your doctor will show you how to adjust it to accommodate the swelling.

It is very important to keep the swelling down. This will lessen pain and help your injury heal. To help reduce swelling:

- **Elevate:** It is very important to elevate your injured arm or leg for the first 24 to 72 hours. Prop your injured arm or leg up above your heart by putting it on pillows or some other support. You will have to recline if the splint or cast is on your leg. Elevation allows clear fluid and blood to drain downhill to your heart.

- **Exercise:** Move your uninjured, but swollen fingers or toes gently and often. Moving them often will prevent stiffness.

- **Ice:** Apply ice to the splint or cast. Place the ice in a dry plastic bag or ice pack and loosely wrap it around the splint or cast at the level of the injury. Ice that is packed in a rigid container and touches the cast at only one point will not be effective.

Warning Signs

Swelling can create a lot of pressure under your cast. This can lead to problems. If you experience any of the following symptoms, contact your doctor's office immediately for advice.

- **Increased Pain And The Feeling That The Splint Or Cast Is Too Tight:** This may be caused by swelling.

- **Numbness And Tingling In Your Hand Or Foot:** This may be caused by too much pressure on the nerves.

- **Burning And Stinging:** This may be caused by too much pressure on the skin.

- **Excessive Swelling Below The Cast:** This may mean the cast is slowing your blood circulation.

- **Loss Of Active Movement Of Toes Or Fingers:** This requires an urgent evaluation by your doctor.

Taking Care Of Your Splint Or Cast

Your doctor will explain any restrictions on using your injured arm or leg while it is healing. You must follow your doctor's instructions carefully to make sure your bone heals properly. The following information provides general guidelines only, and is not a substitute for your doctor's advice.

After you have adjusted to your splint or cast for a few days, it is important to keep it in good condition. This will help your recovery.

- **Keep Your Splint Or Cast Dry:** Moisture weakens plaster and damp padding next to the skin can cause irritation. Use two layers of plastic or purchase waterproof shields to keep your splint or cast dry while you shower or bathe.

- **Walking Casts:** Do not walk on a walking cast until it is completely dry and hard. It takes about one hour for fiberglass, and two to three days for plaster to become hard enough to walk on.

- **Avoid Dirt:** Keep dirt, sand, and powder away from the inside of your splint or cast.

- **Padding:** Do not pull out the padding from your splint or cast.

- **Itching:** Do not stick objects such as coat hangers inside the splint or cast to scratch itching skin. Do not apply powders or deodorants to itching skin. If itching persists, contact your doctor.

- **Trimming:** Do not break off rough edges of the cast or trim the cast before asking your doctor.

- **Skin:** Inspect the skin around the cast. If your skin becomes red or raw around the cast, contact your doctor.

- **Inspect The Cast Regularly:** If it becomes cracked or develops soft spots, contact your doctor's office.

Cast Removal

Never remove the cast yourself. You may cut your skin or prevent proper healing of your injury.

Your doctor will use a cast saw to remove your cast. The saw vibrates, but does not rotate. If the blade of the saw touches the padding inside the hard shell of the cast, the padding will vibrate with the blade and will protect your skin. Cast saws make noise and may feel hot from friction, but will not harm you. "Their bark is worse than their bite."

Use common sense. You have a serious injury and you must protect your cast from damage so it can protect your injury while it heals.

After the initial swelling has subsided, proper splint or cast support will usually allow you to continue your daily activities with a minimum of inconvenience.

Rehabilitation

Broken bones take several weeks to several months to heal. Pain usually stops long before the bone is solid enough to handle the stresses of everyday activities. You will need to wear your cast or splint until your bone is fully healed and can support itself.

While you are wearing your cast or splint, you will likely lose muscle strength in the injured area. Exercises during the healing process and after your cast is removed are important. They will help you restore normal muscle strength, joint motion, and flexibility.

Chapter 61

Returning To Sport After An Injury

If you have had a recent injury one of your main concerns may be how soon you can return to play. The answer to this question is not always easy because each athlete and each injury is unique. Returning too soon can increase your risk of reinjury or developing a chronic problem that will lead to a longer recovery. Waiting too long, however, can lead to unnecessary de-conditioning.

Understanding Injuries

When the body is injured, for instance when you tear a muscle, the body uses a process called inflammation to try to begin healing the area. You know something is inflamed when you see redness and swelling, feel heat and pain, and can't use your body as you usually would. Often it is the presence of these signs that give us the first indication that we have sustained an injury.

Whilst inflammation is an essential part of the healing process it is important to understand that this should ideally be a self-limiting process but often can cause problems when it lasts longer than it should.

There are three phases of healing: the inflammatory phase, the regeneration phase, and remodeling phase. Sometimes the body gets stuck in the inflammatory phase for a long time, this is known as chronic inflammation.

Until the inflammatory phase is complete the rest of the healing process cannot occur.

- **Acute Inflammation:** Straight after an injury you will see the signs of inflammation mentioned above, often the PRICE (protection/rest/ice/compression/elevation) protocol is used to reduce pain and help to speed recovery times.

- **Chronic Inflammation:** Usually inflammation will stop once the tissue has healed and the patient is recovered, sometimes however the inflammation continues for a number of reasons, which causes prolonged time until recovery. One of the causes of chronic inflammation is early return to sport and increasing your training prematurely.

Once you have finished the inflammatory phase it is important that you allow time for the tissues to regenerate and begin remodeling, it is at this time that you can commence a controlled, graduated return to sport.

Common Mistakes People Make When Returning To Sport

- Not warming up prior to a game/training
- Not working on flexibility and muscle tightness
- Playing into fatigue
- General poor fitness
- Not allowing for adequate recovery time
- Not addressing muscle imbalances
- Not addressing biomechanical issues
- Not sufficiently improving strength prior to returning to sport

General Advice To Prevent Reinjury

- Stay in shape year-round
- Pay attention to injury warning signs
- Treat injuries immediately
- Participate in a full injury rehab program
- Know when it's safe to return to sports
- Stay fit while injured
- Keep a positive, upbeat attitude

While your injury heals try to maintain overall conditioning if possible. Try alternate forms of training such as water running, swimming, cycling, rowing, or weight training of the noninjured parts.

Regaining range of motion and strength should be started as soon as possible as directed by your physical therapist. Use discomfort as a guide and avoid movements that cause pain. Once muscle strength and flexibility return you can slowly get back into your sport, working at about 50 to 70% max capacity for a few weeks. During this re-entry phase, functional drills for balance, agility, and speed can be added as tolerated.

Guidelines For Safe Return To Sports

- You are pain free
- You have no swelling
- You have full range of motion
- You have full (90% +) strength compared with the uninjured side
- For lower body injuries you can perform full weight bearing on injured hips, knees, and ankles without limping
- For upper body injuries you can perform throwing movements with proper form and no pain

Even when you feel 100% you may have deficits in strength, joint stability, flexibility, or skill. Take extra care with the injured part for several months.

What do I need to do to return to sport after a soft tissue injury?

Allow adequate healing time. Pain and swelling should no longer be present.

- **Strength:** At least 80% strength when compared to your uninjured side
- **Flexibility:** Full pain free range of movement at the injury site, scar tissue will remain tight for between 12–24 months so you must keep up your flexibility work by stretching the injured area
- **Stability:** It is essential that the joint where the injury occurred is stable
- **Endurance:** Make sure that you are able to use the body part for a similar period and in a similar manner to that of your normal sport otherwise reinjury is likely. You may want to practice starting, stopping, changing direction and speed in a controlled environment before you return to sport

How long until my soft tissue injury will heal?

This depends on the severity or degree of soft tissue damage. The more damage the longer the recovery and the longer the rehabilitation.

Grade I

- Tight discomfort, little or no swelling or bruising
- Minimal pain on resisted movement and no loss of strength

- With appropriate care, about 7–10 days

Grade II

- Some bruising, swelling, and local tenderness
- Loss of the normal range of movement, pain on resisted movements and with use, walking for example.
- With appropriate care, about 3–6 weeks

Grade III

- Severe pain, marked bruising and swelling with some disability, needing crutches for example
- Loss of local muscle power and pain on static contraction of the muscle
- With appropriate care, 6–12 weeks or even longer

What do I need to do to return to sport after a back injury?

If you have sustained a back injury whether as a result of playing sport or not it is vital that you have followed certain measures before returning to sport.

One of the most important things you can do is to improve your core strength, the more dynamic and higher level the sport, the greater core strength you need. Poor core strength predisposes us to back injuries so it is likely that your core strength was insufficient for the level of sport/work you were performing at the time. Unfortunately having lower back pain can actually inhibit these muscles from turning on when needed and this can cause a reduction in strength following your injury.

Depending on the type of sport you play and at what level, you may need to modify your training and game techniques and your physical therapist can help you to determine what movements put you at risk and ways to modify them so you can keep playing

How long will it take to improve my core strength?

As with any new exercise program you can expect to see improvements in your core stability after a few weeks although it may be difficult for you to notice. It is therefore important as an athlete that you commence early core activation exercises so that once your injury has recovered your core stability is already improving.

Chapter 62

Sports Injuries And Arthritis: Understanding The Connection

The Potential Risk Of Arthritis

Americans of all ages are increasingly participating in sporting activities. This is a healthy trend, as sports are well known to be helpful for cardiopulmonary fitness and weight-control. However, with the benefits does come some risk, namely sports injuries. Most sports injuries are mild and temporary, with no long-term effects. Minor sprains and bruises or overuse injuries treated properly may be nuisances but do not necessarily cause any permanent problems. Some injuries, however, may lead to arthritis later in life.

Millions of Americans are affected by arthritis, a potentially painful and debilitating condition. Arthritis is the result of disease or damage to articular cartilage, the white glistening surface of our bones found in the joints. Articular cartilage is found in all major joints of the body, including the hips, knees, and shoulders, as well as the smaller joints of the upper and lower extremities and even the spine and pelvis. When this normally smooth gliding surface is no longer intact, pain, swelling, and stiffness may result. This is what is referred to as arthritis.

Arthritis is usually seen in older people, but is also seen in younger people who either have a less common form of the disease or have suffered an injury. The most common form is osteoarthritis, also referred to as degenerative arthritis. It usually occurs naturally, without any specific prior injury, in older people. However, this form of arthritis is also the type seen after injury. In this case, it may be referred to as post-traumatic osteoarthritis, or wear-and-tear arthritis. Whatever the name, the result is the same—a painful, swollen, stiff, and sometimes enlarged or deformed joint. It can be mild in some people, offering only an occasional reminder of an old sports injury, or it can be severe, causing daily suffering and degrees of disability.

About This Chapter: "Sports Injuries and Arthritis," by William Cottrell, M.D. © National Center for Sports Safety (http://www.sportssafety.org) 2005, reviewed 2012, reprinted with permission.

Injuries That Can Lead To Arthritis

It is important to understand the types of injury that can go on to cause arthritis in later life. The types of injuries that lead to arthritis include direct injury to the cartilage (as in fractured joints) or injuries that alter joint mechanics, increasing the stress on the articular surface. The first type is less common in sports, more often seen in motor vehicle accidents or falls from a great height. In these instances, severe bruising of the cartilage surface may lead to permanent injury and eventual arthritis. It may also occur from a fracture of the bone through the cartilage in the joint. In these cases the joint may heal with irregularity causing the cartilage to wear unevenly and eventually erode, resulting in arthritis. A key factor is that, while cartilage is a living tissue and does respond to injury, its reparative capacity is limited, and any significant damage usually results in a permanent alteration.

The more common way a sports injury leads to arthritis is when a ligament or supporting structure is damaged, causing abnormal mechanics in the joint. This greatly increases the stress on the articular surface, which over time, wears out and causes arthritis. One of the most known examples of this type of this injury is in the knee. With the increased attention of media to the injuries sustained by star athletes, most people have heard of an ACL injury. ACL stands for anterior cruciate ligament, one of the major stabilizers of the knee. The ACL is in the center of the joint and keeps the tibia (lower leg bone) from moving forward on the femur (thigh bone). Commonly an athlete injures the ACL trying to pivot. The result of a torn ACL is generally an unstable knee, one that buckles occasionally, especially with strenuous activities or further participation in sports. This instability abuses the knee, and over time, the articular surfaces are damaged by the abnormal stresses. Once again, the result is eventual arthritis, although the timetable ranges from a short time to many years.

Another knee injury that results in arthritis is torn cartilage. The menisci are a different form of cartilage found in the knee. They are roughly semicircular wedges, two in each knee, that function to cushion the joint, absorbing a great deal of stress, and also more evenly distributes stress across the joint. A torn meniscus alone can be painful and cause swelling and stiffness, leading a patient to seek early surgical treatment. Historically, the entire torn meniscus was removed. We now know that, while this treatment relieves the acute pain and swelling, it eventually predisposes the patient to premature arthritis due to the absence of the protective effects of the menisci. Currently, attempts are made to repair a torn meniscus to remove only the torn part, leaving as much healthy meniscus as possible. Despite these efforts, an injured meniscus may still lead to earlier arthritis.

Preventing And Treating Sports-Injury Related Arthritis

The next issue is treatment of arthritis due to sports injuries. As is true in most cases, the best treatment is prevention of the injuries. There are a few different methods to prevent sports injuries. The first is proper conditioning. When someone is poorly conditioned or fatigued, the muscles do not protect the joints, and an injury is more likely. It is important for athletes at any level to be properly conditioned for their sport, not only with regards to stamina but also strength and flexibility. Proper nutrition and hydration also come into play. The next aspect of prevention is proper form and technique in the specific sport, assured in part by following the rules of the game. Finally, certain sports offer protective equipment, and this may be of benefit in injury prevention.

Once an injury has been sustained, there are still measures that may prevent arthritis. Avoiding strenuous or demanding activities may decrease the chances of arthritis. In many cases, as in the torn ACL, the problem can be surgically corrected, restoring proper mechanics and thereby hopefully preventing arthritis.

If arthritis does result, there are also many ways to treat the symptoms. The first is activity modification. Occasionally, orthotics or braces may help. Medications such as acetaminophen (Tylenol) or anti-inflammatory medicines such as ibuprofen may offer relief. Physical therapy, including exercises, is sometimes helpful. New over-the-counter nutritional supplements have also shown promise. Occasional joint injections may give some relief. When all other measures have failed, surgery ranging from arthroscopy to joint replacement can be performed. Unfortunately, there is no cure for arthritis, and that is why prevention is the best treatment.

Part Five
If You Need More Information

Resources For More Information About Traumatic And Chronic Sports-Related Injuries

Academy for Sports Dentistry

118 Faye Street
P.O. Box 364
Farmersville, IL 62533
Toll-Free: 800-273-1788
Fax: 217-227-3438
Website:
http://www.academyforsportsdentistry.org
E-mail:
info@academyforsportsdentistry.org

American Academy of Orthopaedic Surgeons

6300 North River Road
Rosemont, IL 60018-4262
Phone: 847-823-7186
Fax: 847-823-8125
Website: http://www.aaos.org
E-mail: custserv@aaos.org

American Academy of Otolaryngology—Head and Neck Surgery

1650 Diagonal Road
Alexandria, VA 22314-2857
Phone: 703-836-4444
Website: http://www.entnet.org

American Academy of Pediatrics

141 Northwest Point Boulevard
Elk Grove Village, IL 60007-1098
Phone: 847-434-4000
Fax: 847-434-8000
Website: http://www.aap.org

Information in this chapter was compiled from many sources deemed reliable. Inclusion does not constitute endorsement and there is no implication associated with omission. All contact information was verified in March 2012.

American Academy of Physical Medicine and Rehabilitation

9700 West Bryn Mawr Avenue, Suite 200
Rosemont, Illinois 60018
Phone: 847-737-6000
Fax: 847-737-6001
Website: http://www.aapmr.org
E-mail: infor@aapmr.org

American Academy of Podiatric Sports Medicine

Phone: 301-845-9887
Website: http://www.aapsm.org
E-mail: info@aapsm.org

American Association of Endodontists

211 East Chicago Avenue, Suite 1100
Chicago, IL 60611-2691
Toll-Free: 800-872-3636
Phone: 312-266-7255
Toll-Free Fax: 800-451-9020
Fax: 312-266-9867
Website: http://www.aae.org
E-mail: info@aae.org

American Association of Neurological Surgeons

5550 Meadowbrook Drive
Rolling Meadows, IL 60008-3852
Toll-Free: 888-566-AANS
(888-566-2267)
Phone: 847-378-0500
Fax: 847-378-0600
Website: http://www.aans.org
E-mail: info@aans.org

American Chiropractic Association

1701 Clarendon Boulevard
Arlington, VA 22209
Phone: 703-276-8800
Fax: 703-243-2593
Website: http://www.acatoday.org
E-mail: memberinfo@acatoday.org

American Chiropractic Association Sports Council

246 First Street, Suite 101
San Francisco, CA 94105
Phone: 414-810-9810
Website: http://www.acasc.org

American College of Foot and Ankle Surgeons

8725 West Higgins Road, Suite 555
Chicago, IL 60631-2724
Toll-Free: 800-421-2237
Phone: 773-693-9300
Fax: 773-693-9304
Website: www.acfas.org
Foot Health Facts:
www.foothealthfacts.org
E-mail: info@acfas.org

American College of Sports Medicine

401 West Michigan Street
Indianapolis, IN 46202-3233
Phone: 317-637-9200
Fax: 317-634-7817
Website: http://www.acsm.org

American Medical Athletic Association

4405 East-West Highway, Suite 405
Bethesda, MD 20814
Toll-Free: 800-776-2732
Phone: 301-913-9517
Fax: 301-913-9520
Website: http://www.amaasportsmed.org
E-mail: aama@americanrunning.org

American Medical Society for Sports Medicine

4000 West 114th Street, Suite 100
Leawood, KS 66211
Phone: 913-327-1415
Fax: 913-327-1491
Website: http://www.amssm.org

American Orthopaedic Society for Sports Medicine

6300 North River Road, Suite 500
Rosemont, IL 60018
Toll-Free: 877-321-3500
Phone: 847-292-4900
Fax: 847-292-4905
Website: http://www.sportsmed.org
E-mail: info@aossm.org

American Orthopaedic Foot and Ankle Society

6300 North River Road, Suite 510
Rosemont, IL 60018
Toll-Free: 800-235-4855
Phone: 847-698-4654
Website: http://www.aofas.org
E-mail: aofasinfo@aofas.org

American Osteopathic Academy of Sports Medicine

2424 American Lane
Madison, WI 53704
Phone: 608-443-2477
Fax: 608-443-2474
Website: http://www.aoasm.org

American Osteopathic Association

142 East Ontario Street
Chicago, IL 60611-2864
Toll-Free: 800-621-1773
Phone: 312-202-8000
Fax: 312-202-8200
Website: http://www.osteopathic.org
E-mail: info@osteopathic.org

American Physical Therapy Association

1111 North Fairfax Street
Alexandria, VA 22314-1488
Toll-Free: 800-999-2782
Phone: 703-684-APTA (703-684-2782)
TDD: 703-683-6748
Fax: 703-684-7343
Website: http://www.apta.org
E-mail: Research-dept@apta.org

American Physiological Society

9650 Rockville Pike
Bethesda, MD 20814-3991
Phone: 301-634-7164
Fax: 301-634-7241
Website: http://www.the-aps.org

American Red Cross

Website: http://www.redcross.org

American Shoulder and Elbow Surgeons

6300 North River Road, Suite 727
Rosemont, IL 60018
Phone: 847-698-1629
Fax: 847-823-0536
Website: http://www.ases-assn.org
E-mail: ases@aaos.org

American Society for Surgery of the Hand

6300 North River Road, Suite 600
Rosemont, IL 60018
Phone: 847-384-8300
(between 7:30 a.m. and 5:30 p.m. CST,
Monday through Friday)
Fax: 847-384-1435
Website: http://www.assh.org
E-mail: info@assh.org

American Sports Medicine Institute

2660 10th Avenue South, Suite 505
Birmingham, AL 35205
Phone: 205-918-0000
Fax: 205-918-0800
Website: http://www.asmi.org
Athletic Advisor:
http://athleticadvisor.com

Ann and Robert H. Lurie Children's Hospital of Chicago

225 East Chicago Avenue
Chicago, IL 60611
Toll-Free: 800-KIDS-DOC
(800-543-7362)
Website: http://www.luriechildrens.org

Arthritis Foundation

P.O. Box 7669
Atlanta, GA 30357-0669
Toll-Free: 800-283-7800
Website: http://www.arthritis.org

Brain Injury Association of America

1608 Spring Hill Road, Suite 110
Vienna, VA 22182
Toll-Free: 800-444-6443
(Brain Injury Information Only)
Phone: 703-761-0750
Fax: 703-7610755
Website: http://www.biausa.org

Bicycle Helmet Safety Institute

4611 Seventh Street South
Arlington, VA 22204-1419
Phone: 703-486-0100
Website: http://www.bhsi.org
E-mail: info@helmets.org

Canadian Society for Exercise Physiology

1800 Louisa Street, Suite 370
Ottawa, Ontario CANADA K1R 6Y6
Website: http://www.csep.ca
E-mail: info@csep.ca

Children's Hospital Colorado

Anschutz Medical Campus
13123 East 16th Avenue
Aurora, CO 80045
Toll-Free: 800-624-6553
Phone: 720-777-1234
TTY: 720-777-6050
Online Health Library:
http://www.childrenscolorado.org/
wellness/library/fhlindex.aspx

Christopher and Dana Reeve Foundation

636 Morris Turnpike, Suite 3A
Short Hills, NJ 07078
Toll-Free: 800-225-0292
Phone: 973-379-2690
Website: http://www.christopherreeve.org

Coalition to Prevent Sports Eye Injuries

5 Summit Avenue
Hackensack, NJ 07601
Toll-Free: 866-265-3582
Fax: 201-621-4352
Website: http://www.sportseyeinjuries.com

Coastal Physiotherapy and Sports Injury Clinic

180 Napper Road
Parkwood, Gold Coast, 4215
Australia
Phone: + 61 (07) 55744303
Website:
http://www.coastalphysioclinic.com.au
E-mail: coastalphysioclinic@bigpond.com

Consumer Product Safety Commission

4330 East West Highway
Bethesda, MD 20814
Toll-Free: 800-638-2772
(Hotline; 8:00 a.m.–5:30 p.m. EST)
Toll-Free TTY: 800-638-8270
(Hotline; 8:00 a.m.–5:30 p.m. EST)
Phone: 301-504-7923
(General Information; Monday–Friday
8:00 a.m.–4:30 p.m. EST)
Fax: 301-504-0124 and 301-504-0025
Website: http://www.cpsc.gov

Gatorade Sports Science Institute

617 West Main Street
Barrington, IL 60010
Toll-Free: 800-616-GSSI (616-4774)
Website: http://www.gssiweb.com

Hospital for Special Surgery

535 East 70th Street
New York, NY 10021
Phone: 212-606-1000
Website: http://www.hss.edu

Ian Tilmann Foundation

102 Timberview Drive
Safety Harbor, FL 34695
Website:
http://www.theiantilmannfoundation.org
E-mail:
iantilmannfoundation@tampabay.rr.com

Institute for Arthroscopy and Sports Medicine

2100 Webster Street, Suite 331
San Francisco, CA 94115
Phone: 415-923-0944
Fax: 415-923-5896
Website: http://www.iasm.com
E-mail: surgerycoordinator@iasm.com

MomsTeam.com

393 Totten Pond Road, Suite 202
Waltham, MA 02451
Toll-Free: 800-474-5201
Website: http://www.momsteam.com

National Academy of Sports Medicine

1750 East Northrop Boulevard, Suite 200
Chandler, AZ 85286-1744
Toll-Free: 800-460-6276
Phone: 602-383-1200
Facsimile 480-656-3276
Website: http://www.nasm.org

National Athletic Trainers Association

2952 Stemmons Freeway #200
Dallas, TX 75247
Phone: 214-637-6282
Fax: 214-637-2206
Website: http://www.nata.org

National Eye Institute

Information Center
31 Center Drive MSC 2510
Bethesda, MD 20892-2510
(301) 496-5248
Website: http://www.nei.nih.gov
2020@nei.nih.gov

National Center for Catastrophic Sport Injury Research

University of North Carolina
at Chapel Hill
Phone: 919-962-5171
Website: http://www.unc.edu/depts/nccsi

National Center for Sports Safety

2316 1st Avenue South
Birmingham, Alabama 35233
Toll-Free: 866-508-NCSS
(866-508-6277)
Phone: 205-329-7535
Fax: 205-329-7526
Website: http://www.sportssafety.org
E-mail: info@SportsSafety.org

National Institute of Arthritis and Musculoskeletal and Skin Diseases

Information Clearinghouse
National Institutes of Health
1 AMS Circle
Bethesda, MD 20892-3675
Toll-Free: 877-22-NIAMS
(877-226-4267)
Phone: 301-495-4484
TTY: 301-565-2966
Fax: 301-718-6366
Website: http://www.niams.nih.gov
E-mail: NIAMSinfo@mail.nih.gov

Nationwide Children's Hospital

700 Children's Drive
Columbus, OH 43205
Toll-Free: 800-792-8401
Phone: 614-722-2000
Health Info Library:
http://www.nationwidechildrens.org/
healthinfolibrary

Nicholas Institute of Sports Medicine and Athletic Trauma

Website: http://www.nismat.org

NIH Osteoporosis and Related Bone Diseases— National Resource Center

2 AMS Circle
Bethesda, MD 20892-3676
Phone: 202-223-0344
Toll-Free: 800-624-BONE
(800-624-2663)
TTY: 202-466-4315
Fax: 202-293-2356
Website: http://www.bones.nih.gov
E-mail: NIHBoneInfo@mail.nih.gov

North American Spine Society

7075 Veterans Boulevard
Burr Ridge, IL 60527
Phone: 630-230-3600
Fax: 630-230-3700
Website: http://www.spine.org
Know Your Back: http://knowyourback.org

Orthosports

Website: http://www.orthosports.com.au
E-mail: education@orthosports.com.au

Prevent Blindness America

211 West Wacker Drive, Suite 1700
Chicago, Illinois 60606
Toll-Free: 800-331-2020 (8:30 a.m. to 5:00
p.m. CST, Monday through Friday)
Website: http://www.preventblindness.org

Safe Kids Canada

555 University Avenue
Toronto, Ontario M5G 1X8
Website: http://www.safekidscanada.ca

Safe Kids USA

1301 Pennsylvania Avenue NW
Suite 1000
Washington, DC 20004-1707
Phone: 202-662-0600
Fax: 202-393-2072
Website: http://www.safekids.org

Sport Medicine Australia

Website: http://www.smartplay.com.au

SportsMed Web

Website: http://www.rice.edu/~jenky/sports

SportsMD Media

Toll-Free: 800-679-1765
Website http://www.sportsmd.com
E-mail: contactus@sportsmd.com

STOP (Sports Trauma and Overuse Prevention) Sports Injuries

6300 North River Road, Suite 500
Rosemont, IL 60018
Phone: 847-655-8660
Website:
http://www.StopSportsInjuries.org

University of Pittsburgh Medical Center Sports Medicine

200 Lothrop Street
Pittsburgh, PA 15213-2582
Toll-Free: 800-533-UPMC
(800-533-8762)
Phone: 412-647-UPMC (412-647-8762)
Website:
http://www.sportsmedicine.upmc.com

Chapter 64

Resources For More Information About Fitness And Exercise

Action for Healthy Kids

600 West Van Buren Street, Suite #720
Chicago, IL 60607
Toll-Free: 800-416-5136
Fax: 312-212-0098
Website:
http://www.actionforhealthykids.org

Aerobics and Fitness Association of America

15250 Ventura Boulevard
Suite 200
Sherman Oaks, CA 91403
Toll-Free: 877-YOUR-BODY
(877-968-7263)
Website: http://www.afaa.com

Amateur Athletic Union

National Headquarters
P.O. Box 22409
Lake Buena Vista, FL 32830
Toll-Free: 800-AAU-4USA
(800-228-4872)
Phone: 407-934-7200
Fax: 407-934-7242
Website: http://www.aausports.org

Amateur Endurance

Endurance Media, Inc.
P.O. Box 9799
San Diego, CA 92169
Website:
http://www.amateurendurance.com
E-mail: service@amateurendurance.com

Information in this chapter was compiled from many sources deemed reliable. Inclusion does not constitute endorsement and there is no implication associated with omission. All contact information was verified in March 2012.

American Academy of Allergy, Asthma, and Immunology

555 East Wells Street, Suite 1100
Milwaukee, WI 53202-3823
Phone: 414-272-6071
Website: http://www.aaaai.org
E-mail: info@aaaai.org

American Alliance for Health, Physical Education, Recreation, and Dance

1900 Association Drive
Reston, VA 20191-1598
Toll-Free: 800-213-7193
Phone: 703-476-3400
Fax: 703-476-9527
Website: http://www.aahperd.org

American Athletic Institute

Website:
http://www.americanathleticinstitute.org

American College of Allergy, Asthma, and Immunology

P.O. Box 738
Saratoga Springs, NY 12866
Phone: 518-796-6337
Fax: 847-427-1294
Website:
http://www.americanathleticinstitute.org
E-mail: mail@acaai.org

American Council on Exercise

4851 Paramount Drive
San Diego, CA 92123
Toll-Free: 888-825-3636
Phone: 858-279-8227
Fax: 858-576-6564
Website: http://www.acefitness.org
E-mail: support@acefitness.org

American Diabetes Association

Center for Information
1701 North Beauregard Street
Alexandria, VA 22311
Toll-Free: 800-DIABETES (342-2383)
Phone: 703-549-1500
Fax: 703-739-9346
Website: http://www.diabetes.org
E-mail: AskADA@diabetes.org

American Heart Association

7272 Greenville Avenue
Dallas, TX 75231-4596
Toll-Free: 800-AHA-USA1
(800-242-8721)
Website: www.americanheart.org

American Lung Association

National Headquarters
1301 Pennsylvania Avenue NW, Suite 800
Washington, DC 20004
Toll-Free: 800-LUNGUSA
(800-586-4872)
Toll-Free: 800-548-8252 (Helpline)
Phone: 202-785-3355
Fax: 202-452-1805
Website: http://www.lung.org
E-mail: info@lung.org

American Running Association

4405 East-West Highway, Suite 405
Bethesda, MD 20814
Phone: 800-776-2732 (ext. 13 or 12)
Fax: 301-913-9520
Website: http://www.americanrunning.org

Aquatic Exercise Association

P.O. Box 1609
Nokomis, FL 34274-1609
Toll-Free: 888-232-9283
Website: http://www.aeawave.com

Asthma and Allergy Foundation of America

8201 Corporate Drive, Suite 1000
Landover, MD 20785
Toll-Free: 800-7-ASTHMA
(800-727-8462)
Website: http://www.aafa.org
E-mail: info@aafa.org

Bone Builders

University of Arizona
4341 East Broadway
Phoenix, AZ 85040
Phone: 602-827-8200, ext. 316
Website: http://www.bonebuilders.org
E-mail: bones@ag.arizona.edu

Center for Young Women's Health

Children's Hospital of Boston
333 Longwood Avenue, 5th floor
Boston, MA 02115
Phone: 617-355-2994
Fax: 617-730-0186
Website:
http://www.youngwomenshealth.org

Disabled Sports USA

451 Hungerford Drive, Suite 100
Rockville, MD 20850
Phone: 301-217-0960
Fax: 301-217-0968
Website: http://www.dsusa.org
Email: information@dsusa.org

HealthyWomen

157 Broad Street, Suite 106
Red Bank, NJ 07701
Toll-Free: 877-986-9472
Fax: 732-530-3347
Website: http://www.healthywomen.org
E-mail: info@healthywomen.org

IDEA Health & Fitness Association

10455 Pacific Center Court
San Diego, CA 92121
Toll-Free: 800-999-4332, ext. 7
Phone: 858-535-8979, ext. 7
Fax: 858-535-8234
Website: http://www.ideafit.com
E-mail: contact@ideafit.com

International Fitness Association

12472 Lake Underhill Road, #341
Orlando, FL 32828-7144
Toll-Free: 800-227-1976
Phone: 407-579-8610
Website: http://www.ifafitness.com

Kidshealth.org

Nemours Foundation
Website: http://www.kidshealth.org

LiveStrong

Website: http://www.livestrong.com

National Alliance for Youth Sports

National Headquarters
2050 Vista Parkway
West Palm Beach, FL 33411
Toll-Free: 800-688-KIDS
(800-729-2057)
Phone: 561-684-1141
Fax: 561-684-2546
Website: http://www.nays.org
E-mail: nays@nays.org

National Association for Health and Fitness

c/o Be Active New York State
65 Niagara Square, Room 607
Buffalo, NY 14202
Phone: 716-851-4052
Fax: 716-851-4309
Website: http://www.physicalfitness.org
E-mail: wellness@city-buffalo.org

National Center on Physical Activity and Disability

University of Illinois at Chicago
Department of Disability and Human Development
1640 West Roosevelt Road
Chicago, IL 60608-6904
Toll-Free: 800-900-8086
Toll-Free TTY: 800-900-8086
Fax: 312-355-4058
Website: http://www.ncpad.org
E-mail: ncpad@uic.edu

National Coalition for Promoting Physical Activity

1100 H Street, NW, Suite 510
Washington, DC 20005
Phone: 202-454-7521
Fax: 202-454-7598
Website: http://www.ncppa.org
Email: info@ncppa.org

National Collegiate Athletic Association

Website: http://www.ncaa.org

National Heart, Lung, and Blood Institute

NHLBI Health Information Center
P.O. Box 30105
Bethesda, MD 20824-0105
Phone: 301-592-8573
TTY: 240-629-3255
Fax: 240-629-3246
Website: http://www.nhlbi.nih.gov
E-mail: nhlbiinfo@rover.nhlbi.nih.gov

National Institute of Diabetes and Digestive and Kidney Diseases

Office of Communications
and Public Liaison
Building 31, Room 9A06
31 Center Drive, MSC 2560
Bethesda, MD 20892-2560
Phone: 301-496-3583
Website: http://www.niddk.nih.gov

National Osteoporosis Foundation

1150 17th Street, NW, Suite 850
Washington, DC 20036
Toll-Free: 800-231-4222
Phone: 202-223-2226
Fax: 202-223-2237
Website: http://www.nof.org

National Recreation and Park Association

22377 Belmont Ridge Road
Ashburn, VA 20148-4501
Toll-Free: 800-626-NRPA
(800-626-6772)
Website: http://www.nrpa.org
E-mail: customerservice@nrpa.or

National Strength and Conditioning Association

1885 Bob Johnson Drive
Colorado Springs, CO 80906
Toll-Free: 800-815-6826
Phone: 719-632-6722
Fax: 719-632-6367
Website: http://www.nsca-lift.org
E-mail: nsca@nsca-lift.org

PE Central

P.O. Box 10262
1995 South Main Street, Suite 902
Blacksburg, VA 24062
Phone: 540-953-1043
Fax: 540-301-0112
Website: http://www.pecentral.org
E-mail: pec@pecentral.org

President's Challenge

501 North Morton Street, Suite 203
Bloomington, IN 47404
Toll-Free: 800-258-8146
Fax: 812-855-8999
Website:
http://www.presidentschallenge.org
E-mail: preschal@indiana.edu

President's Council on Fitness, Sports, and Nutrition

1101 Wootton Parkway, Suite 560
Rockville, MD 20852
Phone: 240-276-9567
Fax: 240-276-9860
Website: http://www.fitness.gov
Email: fitness@hhs.gov

Right to Play International

65 Queen Street West
Thomson Building, Suite 1900
Box 64
Toronto, Ontario M5H2M5
Phone: +1 416 498 1922
Fax: +1 416 498 1942
Website: http://www.righttoplay.com
E-mail: info@righttoplay.com

Shape Up America

P.O. Box 149
506 Brackett Creek Road
Clyde Park, MT 59018-0149
Phone: 406-686-4844
Website: http://www.shapeup.org

Singapore Sports Council

230 Stadium Boulevard
Singapore 397799
Phone: 011 65 6500 5296
Fax: 011 65 6346 1842
Website: http://www.ssc.gov.sg

Weight-Control Information Network

1 WIN Way
Bethesda, MD 20892-3665
Toll-Free: 877-946-4627
Fax: 202-828-1028
Website: http://win.niddk.nih.gov
E-mail: win@info.niddk.nih.gov

Women's Sports Foundation

Eisenhower Park
1899 Hempstead Turnpike, Suite 400
East Meadow, NY 11554
Toll-Free: 800-227-3988
Phone: 516-542-4700
Fax: 516-542-4716
Website:
http://www.womenssportsfoundation.org
E-mail:
Info@WomensSportsFoundation.org

World Health Organization

Avenue Appia 20
1211 Geneva 27
Switzerland
Phone: +41 22 791 21 11
Fax: +41 22 791 31 11
Website: http://www.who.int
E-mail: info@who.int

Index

Index

Page numbers that appear in *Italics* refer to tables or illustrations. Page numbers that have a small 'n' after the page number refer to information shown as Notes at the beginning of each chapter. Page numbers that appear in **Bold** refer to information contained in boxes on that page (except Notes information at the beginning of each chapter).

A

athletic trainers, overview 341–43
ATLAS program 67
atrophy
    defined **81**
    described 81
autonomic dysreflexia,
    spinal cord injury 251–52
autonomic nervous system, described 245
avulsed teeth, described 235
axons, spinal cord 243–47

B

back leg swing exercise 98
backstretch exercise 93
badminton, safety tips 138
BAM! Body and Mind, publications
    helmets 107n
    white-water rafting 159n
basketball, safety tips 138
basketball shoes, described 130
beep baseball, described 12
biceps muscle, defined **212**
biceps tendonitis, described 214
bicycle helmets *see* helmets
Bicycle Helmet Safety Institute,
    contact information 370
biopsy, knee problems 306
black eye, treatment 220
bladder problems, spinal cord injury 252–53
blisters, foot health 314
blood-brain barrier, spinal cord injury 247
boating, alcohol use **70**
body protectors, described 104
Bone Builders, contact information 377
bone fractures *see* fractures
bones
    growth plates 197
    shoulder joint 257
bone scans
    knee problems 306
    overuse injuries 185
bowel function, spinal cord injury 253
boxing, safety tips 138–39

braces
    anterior cruciate ligament injury 296
    overview 123–26
    patellar dislocations 300
    protective gear 104
Brain Injury Association of America,
    contact information 370
broken bones *see* fractures
broken jaw *see* mandibular fracture
"Broken Jaw (Mandibular Fracture)" (Zeigler) 223n
broken nose *see* nasal fracture
"Broken Nose (Nasal Fracture)" (Zeigler) 223n
buddy system, drowning prevention 163
bulimia nervosa, described 41–42, 43–45
bunions, foot health 314
burners
    neck injuries 239
    overview 255–56
burnout
    overview 59–62
    prevention guidelines **61**
"Burnout in Young Athletes
    (Overtraining Syndrome)" (Ann and Robert
    H. Lurie Children's Hospital of Chicago) 59n
bursae
    defined **212, 258**
    described 211
    shoulder joint 259
bursitis
    defined **212**
    overview 211–18
B vitamins, energy drinks 31

C

caffeine
    dehydration prevention 27
    energy drinks 29–35
calcium, described 21–22, 24
calf raise exercise 99
calf stretch exercise **328**
calluses, foot health 315
Canadian Society for Exercise Physiology,
    contact information 371
canoe/kayak, safety tips 139

J

jammed finger, described 273

javelin thrower's elbow, described 267

jawbone fracture *see* mandibular fracture

Jenkins, Mark A. 319n

Jersey finger, described 274

joint aspiration, knee problems 306

joints

defined **213**

described **304**

growth plates 197

muscle strength 80

judo, safety tips 142–43

juice (slang) 63

jumper's knee, described 215

K

"Key Tips on Athletic Taping of the Foot and
Ankle" (Durta) 124n

Kidshealth.org, website address 378

see also Nemours Foundation

knee, depicted *214*

kneecap dislocation, overview 296–300

knee capsule, described 305

knee guards, described 103

knee injuries

arthritis 361–63

described **178**

overview 293–308

knee joint

depicted *295*

described 304–5

knee lift exercise 98

knee pads, skateboard safety 151–52

knee tendonitis, described 215

L

lateral collateral ligament, described 305

lateral collateral ligament injuries, described **298**

lateral epicondylitis, described 212, 267–68

leg extension exercise 98

leg pads, football 156

de Lench, Brooke 53n

lidocaine hydrochloride 216

life jackets, unintentional drowning 162

ligaments

ankle sprains 319–20

defined **81, 194**

knee joint 305

neck injuries 238, 239–40

plantar fascia 325

shoulder problems 259, 262

sprains 81

Little League elbow, described 267

LiveStrong, website address 378

Los Angeles Department of Public Health,
skateboard safety publication 151n

low blood pressure, spinal cord injury 251

Lurie Children's Hospital of Chicago

contact information 370

publications

athlete burnout 59n

burners/stingers 255n

heat illness 187n

hip injuries 287n

knee injuries 293n

muscle contusion 209n

luxated teeth, described 234–35

M

magnetic resonance imaging (MRI)

anterior cruciate ligament injury 295

bursitis/tendonitis 216

defined **198**

knee problems 306

overuse injuries 185

patellar dislocations 297

shoulder problems 261

ma huang 75

mallet finger, described 273

mandibular fracture, overview 228–31

"Marijuana: Facts for Teens" (NIDA) 69n

marijuana use, athletes 71–72

massage, sports injury treatment 340

medial collateral ligament, described 305

medial collateral ligament injuries, described **298**

O